CHILDREN AND HIV
SUPPORTING CHILDREN AND THEIR FAMILIES

Other Children in Scotland titles:

CHALLENGING RACISM IN THE EARLY YEARS
The role of childcare services in Scotland and Europe
Edited by Annie Gunner

CHILD WELFARE
Reviewing the framework
Edited by E. Kay M. Tisdall

THE CHILDREN ACT REVIEW
A Scottish experience
Edited by Carolyn Martin

CHILDREN'S SERVICES:
SHAPING UP FOR THE MILLENNIUM
Supporting children and families in the UK and Scandinavia
Edited by Bronwen Cohen and Unni Hagen

FATHER FIGURES
Fathers in the families of the 1990s
Edited by Peter Moss

HIV AND CHILDREN
A training manual
Joy Barlow

PROTECTING CHILDREN
Cleveland to Orkney: more lessons to learn?
Edited by Stewart Asquith

A SPECIAL PARTNERSHIP
A practical guide for named persons and parents of children with special educational needs
Linda Kerr, Liz Sutherland and Joyce Wilson

CHILDREN AND HIV

SUPPORTING CHILDREN AND THEIR FAMILIES

Edited by

Sarah Morton and David Johnson

Foreword by

Esther Rantzen

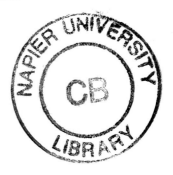

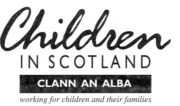

Children IN SCOTLAND

CLANN AN ALBA

working for children and their families

EDINBURGH: THE STATIONERY OFFICE

© The Stationery Office Limited 1996

The Stationery Office Limited
South Gyle Crescent
Edinburgh EH12 9EB

Applications for reproduction should be made to
The Stationery Office Limited

First published 1996

British Library Cataloguing in Publication Data
A catalogue record for this book is available from the British Library

ISBN 0 11 495779 7

About Children in Scotland

Children in Scotland is the national agency for voluntary, statutory and professional organisations and individuals working with children and their families in Scotland.

It exists to identify and promote the interests of children and their families in Scotland and to ensure that relevant policies, services and other provisions are of the highest possible quality and able to meet the needs of a diverse society. It does this with, through and for its members.

Children in Scotland works in partnership with the National Children's Bureau and Children in Wales.

Children in Scotland's programme of work relating to children and families affected by HIV and AIDS is funded by BBC Children in Need.

About the Editors

David Johnson

David Johnson is currently the Director of Waverley Care Trust, a charity providing care and support for people living with HIV and AIDS in Scotland. The Trust manages Milestone House, a hospice for people with HIV and AIDS, and SOLAS, a support and information centre. Educated at Stirling and Edinburgh Universities, he qualified as a social worker in 1977 and practiced in both voluntary and statutory sectors in England and Scotland. Children and family work has always been a major focus of practice alongside an interest in equality issues in social work, education and training.

Sarah Morton

Sarah Morton is currently Development Officer (Children and Families with HIV/AIDS) with Children in Scotland. She has been involved in various activities in this field, including developing local and national fora, work on children's rights, policy and quality issues. Educated at Stirling and Edinburgh Universities, she has worked in a variety of social work settings as well as teaching with both Edinburgh and the Open University.

CONTENTS

ACKNOWLEDGEMENTS

The editors would like to thank all the contributors to this book for their work in drafting and redrafting the chapters. Also thanks to Jennifer Flueckiger and Annie Gunner from Children in Scotland, Fraser Falconer from BBC Children in Need, and Anne Black from the City of Edinburgh Council Social Work Department for their valuable contributions.

We would also like to thank Waverley Care Trust for releasing David Johnson to work on this book, and the children at SOLAS who have produced some of the illustrations.

Children in Scotland would like to acknowledge the grant received from BBC Children in Need for their programme on children and families with HIV and AIDS.

Waverley Care
An AIDS trust

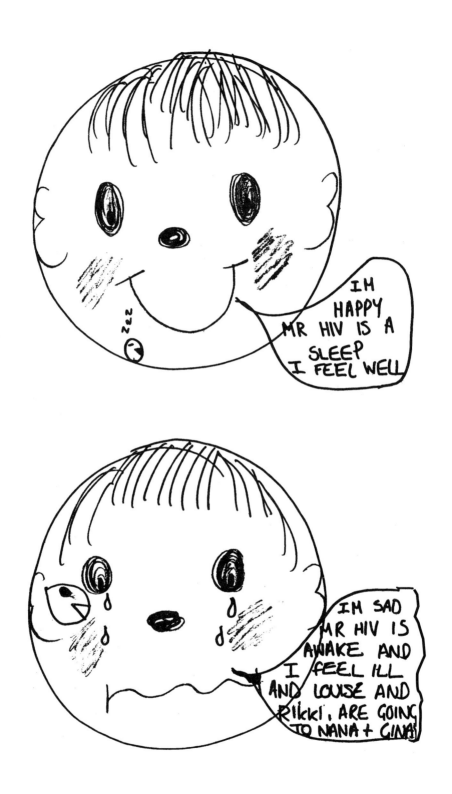

FOREWORD

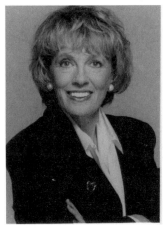

I am glad to be able to contribute a foreword to this important book, which aims to widen our understanding of the skills and experiences of those working with children affected by HIV and AIDS.

While much public debate is focused on the good news that fewer than expected numbers of people in Britain have acquired the infection, those who are living with the virus and its implications are often forgotten. This is particularly true for the children who are living with the secrecy, stigma and taboo that HIV and AIDS can bring into their families' lives.

Working with children who are facing the serious illness and possible death of their parents is always difficult. Working with those who also have to live with the secrecy and fear surrounding HIV and AIDS is even more complex. This book provides insight into ways of tackling this difficult but essential task. Through the eyes of social workers, medical staff and teachers it examines how best children and their families can be supported through the painful and lonely business of living with HIV and AIDS.

I am sure that this book will provide a significant contribution to the development of good practice in working with children and families, and I very much hope that it will offer support and encouragement to others who are engaged in this challenging, vital work. Most of all, I hope it will provide practical comfort and help for children themselves living as they do in the most tragic and painful circumstances.

Esther

Esther Rantzen

INTRODUCTION

David Johnson
Director, Waverley Care Trust
Sarah Morton
Development Officer (HIV/AIDS), Children in Scotland

This book brings together some of the experiences of those working with families affected by HIV in Scotland, where work with affected families has been pioneering, and continues to take a leading role. The aim is to give insight not into systems that have been developed, or service structures, but into the detail of work that goes on between children, families and those who work with them in a range of settings. The work presented is varied and covers a wide range of settings. It is therefore not necessarily a book to read from cover to cover, but to dip into, selecting what relates to one's own interests and role.

This introduction considers the particular circumstances which led to the development of work with affected children in Scotland, and some of the issues which make this area of work both difficult and rewarding.

HIV and families in Scotland

HIV is usually associated with adult issues, adult lifestyles and risks. Whilst concern in the early days of the epidemic focused almost exclusively on gay men, drug-users and sexually active heterosexuals, the potential impact on families and children was overlooked. It was not until the mid-eighties and later that the issues for families started to emerge, with parents, siblings, grandparents and children of all ages coping with the implications of dealing with an incurable and highly stigmatised disease in their families and communities.

In Scotland, the epidemic had been predominantly a heterosexual one from the start, with large numbers of drug-users as the main group affected. In December 1995, 45.7 per cent of people with HIV had acquired their infection through drug use, and a further 15.7 per cent through heterosexual sex (Scottish Centre for Infection and Environmental Health 1995).

It became apparent from the late eighties that the number of children who were HIV positive was going to be relatively small, but that there would be a large number of children affected by the virus due to the infection of one or more family member, including a large number whose primary carer was HIV positive. It has been very difficult to ascertain the number of children affected as details of parental status are not collected with other material at diagnosis. Various studies have tried to estimate the number of affected children. Research in 1993 in Edinburgh indicated that a group of 1034 HIV positive individuals had between them 500 children (Ronals et al. 1993).

More recently, Barnardo's commissioned research to estimate the number of affected children in the UK. Using a model based on the mother's infection, it estimates that in 1995 there were 691 affected children in Scotland (Imrie and Coombes 1995). This number does not take into account children affected by their father's HIV status, including the children of gay and bisexual men. It also ignores children affected by a sibling with HIV. It is a figure based on known infection, and so cannot account for the real, unknown numbers of people with HIV. For all of these reasons it is safe to assume that this is an underestimate.

The difficulty in ascertaining the number of affected children causes a variety of problems. Whilst infected children are formally counted and documented, this much larger group remains hidden because of the nature of the disease, and the concerns of parents and agencies about confidentiality. It is difficult to plan and raise funds for services which have no access to confirmed numbers of potential clients. It may also reflect the lack of priority given to this group that moves have not been made to obtain accurate figures. When an individual presents for an HIV test, they are asked a huge range of intimate questions. Surely it would be a simple exercise to find out whether they have children during this process.

A large proportion of the families affected, in Scotland and many other parts of the UK, are also living with poverty, poor housing and associated problems and are often perhaps the least well equipped to deal with the complex cocktail of issues associated with HIV. Those who are drug-users or ex-drug-users may have particular fears about asking for help with their children, as they may have a suspicion of those in positions of authority, and may have concerns about social workers seeing them as unfit parents.

In Scotland, following the recognition of children's issues within HIV services, there was a relatively speedy response, and services were developed for families from the mid-eighties. In Edinburgh, flexible care systems were developed by the social work department, and a family clinic was developed at the main infectious diseases hospital (Batty 1993). Voluntary organisations started to respond to the needs of parents by setting up crèches and childminding services. Some social workers began to work more intensively with families, supporting parents as they made care arrangements for their children and as they worked out the best ways of supporting and communicating with those children.

It is important to note that the experience of family work in Scotland has been exclusively with the white community – unlike in other parts of the UK, as far as we know. This reflects partly the difference in racial mix north of the Border, but also that the epidemiology of the infection in Scotland has not included the equivalent black refugee population that has been a major part of family work in London and the surrounding areas. For this reason there is very little experience of racial issues in relation to HIV work, and this is reflected in the content of this book. We therefore invite the reader to consider the implications of race issues on the work described in this book, and hope that those working with different racial groups will use their own experience to consider the extra dimension this might add to the issues described. For further discussion of racial issues see Tan (1993) 'Issues for black families affected by HIV infection and AIDS'.

We also acknowledge that the practical limitations of this kind of book mean that we cannot reflect every single setting and every point of view. In particular we have been unable to provide a carer's or parent's voice here. Neither have we provided a child's perspective, but we hope to have reflected some children's views through their drawings.

Issues for families

As the consequences of HIV infection began to emerge, it slowly became clear that children of all ages were going to have to deal with a myriad of complex and taboo issues. It seemed likely that many infected parents would not live long enough to see their children into adulthood, and many children would have to deal with bereavement at a young age. Families would have to face up to the complex issues of how the virus was acquired, often with associated feelings of parental guilt, and involving subjects we least like to talk to children about: drug use, sexuality and death. All of this is within a climate of stigma, where families live in fear of potential reactions provoked by the disease amongst those around them, making it less easy to ask for help, and causing increased concern about what children might do with any information they acquire. A child whose mother has cancer might expect to receive sympathy and support from teachers, neighbours and friends. Parents with HIV know that this cannot be expected when HIV or AIDS is mentioned. In addition, many of these families are already dealing with the prejudice associated with poverty and drug use.

It should be stressed that the process of developing support systems for parents was not simple. For a parent to face up to the issues their HIV infection may have for their child is extremely painful. While parents feel well, they may decide it is better not to talk to their children about their disease and its implications, particularly given the level of stigma and prejudice they know they – and their children – will have to face. They may fall ill and start to make preparations, only to abandon them when they feel well again. The episodic nature of the disease may be particularly difficult for children too, who can understand that mummy is very ill and may die, but are confused and insecure if she becomes well again. Parents also have to balance the effect that knowledge may have on their children with the effect that ignorance may have. It may be impossible for young children to understand the long-term nature of this complex disease and information may create unnecessary insecurities. On the other hand, for a child to be aware of problems and secrets in the family but not know what they are may cause serious distress. While parents grapple with these issues, children's workers tread a delicate path between supporting the child and ensuring their rights are respected, whilst not alienating the parent by working too fast, and risking losing contact with the family altogether.

Issues for practitioners

It is clear that working with affected families requires careful practice. The multiple issues involved demand the very best practice from workers. Experience has been drawn from a variety of related fields: bereavement work with other illnesses; social work with families with complex problems; HIV expertise; and child psychology. It has demanded an unprecedented level of multi-disciplinary and multi-agency co-operation. This book brings together some of the experiences of this work in the fields of medicine, social work, education and criminal justice within both voluntary and statutory sectors. It aims to give insight into the detail of practice issues and inform the development of future work by allowing the reader to be a 'fly on the wall' in a variety of practice settings. The work described looks at one-to-one interactions with children, whole family groups and group work. Although children have not been asked to contribute directly, their views are reflected throughout the chapters, and in the artwork which illustrates them.

The development of work with children affected by HIV has presented a number of particular challenges for practitioners. Those in the adult HIV sector often feel de-skilled when faced with children's work, particularly child protection, while those with extensive experience of working with children often feel they need some specialist skills to work with HIV. It is only through dialogue and exchange between these two groups that this gap can be bridged. We hope this book goes some way towards informing both of these groups and addresses this perceived lack of skills. What becomes apparent is that the best practice from children's work is what is required from workers when dealing with families affected by HIV, and that there are no special solutions for those affected by it.

Workers are consistently faced with clashes between parents' and children's rights in the families they work with and this is reflected in some of the contributions. There is a tightrope to be walked when you feel that a child has a need for information which a parent is not ready to give. Both parents' and children's trust must be maintained, whilst their needs may be in conflict. Holding on to and working with this kind of professional dilemma requires great strength and perseverance, and is the day-to-day work of many of the contributors to this book.

We hope that this book will bring some recognition to those involved in this work. While the skills involved are common to much work with children, the issues are particularly sensitive and complicated. Often those working with children are not involved in the power structures of their organisations, and their input may be seen as the 'soft' end of the organisation's overall role. Children's work in general has been traditionally devalued, and we hope that what is described here will throw light on the extreme skill and sensitivity with which difficult issues are being addressed in this field.

A group of parents was asked to contribute a chapter, but for many reasons felt unable to do so. One man, a father of two children, did however give us a very clear picture of some of the complex issues which can be around for the adults which impact on their children:

> When I was diagnosed as HIV positive it came as a shock and I did not want to talk about it. I became very depressed, could not sleep and ended up taking a high dosage of tablets to help me through the day. I did tell two of my sisters that I was positive and they, in turn, told their families as they thought I was a risk to them.
>
> I then thought it was about time I told my parents I was gay. It was the hardest thing I have ever had to tell them. I had to let them get used to their son being gay before I could tell them I was positive. Is there ever a right time to tell anyone that kind of news?
>
> I see as much of my children as I can, and do as many activities with them as possible. Even without the virus I would be there for my kids. I will be there for them, to love and care for, as long as I live. It is not necessary for them to know my status as this will unduly concern them. I will tell them when the time is right.

The themes of what to tell and when to tell the children appear throughout this book.

The sequence of the contributions in this book is intended to mirror, as far as possible, the potential progression of HIV disease and the accompanying work with families. It starts with general issues and works through communicating about illness and preparation for bereavement, and concludes with supporting bereaved children. The nature of the work means that there is some overlap of issues and material between contributions.

We would like to thank all of the contributors for grappling with the difficulties of describing their practice in detail. It is not easy to know where to begin in describing work in this way, and it is a brave step to throw open the detail of your practice, 'warts and all', to the scrutiny of readers.

Outline of chapters

In Chapter 1, 'Key issues in working with children and HIV', Ann Sutton provides an overview of HIV issues as they affect families and children and looks at some of the issues common to all of the following chapters. It considers the principles and practices of confidentiality in relation to families and discusses how child development needs to be taken into account. She also highlights the stress that this kind of work may have on workers, and discusses the need for good support and supervision systems.

In Chapter 2, Hazel Robertson looks at working with families from a statutory social work perspective, based on the experience of a specialist social work team in Dundee. She considers the role of the social worker in relation to this area of work, and looks at problems affecting families, considering appropriate social work interventions, taking into account that the parent is usually the main client.

The book moves on to consider the process of supporting individual families through the process of disclosure in Chapter 3, where Ingrid von Arnim describes her work with affected families in a hospice setting. This chapter provides useful insights to the process of disclosure for women, their children and extended family, and looks at the kinds of support needed throughout the process.

Staying within the residential setting, in Chapter 4 Joy Barlow and Isobel Hamilton of Aberlour Child Care Trust provide an insight into a rehabilitation project for women and their children, where the issues of HIV as they affect families have been apparent since the early days of the infection in Edinburgh. Here workers have the opportunity to carry out intensive work with women and children over a period of months and sometimes years. In this chapter the implications of drug use in families are more fully explored, and some of the interactions with children, both individually and within a group, are described.

Children who themselves have HIV are considered in Chapter 5, where Jacqueline Mok and Fiona Mitchell describe some of their practice in dealing with HIV positive children and their families. Their experience is based at the City Hospital in Edinburgh, where their team is responsible for visiting and following up all children born to HIV positive mothers in Edinburgh. This chapter looks at ways of communicating with children about medical procedures, and dealing with family anxieties in the clinic setting.

Continuing in a medical setting, a team of hospital play specialists at the City Hospital in Edinburgh consider how play techniques can be used with children undergoing treatment themselves, as well as children who are anxious about their parent's illness or treatment. Chapter 6 considers a variety of play techniques and the situations they can be applied to, and includes a list of activities which could be used in other settings.

Chapter 7 looks at working with women to consider what they need in order to discuss their HIV status and its implications for their children. Jan McClory, from the Women and HIV/AIDS Network, describes how she was involved in planning and setting up groups where women could come together to address these difficult issues.

Turning to education, in Chapter 8 Eleanor Carr and Liz White describe their work as teachers supporting affected and infected children in the classroom and school in the earlier days of the infection. Both are teachers working in one of the peripheral housing estates of a Scottish city and their chapter raises a number of important issues for education staff.

In Chapter 9, Jean Raeburn considers the issues of HIV and children in the children's panel system. She looks at the implications for practice as more affected children come into contact with the panel, and considers how best to respond. Here again, good practice relevant to other issues is highlighted.

The final two chapters consider the needs of children who have been bereaved and how they can be helped to come to terms with their experience. In Chapter 10, Judith Morkis from Barnardo's Riverside Project describes her work in preparing children for bereavement and supporting them through the process. She considers how theory can be used in practice to support children, and looks in detail at the issues that might arise. She also considers the role of the workers, and how we can deal with our own feelings in the process. Chapter 11 looks at another kind of support for children who have been bereaved. Daryl Cuthbert describes some group work in which children who had suffered bereavements due to various causes came together to work through their feelings.

The work described in each chapter took place before local government re-organisation in Scotland on 1 April 1996.

Conclusion

Whilst there are many books published on HIV, there have been very few on children's issues. We hope that this book will provide some impetus for addressing this gap, as well as some material for those who want to take a closer look at work with this client group. We hope it will be useful for those already engaged in work and planning in the HIV sector, but that it will also be read by the many thousands of children's workers in all settings who may at some point be in the position of working with a child or family affected by the virus. We also hope that it will provide some recognition of the skills and expertise needed to carry out this kind of work.

References
Batty, D., (ed.) (1993), *HIV Infection and Children in Need*, London: BAAF.
Imrie, J., and Coombes, Y., (eds) (1995), *No Time To Waste: The Scale and Dimensions of the Problem of Children affected by HIV/AIDS in the United Kingdom*. London: Barnardo's.
Ronals, P., Robertson, J., Duncan, B., and Thompson, A. (1993), *Children of Parents with HIV in Lothian*, BMJ V306, 6 March.
Scottish Centre for Infection and Environmental Health (October 1995), *HIV infection and AIDS: Quarterly Report to 30 September 1995*.
Tan, H. (1993), 'Issues for black families affected by HIV infection and AIDS', in Batty, D. (ed.) HIV *Infection and Children in Need*, op. cit.

Chapter 1

◆

Key issues in working with children and HIV

Ann Sutton
Scottish Adoption

Introduction

There are certain key principles and issues underpinning all work with children and families affected by HIV and AIDS. These are:

- the need for the welfare of the child to be considered as paramount;
- the need for collaborative working between agencies;
- a flexibility in the approach to planning;
- a code of confidentiality;
- a theoretical framework to underpin our work, including loss and bereavement, attachment and child development;
- the issues of isolation and discrimination; and
- good support systems for workers.

These are not unique to this area. They are fundamental to good social work practice with all families. However, there is a need to re-evaluate them in light of some of the other issues impacting on families where illness and death through HIV features.

For many affected families, HIV infection is not limited to one family member, but rather whole generations, as well as friendship and social networks. Many have to face not just the stigma of HIV and AIDS, but often social isolation and discrimination, stemming from drug use or racial heritage. For those who have a history of using illegal drugs, there are further wide-ranging issues for both children and families.

Recent legislation has helped consolidate the framework within which good social work practice with children and families occurs. The rights of children, as incorporated in the UN Convention on the Rights of the Child and the European Convention on Human Rights, are now reflected in the Children (Scotland) Act 1995, as they have been in the Children Act 1989 in England and Wales.

Good practice principles include:

- The child has the right to express their views if they so wish.
- Parents should normally be responsible for the upbringing of their children and should share that responsibility.

- The child has the right to protection from all forms of abuse, neglect or exploitation.
- Every effort should be made to keep the child in the family home in decisions relating to the protection of a child.
- Any intervention by a public authority in the life of a child should be properly justified and should be supported by services from all relevant agencies working in collaboration.

Thus, throughout the Children (Scotland) Act 1995, the welfare of children is the paramount consideration. The Act also recognises and highlights the need for agencies to work in collaboration (The Scottish Office 1995).

What will emerge throughout this book is that for children and families to receive the services they need and deserve good collaboration is essential. Inevitably there is multiple-agency involvement, including statutory and voluntary agencies with health, social services and education all playing a potential role.

Good collaboration implies mutual respect and understanding, but such understanding needs to be developed and can be helped by joint training and honest communication. Where there are differences of policies these need to be explored. There should be clarity of boundaries and roles. Some services will be adult-centred and good communication between these agencies and children's services would help adult-oriented service providers to take on the implications of good child care practice, including child protection issues and the needs of children.

Confidentiality

Confidentiality is one of the core themes for all practice in this area and one which potentially requires the issues of inter-agency working to be addressed. Setting aside the issue of HIV and AIDS, it can be hard for families and individuals who are involved with social work, benefit agencies and public housing authorities to maintain or achieve any sense of control or power over their lives. In such circumstances it is hard for people to believe they have the right to confidentiality. Many of the families with whom practitioners work will already be vulnerable and will not have any internalised sense of their right to confidentiality. Workers will need to continue to clarify differences between confidentiality and secrecy. While the stigma associated with HIV and AIDS causes workers to be especially sensitive to sharing information, they also need to balance this with the 'need to know'.

All professionals and statutory and voluntary agencies will have a code of confidentiality, and professionals are also bound by professional and legal codes of practice. There is a need for people working in this field to check that they are clear about their own agency's policies, and have an understanding of the policies of others with whom they are working. When working together, the boundaries of confidentiality should be negotiated and understood at the outset. The following questions can provide a helpful checklist:

- Is disclosure of HIV status necessary in order to receive the service?
- Does the individual whose status is being revealed give consent?
- Does that individual understand the implications of giving consent?

Increasingly the rights of children to have appropriate information challenges all of us working in this field to re-examine codes and practices. Working in partnership with parents leads us to advocate for their right to decide when and what to tell their children, but also requires us actively to advocate on behalf of children and young people. Differences in perception of need can be acute and will be discussed in other chapters in this book.

Discrimination and isolation

HIV and AIDS have isolated and stigmatised people who were already often discriminated against and isolated within society. For example, most of the families who have previously used, or are currently using drugs, will also be affected by poverty, poor housing, and may not have had a positive experience of education and employment. Many adults will have experienced judgemental attitudes from service providers because of their drug use. Many will be experiencing isolation or difficult relationships within their extended families because of their behaviour and its effects on the family.

Women in particular will often be more openly and negatively judged if they chose to have children knowing they are HIV positive. This is often a qualitatively different experience from parents who may be at risk of passing on some other genetically transmitted condition. One reason for this is that HIV is often seen as a condition brought upon oneself by behaviour for which society has little sympathy or understanding. Drug use or sexual activity are often incorrectly equated with prostitution and promiscuity, when the underlying issue might be one of poverty. Another reason is a lack of understanding of the availability of counselling and assessment of risk in relation to mother-to-child transmission which can help pregnant women make choices, as with other genetic conditions.

There is also, I suspect, a combining and confusing of two separate strands. One is powerfully positive, that is, the feelings of regret and sadness about a parent who will die before a child reaches maturity and the position in which that leaves the child. The other is a harsher judgement, that is the woman who has 'allowed' herself to become HIV positive is considering becoming a mother and will then leave her child motherless. She is seen as not deserving of being a mother. It touches on the 'right to have a child' and what seems to be that inevitable human response of assessing some as 'deserving' and others as 'undeserving'.

Many children and young people whose parents have used drugs may have experienced a chaotic lifestyle with many basic needs being at best erratically met. Many may have taken on a caring and parenting role both for siblings and their parent. Family patterns and behaviours will have adjusted to contain and manage the behaviour of the drug-user. This may include children isolating themselves from their peers because of embarrassment at their differences and protecting themselves from hostile community responses.

Children may have experienced actual emotional and physical neglect and almost certainly a lack of consistency in who takes care of them. They will often have witnessed conflict amongst the adults surrounding them and bouts of illness in their parents. They may have had the experience of multiple losses through separation, divorce, imprisonment of a parent and periods of being cared for by foster carers. They may not have been able to move through appropriate developmental stages of trust, security, autonomy and so on. There may have been sporadic good parenting, but the reliability of this will have left them vulnerable, without basic coping strategies. They may be very self-sufficient and also intensely loyal to their parents.

It is therefore necessary for workers from helping agencies to have an understanding of the very complex feelings and needs of the children with whom they are working. There is enormous concern about the lost childhood of the young people who become 'carers' for their parents or siblings. Attempts to help children and young people with these experiences will need to be undertaken with care and, as new opportunities for helping arise, there will need to be an understanding of the feelings of loss and vulnerability associated with the loss of old strategies and ways of coping, and the development of new ones.

Loss, separation and bereavement

There is much material available on the impact of loss and separation on children and adults and of how these experiences affect attachment and behaviour (see works by Fahlberg (1994), Dyregrov (1990), Parkes (1983) and Kubler-Ross (1969)). However, our society does not in general deal well with death and we have lost mourning patterns and rituals. For any family, talking to children about the death of a mother, father or sibling is not straightforward or easy. For families and children affected by HIV and AIDS there is the added possibility of multiple loss, and the stigma and prejudice surrounding the illness can often rob families of the usual sympathetic public responses to family crisis and tragedy.

Many families affected by HIV turn to statutory and voluntary agencies for help in considering options and making longer term plans for their children. The final loss, through death, for children and parents is rehearsed through foster and respite care placements. If these experiences are to be a positive contribution to families, then carers and workers need to be able to work in partnership, even where there are other major issues like child protection.

To help adults and children cope with new losses, it is essential for workers to have a sound theoretical base. A knowledge of bereavement theory is vital, and it will also be helpful to gain as much knowledge of an individual's and family's previous experience of loss as possible.

The following is a list of needs that will have to be met for children as family members become ill. It draws heavily on Dyregrov's work (1990). Children need to:

- have a well-trusted person to talk to;
- have access to good, age-appropriate information;
- be prepared for the death of a parent or sibling and not be excluded from the process;
- not be made to feel guilty or responsible for the death;
- be helped to take appropriate responsibility, but no more;
- be talked to about the future and possible plans and to be involved; and
- have good information about personal and family history.

At the time of death children need to:

- be included in the rituals, such as funerals;
- be offered stability and as much continuity as possible at home, school, nursery, and so on;
- suffer as few separations from important people as possible;
- be able to share and witness the emotions of others;
- be allowed to play and have 'time out';
- be able to share their fears and anxieties about what might happen and who else might be lost;
- receive clear, concrete explanations, for example death is not sleep; and
- be helped in keeping memories alive.

Adults will need to be helped to understand that at different ages children have different levels of understanding. Pre-school children will have heightened anxieties about all separations. They might talk about the dead person 'being back in time for tea tomorrow' and they will not have a concept of 'forever'. School-age children will find it hard to concentrate. They may plan how not to let this happen again, and have elaborate fantasies. Adolescents can revert to the magical thinking of earlier childhood and feelings will be intense. Many adolescents will be afraid of losing control of their emotions and becoming caught in conflicts as a result of the intensity of their unexpressed feelings.

Most professionals and volunteers will have knowledge of grief reactions – denial, anger, sadness, resignation, eventual acceptance and resolution. However, people do not always progress neatly through the grieving process, nor do they always visit all of the stages that we know can exist. Sometimes people surprise us by their acceptance and this can mean, for example, that they have completely missed out feelings of anger or despair. This may have been their way of coping at the time, but when a subsequent loss occurs the response may be very different. Some people never seem to pass beyond sadness and struggle to reach acceptance or resolution. Moving through the various reactions, or 'stages of loss', and reaching resolution or acceptance does not mean that we cease to have feelings about those losses and events, but that we are able to live in the present and view the future positively.

To mourn and grieve appropriately, people need a level of security, support and nurturing. We need to respect boundaries. We need to respect individual patterns of grief whilst facilitating exploration, taking care not to dismantle existing coping strategies without being able to provide the security and space to allow others to develop.

In this area we are faced with the challenge of working with people who are multiply affected and may have been in the past. Workers need to acknowledge that sometimes this work will combine with personal issues and there will be a need to acknowledge personal vulnerability and the need for support.

Support for workers

Good practice should dictate that all agencies, statutory or voluntary, have in place systems for consultation, supervision and support. However, there are particular stresses involved in supporting children and families in this area of work. Working with children who are coping with a terminal illness or the loss of parents, siblings, other family members or of members of friendship networks is particularly painful and stressful. Workers are inevitably working with complex family dynamics and within complicated inter-agency situations and agreements. They are often balancing the conflicting needs and rights of children, young people and parents. In these complex situations, where the aim is to work in partnership, workers are holding on to child-centred policies, child care legislation and child protection issues. They are communicating about extremely sensitive issues – HIV, sex, sexuality, drug use and death. Finally, they are working with people who are young and in the natural course of things would not be facing death.

Support systems begin with good basic and on-going training. This should include:
- how to identify support needs;
- the principles and issues of inter-agency working;
- the principles of working in partnership with families and carers;
- child care legislation;
- child protection issues;
- principles underpinning a child-centred approach;
- confidentiality and specific HIV issues, including testing of children;
- techniques for working and communicating with children about HIV, sex, sexuality and drug use;
- family therapy techniques; and
- bereavement and loss.

Workers, carers and volunteers need to be continually helped to identify their professional and personal support needs. This should include well-structured management, supervision and consultation; access to specialist consultation where the direct manager does not hold the necessary experience; the right to consultation outside line management structures to help with personal issues and impact; and some level of peer group support.

Child development

A good understanding of child development helps underpin work with children, young people and their families, in this complicated and stressful area. It helps workers to understand the impact of experiences like separation, loss and children's reactions to these. It helps workers to appreciate the need for children and young people to re-work and re-visit earlier experiences in order to provide opportunities for them to redress any gaps in developmental progress.

Vera Fahlberg (1994) provides a useful framework for looking at developmental tasks in relation to age, suggesting the consequences of interrupted development and how these consequences might manifest themselves in behaviour. She helpfully offers advice on how these children's needs might be met.

When working with children and young people about death, it is important to realise that while grief reactions across the age range will have many similarities, the way children attempt to master what has happened to them will depend on their age, level of maturity and earlier experiences. Using Fahlberg's work as a theoretical base, it is helpful to see how children and young people's development builds on earlier experience and how parents, workers and carers can be helped to give opportunities for re-building and re-parenting to help with any missed stages. Some children and young people will have a real need to learn more appropriate ways of managing and coping.

If parents have themselves received poor parenting, or had disturbed or disrupted childhoods, then they too will need not just help with how they parent, but also the opportunity to have some of their needs met, and an opportunity to reconsider their childhood experiences. Sometimes parental needs will be so great that it will be difficult or impossible to address them or for them to have time to develop the skills required to become more supportive parents. Services need to focus on helping them achieve enough progress in a time scale that is realistic for them and their children.

Conclusion

At the beginning of this chapter I mentioned the need for flexibility. Helping parents plan, working with children and helping extended families, partners and friends work through and re-work possibilities, hopes and anxieties does involve holding open as many options as possible, for as long as possible. For workers this can mean helping those involved accept what is not going to be possible as well as holding on to possibilities that seem remote. I think this means not rushing to plan irrevocably to relieve anxiety either in the family or in ourselves.

We need to be able, when necessary, to act decisively for children if their needs demand it, while recognising that, as workers, we need to keep doors and opportunities open and be flexible. Agencies need to work together with a lack of preciousness and without any sense of rivalry and competition in order to hold central the needs of children, young people and their families.

References

Dyregrov, A. (1990), *Grief in Children: A Handbook for Adults*, London: Jessica Kingsley.

Fahlberg, V. (1994), *A Child's Journey through Placement*, London: BAAF.

Kubler-Ross, E. (1969), *On Death and Dying*, New York: Macmillan.

The Scottish Office (1995), *Scotland's Children: A Brief Guide to the Children (Scotland) Act 1995*, Edinburgh: HMSO.

Parkes, C. M. and Weis, R. S. (1983), *Recovery from Bereavement*. New York: Basic Books Inc.

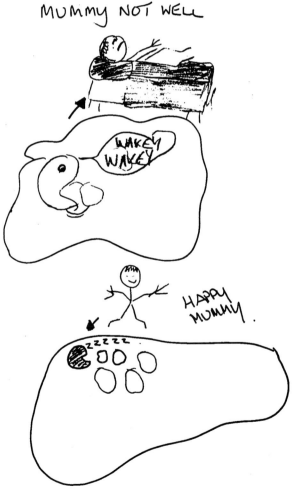

Chapter 2

◆

WORKING WITH FAMILIES AND HIV
A SOCIAL WORK PERSPECTIVE

Hazel G. Robertson,
Senior Social Worker/Senior Care Manager, Tayside Regional Council

Introduction

In its commitment to HIV and AIDS, Tayside Regional Council Social Work Department services established a specialist social work team in 1988 to address the needs of people who are HIV positive, their families, carers and those concerned about HIV infection. The team is an integral part of a multi-disciplinary immunodeficiency service based at Kings Cross Hospital, Dundee, where, between team members, efforts are made to provide a comprehensive health and social care service to people who are HIV positive.

In looking at how social work has responded to HIV and AIDS, this chapter examines the problems which can and often do confront families and how specialist knowledge has informed practice.

To assist this process, it is necessary to begin by focusing on:
- the social work role;
- co-ordination of care;
- challenges in working with children;
- permission to grieve;
- breaking bad news; and
- access to services.

Finally, many of these issues are brought together in the form of a case study, which it is hoped will bring meaning to the preceding text.

Statements and scenarios

The following statements and scenarios are intended to illustrate some of the many dilemmas faced by families where HIV infection exists:

> 'I will never forget that haunting wail coming from the doctor's room; it was horrible and told me everything I didn't want to hear.'
>
> (a mother on finding out her daughter was HIV positive)

'I'm really scared and I don't know what to do; my mum's changed – she used to be so strong and we could depend on her and now she is really weak.'

>(A 16-year-old girl facing her mother's terminal stages of illness and who has been told by her big sister not to cry in front of mum – or to speak about HIV to anyone)

An HIV positive man resists contact with any specialist medical service as he feels people will view him as 'gay' or a 'junkie' and fears how this may impact on his daughter and family.

A 10-year-old boy is physically sick at the thought of life with alternative carers. His mum, a single parent, is terminally ill.

An 8-year-old girl, whose dad died when she was an infant, is told by a 'friend' in the street that her mum has AIDS.

All of these situations clearly require an individual response but they share a common element in that they highlight the sense of stigma and isolation confronted by people affected by HIV and AIDS. HIV does not in itself create social inequality and injustice, but it can and often does compound it. Therefore, for many people, HIV is yet another disadvantage to contend with and brings with it great anxiety and fear.

The social work role

Social work, as a profession, accepts the necessity to work with uncertainties, and social workers repeatedly face dilemmas about how and when to intervene in the lives of other people. Consequently, the principles which govern the nature and delivery of service become vital in providing a firm foundation from which to work.

The following principles therefore apply:

- It is essential that a clear definition of role is established, thus leaving no illusions or misconceptions regarding responsibility.
- Workers must aim to identify and resolve any immediate problems with minimum intervention.
- It is necessary to recognise one's own feelings and ability to work with the situation and individuals involved.
- Workers must:
  communicate clearly, verbally and in writing;
  be able to negotiate, network and work in partnership;
  assist the individual to reach decisions and maintain their right to choose;
  and be able to assist, care for, counsel and supervise individuals and families in difficulty.

In developing this further, the role of the social worker in HIV and AIDS can be described as multifaceted and is underpinned by basic principles which include:

- respect for people as individuals, safeguarding their dignity and rights;
- the development of knowledge and skills;
- no prejudice in self or tolerance of prejudice in others;
- the empowerment of clients and their participation in decision-making and in defining services;
- responsibility for standards of services and for continuing education and training; and
- collaboration with others (BASW 1986).

In recognition of the prejudice and discrimination which exists around HIV, it is vitally important that all social workers acquire knowledge, skills and values necessary to work with people who are HIV positive. These qualities are transferable from other areas of social work practice but it is essential that workers acquire sufficient knowledge of HIV in order to provide an effective service.

The advantage of having a specialist social work service as part of the multi-disciplinary team is that contact with families can be integrated and timed to reduce the sense of being overwhelmed while providing an opportunity to allow important decisions to be made in a planned, calm, participatory manner, empowering people to make the choices they feel comfortable with.

Confidentiality and recording of information

> Confidentiality is a basic tenet of good practice, social workers have had no need to theorise about the nature of the ethical obligation because their consciousness of being professional persons always inclined them to accept confidentiality wholeheartedly. (Biestek 1961)

In Tayside Regional Council Social Work Department, in recognition of the particular issues around HIV infection, a strict confidentiality policy has been established highlighting the repercussions if this is breached. The recording in case records of any information concerning an individual's HIV status will only be made if it is directly relevant to the service being received. No information will be given to a third party without written consent from the individual and this will be used only for the specific purpose for which it had been requested, for example to refer for another specialist service or to write to an HIV-specific charity.

It is rarely necessary to share information regarding an individual's HIV status, but if this has been agreed by the individual and written consent has been given, this is recorded as restricted information. Furthermore, should the need for this information arise on subsequent occasions, formal written consent would again be required prior to any disclosure. The only exception to this being when there is a specific legal requirement for the information, such as the Boarding Out and Fostering of Children

(Scotland) Regulations 1985, where if an HIV positive child is being placed with foster carers, the carers would be informed of the child's diagnosis in order to ensure relevant and appropriate care. However, if the child's parent is known to be HIV positive, the foster carers would have no automatic right to know.

Clearly there is an argument to support carers having access to this information in order for them to continue supporting the child and providing appropriate care. It is however vitally important that any information concerning the HIV status of a parent is only shared with the consent of that parent and that any discussion with a child regarding this matter is fully supported by the parent. Help and support must be made available to assist parents and families discuss these very difficult issues as this, in turn, will ensure that the child hears the information from someone they trust and can believe.

Co-ordination of care

In addressing HIV, social work, health and voluntary workers have learned to work together. This multi-agency challenge highlights the need for mutual trust, respect and understanding amongst practitioners in order to provide the care and support required. However, despite this acknowledgement, fear of potentially negative reactions prevents many families accessing services or utilising existing supports, for example home help, district and community nursing, social work, specific voluntary groups, and so on, and has been a major factor in the emergence of young carers who, in essence, are providing the practical and often emotional care for a sick parent.

With the development of care in the community under the NHS and Community Care Act 1990, care managers and social care officers have been employed to assist people who are HIV positive to maintain their independence at home in the community.

A care manager, will, in consultation with the individual, gather comprehensive information in order to identify needs. This will include, as appropriate, specialist assessments from other professionals – for example, medical, nursing, occupational therapy, dietetics, and so on – following which a care plan document will be compiled and circulated to the individual and all those involved in their care, thus ensuring clarity of role and minimising the potential for duplication. The care will then be regularly reviewed and the individual made aware of the choices and options available to meet their specified need. This system helps ensure services are well co-ordinated and sensitively offered, enabling the individual to remain in control of the services they receive. A social care officer can be employed to relieve carers and assist individuals in a practical way in order to allow them to remain at home. This may include help with personal care, budgeting, shopping, preparation of food and social and recreational outings. In Tayside, as this is a specialist resource and part of the Social Work Department HIV Team, this has been well received and has helped alleviate some of the stress for many families.

It has been important that prior to commencing work with an individual or family, and following initial contact, that the worker considers an action plan in order to remain clear about their role and level of input. This should include:

- expectation of role, that is:
  what is the purpose and value of my job?
  what do I plan to do?
- what resources do I have access to?
- what can I help to change or improve?
- what is possible to change?
- how can this best be done?

In sharing this with service users they remain in control of the process and are clearer about the opportunities and limitations of contact from a wide range of services. Equally important in this process is that responsibility and power remains invested in the individual service user. Consequently, in order to achieve this objective, collaboration, mutual trust and respect must be given credence to enable services to be comprehensively and effectively used by the families who need them.

Challenges in working with children

In discussing HIV and AIDS with children many parents have commented that they find 'AIDS' an extremely emotive term, which for some people conjures up pictures of a skeletal 'victim' unable to help themselves. Many parents have therefore chosen to avoid using this term and refer to their illness solely as HIV, thus softening the impact and giving more time for explanation.

Having been given this information, a child needs time to assimilate this and then be given:

- an opportunity to express any immediate concerns;
- help to identify how these can be addressed;
- help to find or locate 'safe' people;
- an opportunity to reflect on what HIV means to them;
- a chance to consider, if appropriate, to tell other people; and
- regular and easy access to people who may be a support.

Fear and suspicion can distance children from accessing support. This may be a fear of having their parent taken from them or of being received into care themselves or it may be as a direct consequence of the stigma and prejudice associated with HIV.

In supporting children to make decisions about their lives and their family and in order to encourage them to feel confident enough to ask for help, it is important that the child can trust the adult(s) involved in their care.

When working with children regarding HIV and the implications of this, it is important that an individual is identified with whom the child can address their specific needs.

A potential drawback in undertaking this work is the amount of time involved in developing and nurturing a positive relationship with a child. It is therefore important for workers to ensure that this is agreed upon prior to embarking on any work with an individual child. Timing is extremely important and it may be that the afternoon/ evening set aside to spend time with a child or young person is not when they feel able or willing to address complex issues. As a consequence of this it is almost always better to utilise existing support within the family, for example an aunt, uncle, grandparent and so on, as this is likely to be longer lasting and more accessible to the child. Alternatively, if this is not possible, the child must be given the opportunity of having 'protected time' with a professional worker with whom they feel they can be honest and open.

Recognition that children are relatively powerless to make demands on services or to insist on their rights will influence the way services are offered. However, in order to gain trust and mutual understanding, workers must make a firm commitment to prioritising this work and not allow themselves to be diverted. This may entail arranging emergency cover to ensure that this work can go ahead uninterrupted.

The feeling of impotence which children and young people experience can result in children accepting their family situation as a *fait accompli*, regardless of the burden it places on them. This may include whether they have any opportunity to play, attend school, be adequately cared for or whether they feel the need to fulfil household chores, accept responsibility for the home and other siblings and so on. Consequently children and young people will often attempt to develop strategies to cope with these difficulties and may attempt to minimise the strain this places on them and their families.

Within social work there is a responsibility to approach and identify the needs of these young carers in a sensitive and supportive manner and to acknowledge that very young children can and do adopt a 'caring role'. With this in mind, it is crucial that families receive a supportive, helpful, effective and accessible service which addresses the needs of the children as well as those of the adult(s) involved. This, in turn, can reduce the potential for family dysfunction and distress and empowers the children to begin to make positive changes within their families.

Permission to grieve

Often it is assumed or privately wished that the children or young people living in a family with HIV infection are unaware of the illness and the possible repercussions, when in reality there is an unspoken rule that illness and death will not be mentioned. This conspiracy of silence creates its own difficulties as children are unable to grieve or begin to step into the cathartic process where mutual trust and a supportive environment make it possible to express fear, anger, guilt, sadness, and so on. This enables them to explore and begin to understand some of the problems, but will not assist in helping them come to terms with the stigma and social isolation of HIV.

Adults often expect children to talk about their feelings rather than express them. When children cry, shout, act up, and so on, they can be told to stop and sometimes assume that this instruction is to 'stop having the feelings'. Children need permission to express feelings, for example talking about other children or other situations and then relating these to the present situation, or allowing young children to express their feelings by using their hands or by using a game in which children use drawings of emotions.

Vera Fahlberg (1988) in *Fitting the Pieces Together* suggests that if children become aggressive and this is directed towards another individual, this must be channelled more appropriately, for example: 'You are right to feel angry, but you must not hurt Jim – you can thump this pillow instead.'

Other means of venting sadness and anger include: tearing newspaper, playing with clay/play dough, using cardboard or foam, hammer and nails and scribbling with red crayons on paper. All of these 'safe' alternative means of expressing anger provide a feeling of control and can work effectively in controlling aggressive behaviour.

If these feelings are suppressed and the child is prevented from processing emotion, they will not 'simply disappear' and may be the reason for aggressive or difficult behaviour some years later.

Unfortunately, because of the level of ignorance about HIV and the resultant stigma it attracts, there are some young people who refuse to access specialist services, despite having lost several members of their immediate family and whilst continuing to live with chronic illness in their home. The importance of life story work with these children cannot be overstated as this provides them with facts about their families, assistance to understand this information and the opportunity to come to terms with it. It is also important that they have positive memories, this being the basis on which they can build their futures.

Social workers are both experienced and skilled in working with children regarding issues of loss and change. The necessity to have a thorough comprehension of 'who I am' and 'where I have come from' is the foundation on which we grow. Without this a child may find it difficult to develop emotionally and socially and may believe that all their past is very bad. Helping a child develop their own life-story book helps remove the mystery and can establish a positive sense of identity, which is ultimately very rewarding and effective. Many parents can become involved in this process and this has a therapeutic role in reconciling relationships and leaves both the parent and child with the satisfaction of having dealt with 'unfinished business'.

The social worker, in carrying out this role, must be able to spend time establishing a trusting relationship with the child and family in order to allow this work to proceed. If possible, it is always best to commence at an early stage when a parent is well and able to participate as this allows for full and frank discussion and ensures access to a wider source of information for the child.

Breaking bad news

As a direct consequence of the nature of the work we do as professionals, we may have to initiate the process of grief by helping parents to impart bad news to their children. This inevitably causes pain and needs to be carefully planned. Many practitioners avoid the issues, unable to cope with their own discomfort, and will justify this by claiming it is too painful and distressing for the child.

Buckman (1993), in *How to Break Bad News*, gives a framework which can be usefully employed. He suggests:

- Get the physical context right.
- Find out how much the individual knows.
- Find out how much the individual wants to know.
- Share information.
- Respond to feelings.
- Plan and follow through.

Clearly, preparation for this complex piece of work is fundamental to its success. However, the relationship between the worker and the child and/or parent, once again, becomes vitally important and can, in turn, create the positive environment required to carry out this task.

If information is to be given, it should be given in small pieces allowing time for this to be absorbed and then checked out, avoiding saturation but reinforcing the important aspects of the discussion. Language must be kept clear and simple and feelings validated. It may also be important at this stage to reassure children that they will always be cared for and, if appropriate, identify who this will involve. A discussion of this nature must be planned and carefully considered with on-going support, and easy access to information is essential.

In counselling young people who are reluctant or unable to begin discussing the nature of their own exposure to HIV infection or their feelings about a parent or relative's ill health, I have found that I am occasionally faced with a series of 'don't know' responses. This usually means 'I don't want to discuss this'; rather than simply accept and/or ignore the issue, I endeavour to ensure this statement is made and acknowledged by the young person, otherwise this can create on-going barriers in communication and can prevent the young person from changing their mind about participation. Timing, venue, personality and skill or expertise influence the response and some young people need time to adjust to this relationship and develop confidence and the ability to share their concerns.

Access to services

Although many people who directly access the specialist social work service do so under a veil of disguise, citing practical problems as the focus for intervention, when confidence grows and they feel a little more comfortable, they inevitably seek guidance, support and counselling in respect of personal fears regarding their health, future or the ultimate care of their child(ren). As this service is adult focused, much of the time is spent addressing needs identified by the parent, and it is incumbent on the social worker involved to identify the need for specialist child-centred work and seek out the most appropriate resources.

Case study

Jennifer was 36 years old when she discovered her HIV status, having been infected sexually by a former partner whom she had been unaware was injecting drugs and sharing needles. In discussion with her consultant at the local genito-urinary clinic, she accepted that she would need advice, support and assistance to work through her anxiety about the immediate future and explore the issues regarding her relationship with her partner. She also needed the opportunity to consider plans for the care of her children in the event of her health deteriorating.

The consultant explained that there was a specialist social work team available to discuss these matters with and help her reach a decision. With this knowledge, she agreed to be referred to the social work department.

Within a few days Jennifer was contacted by letter with an arrangement made to meet her at home. On meeting Jennifer, I explained that the HIV team was a specialist resource and that any support and assistance required would be dictated by her. The policy on confidentiality was explained and thoroughly explored as this was a major concern for Jennifer and she was advised she would have access to any information recorded by me and stored in her file. We discussed some of the initial services and facilities she would have access to and what she felt was most appropriate at this stage. As Jennifer relaxed a little she offered to make a cup of tea and began to explain the circumstances around her becoming HIV positive and her grave concerns for the future. She explained that she had five children between the ages of 10 and 16 years, all of whom were a product of her marriage which ended when her youngest child was 3 years old. Her current relationship was described as strong and her partner, David, had been aware of her decision to be tested and was supportive and wanted to maintain their relationship of almost two years.

Jennifer's immediate concern on discovering her HIV infection was for her children and who might be available to care for them if she was unable to do so. She fully appreciated that it would be difficult, if not impossible, for any member of her family to accommodate five children and she was unsure how David would manage, given he is ten years her junior and not experienced in caring for children.

After several weeks of visiting Jennifer at home and after meeting David and the children, Jennifer felt more comfortable about exploring the possible options for care of the children and it was tentatively agreed that should the need arise, a carer would be found to help David care for the children within their own home, thus avoiding the need for them to be separated.

As a consequence of many families facing similar difficulties regarding finding suitable and appropriate care for their children, Tayside Regional Council Social Work Department in partnership with Barnardo's established a Flexible Care Service in 1993. This service is only available to families affected by HIV and the project matches carers to a family affected by HIV, allowing time for relationships to grow, and relieving a great burden on parents who know if they require a break from constantly caring for their child, or if they require in-patient hospital treatment, that their child will be cared for by the same carer who is then known to the child and parent.

As Jennifer maintained good health, she made a decision to keep specific information concerning her HIV status to herself and David, and chose at this time not to share this with any member of her family. Jennifer described me to her family as her health social worker and, as the counselling relationship developed, we were able to discuss in great detail the issues around HIV and the impact this had on both Jennifer and her family. After several months she moved to deciding it was time to share this difficult information with her two eldest children, who were now 17 and 16 years. They had a notion all was not well with their mum's health and they needed an explanation. Jennifer felt they would be able to understand and would also respect her wish for confidentiality, but she also wanted to share this information with them while she was still well enough to offer them support to cope with the implications of what HIV would do to their lives.

We discussed at great lengths the options available to Jennifer about how to deliver the information and in what format. We considered the setting, timing and access to support and information for both Brendan and Sarah if they felt they needed this. We also examined potential negative reactions and how best to handle the inevitable emotion. Jennifer went ahead apprehensively, but none the less bravely, and succeeded in breaking the 'bad news'. Both children had recognised something was wrong, but having learned only a little about HIV from school and the media, they now wished to learn more. Their immediate concern was whether mum was going to die and both cried and hugged their mum. At first neither accepted this was true and responded by denying the facts. Brendan became very angry and this was directed at his mum's former partner. Ultimately both accepted their mum was ill and needed their support, particularly emotionally. Both Brendan and Sarah became very protective, but felt ill equipped to cope as they had insufficient information.

With their consent, a meeting was arranged with the consultant, Brendan, Sarah and me to enable them to ask questions and receive frank and honest information. There was an open offer that this would continue to be available for as long as required.

Inevitably, within a short space of time, Michael the 'middle child', who was aged 14 years, began to present problems both at home and at school. It was fairly apparent that he, too, suspected something was wrong with mum, but was not sure what this was. Jennifer remained adamant that she did not want him to know her diagnosis as she felt he was too immature and unable to handle the information. She opted instead to tell him she had a blood disorder which made her very tired.

This began to get dangerous as Jennifer was prepared to be open and honest with Brendan and Sarah but was deviating from the truth with Michael, who clearly suspected he was being kept 'in the dark'. Sally and Patrick, at 12 and 11 years respectively, were considered too young to be told and were very involved in activities outside the household. Jennifer did not wish them to be 'burdened' with information about her health while she was still relatively well. We discussed the need to share information gradually and I explained this was not a one-off event and that details can be provided in a gentle and gradually increasing way, thus helping the children prepare. Jennifer was able to acknowledge this, but still found this too difficult.

As time passed, Michael became more persistent in enquiring about his mum's health, but this was interspersed with minor, and some major, disturbing episodes at home and school, thus creating an uncomfortable atmosphere to discuss Jennifer's health and future. Both Jennifer and David began to feel stressed by Michael's behaviour, but could not accept that his feeling of being excluded from important information about his mum might be contributing to his behaviour. Finally, after a great deal of soul-searching and after considerable negotiation with Michael and his uncle (from whom Michael sought support), it was agreed that Jennifer would share more information regarding her health.

The family did not feel able to read books together or use other methods of communication, such as drawing or educational games, as this had never been part of their routine and would have been alien to them. Usefully, however, they were comfortable and familiar with the concept of a family meeting to discuss issues concerning them all and felt this was the best means of addressing this issue.

This was particularly difficult as it was accepted that there were no right answers and Jennifer rehearsed with David and me how she might approach this difficult subject. We acknowledged that Michael might require factual information and need to know with whom he could share his concerns and fears. His brother and sister were felt to be key people who might share his perspective, and he would undoubtedly receive support from his uncle, who would also be present.

Despite the availability of literature on death and loss and the countless papers on HIV prevention, care and treatment, there was little to refer to for parents who decide to share this difficult information with their children or suggestions and ideas on how this can be done. Naturally it is very difficult to tell a child that someone important to them has a terminal illness, but, from experience, the most important factor to consider is how to offer reassurance that they themselves will be cared for and for the adults to provide physical contact to reinforce the fact that the child is loved. If a young person wishes to do so, they should have access to a doctor or nurse, who can explain some of the medical details, but this will be a secondary concern to the emotional impact of beginning to come to terms with this information.

It is appropriate in counselling children and young people that a client-centred approach be employed, reflecting back feelings and thoughts, checking information has been understood and assisting the child to identify strategies to deal with the difficulties which may arise. Honesty is generally the best policy and Jennifer finally decided that information concerning her health might be best communicated while she was still relatively well. This would then provide opportunities to share feelings, thoughts and memories. We discussed that seeing an adult cry can be an unusual occurrence, but this can also give the child permission to cry. It was agreed that it was important that such bad news came from someone the child knew and trusted and, with this, Jennifer explained her circumstances to Michael.

Michael reacted very badly to the information that his mum had HIV infection. He was very angry and felt he had been lied to and that his mum was to blame for her HIV status. He stormed out of the house and ended up in a park across the road where, after a short while, he was met by his uncle, who encouraged him to stay at his house for the evening. Jennifer felt terrible and was very upset as this, for her, reinforced a belief that she should not have told Michael and she feared what he might do with the information.

Michael did tell other people, against his mum's wishes, and the family were faced with the dilemma of how to respond. David feared he would be discriminated against at work if it was discovered that his partner was HIV positive and Jennifer was still unwilling to let her family and friends know, so, despite the stresses, they continued to deny Jennifer was HIV positive. Michael, although still very angry about his mum's diagnosis, settled at school and was much more responsive at home.

Two years later Jennifer became increasingly unwell and began to require regular hospital treatment. She now felt able to share information about her HIV infection with her immediate family, David's family and selected friends. She was remarkably candid about her future and, throughout this time, we sought and obtained legal advice on guardianship for the youngest child and discussed in detail her plans for her death and her funeral. All of the children were now aware of her HIV status and Jennifer retained control of this process.

The support services required had grown considerably and Jennifer now had a need for input from various agencies (see Figure 2.1). This required careful co-

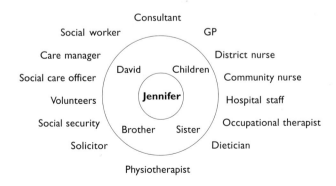

Figure 2.1   Support service for families.

ordination as each person was required to carry out a specific task, but there was potential for duplication, thus overwhelming the family with services which was a situation they desperately wanted to avoid. The need for care management became more apparent as the need for services grew and I therefore adapted my role to include that of care manager and to co-ordinate Jennifer's care.

Jennifer spent several happy months at home with periodic admission to hospital for treatment. Her philosophy was to laugh in the face of adversity and she gave her partner and children the strength to cope with her illness. She wanted her family to be with her when she died and this was exactly what happened. In the hours before she died, Jennifer laughed and was able to joke with David and the children. She died peacefully in hospital surrounded by all those she loved.

In the immediate aftermath the children supported one another. Their concern for each other was strongly reinforced by a common understanding of their mum's wishes and what she wanted for them. All fondly touched photographs of their mum taken when she was well. She had ensured that they all had a photograph of her looking well as this was how she wanted to be remembered.

Despite their ups and downs, all five young people remain close and rely on one another. Six months on, they continue to cry and feel angry about her death. Sally feels resentful of other girls she sees with their mum and asks why this happened to her mum. Life is complex and difficult to understand.

All the family need to meet regularly to discuss problems they are experiencing and in order to have what they feel is a legitimate opportunity to talk about their mum. I have continued to invite them to meet and almost all attend, whenever this is planned. We have used meetings to discuss 'if only' situations, 'favourite memories', 'things that make me angry' and lots of other subjects concerning their mum. Understandably, this is not always comfortable or easy for them to participate in and we inevitably face difficulties and great sadness, but all have benefited in some small way and willingly co-operate.

None of the family have wanted to meet with other young people who have experienced a similar loss and they feel the opportunity to share their feelings and experiences with one another is sufficient for the time being. All find it difficult to discuss their feelings when they are together, unless this is planned, but Sally and Sarah often meet and support one another.

The social work role here was to help this family through a very stressful and emotional period, help them to develop coping mechanisms and recognise their unique qualities and skills in being able to support one another. As time has passed and they have begun to rebuild their lives, they are now reaching a stage where they have less need for me to help them organise and facilitate their 'family meetings' and they are beginning to develop confidence in their ability to manage alone, with the love and support of one another.

Conclusion

Unfortunately, not all children have the luxury of a supportive familial response to the need for care and some require parents to explore alternative methods, for example guardianship, private fostering, custody or formal fostering or adoption. This is an extremely important factor to most parents and requires a sensitive and professional approach. In addition to this, families are constantly confronted by prejudice and discrimination as a consequence of the illness affecting them and face great fear and apprehension about the future.

For the practitioners involved, it would be easy to be seduced into believing that the stronger the individual or family's dependence on the worker, the greater the influence for any positive change. This attitude is extremely unhelpful and can have negative repercussions resulting in the person concerned feeling used and angry. All responsibility, credit, disappointment and joy must be 'owned' by the individual, thus reducing dependence on services to a minimum and enhancing self-esteem.

For practitioners in acknowledging the great sense of grief and sadness involved in this work, questions often arise :

- Was I able to do enough?
- Should I have done more?
- Why didn't/couldn't the parent take my advice?
- How could the situation have been better handled?
- What can I do to support those who remain?

The importance of quality supervision and access to support networks cannot be overestimated. It is essential that this is provided as structured support allowing additional time, if desired, for workers to access some informal support. This in turn gives the opportunity to consider professional practice, examine viable options, restore confidence and allows for professional and personal development, which will ultimately enhance the service provided.

In considering the issues to be addressed when working with families and HIV from a social work perspective, this chapter has considered the framework I have found to be most helpful. This has included the importance of the social work role in assisting families to cope with extremely complex circumstances and emphasising the positive effect individual practice can have when this is achieved in conjunction with the individual and their family. Ultimately, in providing an appropriate social work service to families in need, it is essential that social workers approach each situation with the utmost sensitivity, consideration, care and sincerity, thus ensuring that families affected by HIV receive a high-quality service.

References

BASW (1986), *A Code of Ethics for Social Work*, London: BASW.
Biestlek, F. (1961), *The Casework Relationship*, London: Unwin/Hyman.
Buckman, R. (1993), *How to Break Bad News*, London: Papermack.
Fahlberg, V. (1988), *Fitting the Pieces Together*, London: BAAF.

Chapter 3

◆

WORKING WITH FAMILIES IN A RESIDENTIAL SETTING

Ingrid von Arnim
Milestone House

Introduction

Milestone House opened in February 1991. It is Scotland's only hospice specifically offering care to people with HIV and AIDS. It offers, along with convalescent and palliative care, the opportunity of regular respite care to people who are physically well, as well as those who are ill, recognising the extreme psychological and social pressures placed on people who are HIV positive. HIV infection is a chronic, socially isolating and stigmatised condition, as discussed in Chapter 1. In such a situation, Milestone offers true 'asylum': the opportunity to escape the daily hassles of life for a period of time, to regain lost energy, and the opportunity to address issues in a peaceful, supportive environment.

Milestone offers family care and support, recognising that HIV affects the whole family, and that the hospice has a crucial role to play in helping parents to care for their children for as long as possible, by enabling children and other family members to stay in Milestone with the parent. Nearly two hundred children have either stayed in Milestone or visited a parent or other relative. With this level of contact, we clearly needed to be able to offer parents the opportunity to address the needs of their children.

It was apparent from the outset that for many parents, however caring, addressing these particular needs came quite a long way down a compelling list of family needs. It is almost impossible to focus your emotional energy on such issues if you are homeless, living in appalling conditions, if you are in deep debt, living in a violent and chaotic relationship or suffering persistent harassment or worse as a result of HIV. Assisting parents to achieve some stability in their lives was often a lengthy prerequisite, allowing them to move on to address their own and their children's emotional needs. As the social worker in a multi-disciplinary setting, it was part of my remit to offer a service to children and families, and throughout this chapter I will draw on practice examples to illustrate this work.

Working with Kim

Through years of hard work Kim had already achieved this stability when she began to use Milestone for regular respite. She had two children, aged five and seven. She approached me in some distress about her children, who had never visited Milestone. Being HIV positive meant that she was already leading a life full of secrets not shared with her children. She could not tell them why they had to stay with a carer while she regularly 'disappeared' for respite in Milestone, or why she made regular visits to the clinic. She felt that the very presence of the secret, that she had HIV infection, that she would become ill and might die, was inhibiting and impoverishing her relationship with her children, at the very time when she wanted to enrich that relationship and to give her children as much love as possible in the limited time available to her. She was also aware that the secrecy and changes being experienced by her children were beginning to have an impact on them, as evident through their behaviour. The younger child in particular was becoming both clingy and aggressive. She lacked concentration and was already underachieving at school, where staff had expressed concern about her aggressive behaviour.

Kim decided that she needed to begin telling her children what was happening. She was, however, terrified. Could she actually tell them, and how would she do it? How would they respond? Could her children cope possibly for years, with the pain of knowing she would die? Could she cope with their responses? Would such disclosure actually enrich their relationship or would it wreck it? Would the children blame her? Could they keep the secret? She did not want to risk the local community, including the school, knowing that she was HIV positive.

Above all Kim recognised that her fear came from her own fear of dying. To tell her children that she was going to die meant she had to accept that this was indeed the case. Until she accepted this reality she could not begin to tell them.

Kim spent nine agonising months exploring these issues, particularly her fear of accepting that she might die, and associated feelings of guilt, shame, anger and loss. She needed, in effect, to grieve for herself, and only having passed through an intense period of mourning could she move towards a greater focus on the children. I gave her as much information as possible about what we know of children's developmental needs, their emotional capacities and ability to understand the concept of death and dying. With this information we explored the possible range of responses the children might make and how they might express themselves cognitively, emotionally and behaviourally. We explored her coping mechanisms and how she might respond appropriately to any evidence of distress. We explored ways in which she could minimise the impact by providing a physical and emotional environment which remained as stable, secure and consistent as possible. We mapped her support network, and the pros and cons of informing members of her family and the school, for instance, about her infection and what she might be telling the children.

Kim finally decided it was time to act on her decision to tell the children. At this point she had yet more decisions to make. What exactly was she going to tell the children, and how was she going to give them this information in the safest and most age-appropriate way? Did she wish to be on her own when she did this, or with me or someone else? Kim decided that she wished to do the work jointly with myself. We planned two sessions with the children, and arranged for her to come into Milestone with the children for two weeks, so that I could get to know the children informally beforehand, and the work could take place within a supportive, contained and safe environment.

We had six 'planning and rehearsal' sessions. Kim had decided that she wished to tell the children about her HIV infection, and that she might become ill, and give them clear information about the lifestyle changes this would entail. She did not, at this point, want to tell them she would die. We devised a way of communicating this information in a way we thought the children would understand, using their own experience of illness as a starting point. We needed to focus on what would change in their lives, and what would not change, to be both factual and reassuring. We needed to be able to convey a concept of time to account for the chronic nature of HIV, and that not everyone who had the virus was ill. We spent a session attempting to anticipate all the possible questions the children might ask, and exploring how she would respond, including the question 'Are you going to die?' We needed to work out a way of addressing the issue of confidentiality with young children without encouraging them to keep 'secrets'. We were unable to do this at the planning session, but did in fact address it in the first session.

The importance of rehearsal became clear. During these sessions Kim frequently broke down. During the sessions she would need to be sufficiently familiar with the process and the information to focus on her feelings and those of the children. She would need to be able to express her feelings, but not loose control to the extent that the children would feel unsafe.

Kim described the moment she entered the room to begin the session as 'jumping off the cliff'. Of all the decisions an HIV positive person has to make, this is surely one of the most painful. There is no going back. This can feel like losing control, but alternatively be a moment of taking control.

Over the previous days I had met the children. We had the opportunity to eat meals and play together. I had found out important information: who they considered to be the important people in their lives, what they thought of school, how they perceived secrets (birthdays and presents were high on the agenda), what their favourite television programmes were. I had also had an informal opportunity to assess their personalities and cognitive ability.

We began by asking the children to draw a huge 'map,' on paper on the floor, of all the places in Edinburgh that were part of their lives. On to the map came their home, school, friends' homes, grandmother's house, the foster carer, the doctor, hospital and Milestone. The children were allowed to talk and draw in people and I asked questions: who was who, why did they stay here, or there, and when? Why had they drawn in the hospital, Milestone?

Unsurprisingly, we elicited that the children knew their mother was ill sometimes. I asked them if they had ever been ill. They had both had chicken pox, and we talked about how that made them feel, and what happened when they were ill. The children drew pictures of being ill and in bed. We explained to the children the concept of a 'bug' (virus or bacterium) entering the body and causing the reaction which makes them feel ill, and more important, leaving the body again, so that they feel better. We described the 'chicken pox bug' using the wings of a chicken as the metaphor, and the children drew pictures of the bug as they imagined it.

Kim described the HIV bug in the same terms, flying into the body. Only this bug is different. It sheds its wings and can never leave. A lot of the time it sleeps, at other times it wakes up and feels very hungry and energetic. It races round mummy's body. It's very exhausting rushing round like that and it makes mummy feel very exhausted and ill. Everyone drew pictures of the HIV bug asleep and awake in the body, and compared it with the pictures of the chicken pox bug. Kim explained that, while there are medicines that make other bugs fly away, no such medicines exist yet for HIV. She explained that the bug will get hungrier and hungrier, and make her more ill over time, and used birthdays and Christmases as benchmarks.

Kim then went on to explain that it was when she was feeling tired or ill that she needed to come into Milestone for a rest, and the children had to stay with their carer. The younger child told Kim that she didn't really like being with her carer. She wanted to stay with her mother. Kim told her that she felt the same way, but explained why this could not always be. We moved back to the map and looked at the things that were changing in their lives as a result of their mother's HIV infection, and all the things that would not change, such as school and family members.

Kim made it clear that the children could ask her questions at any time and she would endeavour to answer them. She might not be able to do so, but she would always tell them what was happening. I asked the older child who else he felt he could talk to if he needed to ask questions, or felt worried about what he had been told today. The list he gave included myself, his aunt and his grandmother. I asked him who he might feel uncomfortable talking to, and he listed his school friends among others. We put the lists on two separate sheets of paper. Children, it appears, can have a highly socialised sense of what is private 'family' information and what may be public. The session ended with card making for each other and lots of cuddles, time for questions and an opportunity for distress to arise. Nothing happened.

It was a year later, following a number of further sessions that focused, through play and drawing, on giving the children permission to express their feelings that Jane, the younger child, asked Kim, at home, whether she was going to die. By this time, Kim was well prepared and able to respond honestly. She confirmed to Jane that, yes, she would die eventually, but she could not tell her when or how it would be. She told Jane that all she could do was continue to be honest with her and keep her informed.

Kim asked Jane whether she wanted another session with me. The three of us met together. It was a dramatic session that again took place within the safety of a respite stay at Milestone. Jane needed to pour out her grief. She was held by Kim while she did so, and later fell asleep. Later that evening, Jane needed to pour out her anger, which she did with the help of a nurse and lots of cushions to hit and newspapers to tear.

Over the following months, we continued to focus on Jane's feelings. Kim and the children also began to compile a life-story book together, and created 'memory boxes'. These were filled by all three with great excitement, enthusiasm, sadness and happiness with photos, diaries, short stories, poems, paintings, and knick-knacks.

Jane's behaviour at school had been a cause for concern for some years. Her class teachers had not responded sympathetically, but were also unaware of her situation. Kim knew that there might be a relationship between the continual stresses at home and Jane's school behaviour. She now found the courage to inform the head teacher and the class teacher that she was HIV positive, and to address Jane's behaviour at school and at home. The school responded positively, arranging a weekly meeting between the head teacher, class teacher, Jane and Kim, which focused on both Jane's academic achievements and a behavioural star chart, kept at home, which we constructed together with Jane. Jane's behaviour and achievement level showed an immediate and sustained improvement. It was clear that she was aware of, and responding to, the consistency, understanding and support developing around her.

As she became more ill, Kim began to focus on the painful question of where the children should live after her death. She left this until last, she said, because she felt once this was done, everything would have been achieved and she would have to 'give up and die'.

Discussion

I have described the work with this family in great detail to illustrate some of the factors that need to be considered when helping parents to prepare their children for bereavement and its consequences. There is no one way and it is important to recognise that information can be dangerous. Not every child needs to know from the beginning that their parent has HIV or that they are dying. A burden is being placed on the child and it must be carefully weighed. On balance, it must be for the child's benefit and not the adult's. Major changes in lifestyle resulting from illness or emotional or behavioural evidence of fear, insecurity and distress might indicate that even very young children should be given sufficient information to make sense of their experience.

As a child becomes older, the question of the right to know may become as important as the need to know. Each situation must be considered individually. What has the family already experienced, what developmental stage is the child at, what is the parent's state of health, what losses is the child going to experience in addition to the death of the parent, where is the child going to live, what is the strength of the child's support network, the parent's network, the future carer's network?

It is not always necessary or desirable for a professional to work directly with the child. The most important legacy children will have is the memory of the quality of their relationship with their parent, to know they were loved and not abandoned, to know they were not to blame for their parent's death, to have a sense of continuity and identity that stems directly from the parent. Life story books and memory boxes are important instruments for conveying this information, but they are less important than the process by which they are constructed. Parents who engage in this process with their child can say these things directly. A professional worker or substitute carer is a poor substitute.

On this basis, I worked most frequently with parents rather than directly with children at Milestone, supporting the parents to prepare their own children, enabling them to overcome their own fears, equipping them with both the information and tools they needed, helping them to plan, monitor, respond and provide a safe place for them to express their distress.

Working with Nikki

Nikki came to see me nine months before she died. She knew she was dying. Her son John was six years old and had, up until then, been told nothing. Nikki knew she had to begin to tell John she was dying and wanted to know how to do this. She was clear that he did not need to know that she had AIDS. She had made her own plan for John's future, but had not told anyone, nor attempted to make it a reality. Although her mother and sisters knew what was happening, nobody was prepared to discuss John's future, least of all Nikki, who wanted to make her current partner John's carer. Her partner was not John's father, and there had been little contact over the previous two years as he was in prison. Nikki knew her family would be upset and furious. She wanted to know how to secure John's placement legally.

In just two sessions Nikki realised that her plans were the result of her own needs, not those of her son, and changed her mind. Together we had explored John's current and future needs and used a genogram and ecomap[1] to explore the strength and quality of John's relationships. Nikki decided that John would be better placed within her own family, and identified a close sister who was married with two children of her own. She called a 'family meeting' and was astonished to discover that the family had already discussed this. Nikki's sister had already volunteered herself as John's future carer.

I became involved in further meetings with Nikki, her sister and brother-in-law. Nikki wanted to be sure they understood the commitment they were making and the difficulties they might face in the future. She also wanted to explore the legal options available to secure John's future, but ensure he maintained his identity as her son until he was able to decide for himself.

Nikki did not forget John. She demonstrated astonishing creativity and attention to his needs. Before contacting a solicitor, the family held a Sunday lunch. They went round the table asking, 'If anything happened to me, who would you want to live with?' John chose his aunt, uncle and two cousins.

Nikki then began the process of telling John that she was very ill and she was going to die. She chose to do this on her own and met regularly with me for support. She created a 'special time' when she and John could say anything they wished to each other. She begun by reading to him *Waterbugs and Dragonflies* (1992), exploring losses and deaths he had experienced and his concept of death. Eventually she told him that she too would die soon. She encouraged him to cry if he needed to, and ensured she was there to give him physical affection. They began a memory box together. She told him of the plan for his future and together they planned for him to spend time gradually with his aunt and her family. By the time Nikki entered Milestone for terminal care, John was spending all his time in his new family.

Giving parents the confidence to involve their children and their extended families and the information to understand their children's needs, as well as the tools to help them to work together, is essential. But not all parents are able to overcome their own fears and pain sufficiently to do so. I have worked with children individually on their own at the parents' request, although I will only do so if the parent is prepared to continue to work with me separately, and if we have identified sufficient supports for the child. Such supports may be identified within the extended family or in other agencies.

Working with Sarah

Sarah was a parent who clearly recognised her children's needs to express their grief and worries, but was unable to cope with them herself. Susan, her daughter, was 12. Her father had died four years earlier and she knew her mother was HIV positive and what this meant. She had not attended her father's funeral, but began to attend the funerals of her mother's friends as they died of AIDS. Following one such funeral, Susan asked her mother if she could meet with me: she was too fearful of hurting her mother to speak to her.

Susan needed to talk and cry. She recognised that she had never grieved for her father. She wanted to hear the details of his funeral. She was also terrified that she would wake up one morning and find her mother dead. She needed factual information on the course of HIV-related illness, and to know that, while it was possible, it was unlikely that her mother would die a sudden death. Susan spoke about how isolated she felt at school, and her frequent feelings of overwhelming anger. She said that if she could grieve now for her mother's future death, she might be able to get on with her life until it actually happened, and somehow be better prepared. I asked her what would help her to grieve. She wrote an obituary for her mother, which was to be placed in the Milestone memorial book after her mother's death.

Sarah's other child, Nicola, was eight years old when her second partner died in Milestone. Sarah herself became deeply depressed and terrified by the reality that was awaiting her. Nicola became withdrawn and tearful and Sarah was sure that she was grieving for her stepfather. Sarah asked me to undertake grief work with Nicola. When I arrived, Sarah was panic-stricken. The previous night Nicola had asked her mother whether she had AIDS. Sarah had been unable to answer, and had asked Nicola to ask me the following day. Sarah said I had permission to discuss this honestly with her. Nicola not only wanted to know whether her mother had AIDS but what HIV and AIDS were and whether she herself was infected. She wanted to know whether her mother was going to die, and whether she herself was going to die. After giving her the information she needed, we spent some time drawing and talking about feelings. Nicola was finally able to cry. Her mother came in but was unable to hold her or comfort her, and was extremely distressed herself. Nicola finally calmed down and drew her mother a picture. On it she wrote, 'It's okay to cry'.

Further work with this family focused on addressing their isolation and finding supports appropriate to their different needs. I continued to work individually with the children. It also focused on helping them to communicate with each other in a way that was safe for all of them. They began to attend the sculpture workshops at Milestone as part of this process.

Discussion

For the majority of parents, preparing their children for bereavement and loss, and consciously planning for their future, was to think the unthinkable and the unbearable. Most parents recognised their children's needs but felt unable to address them, such was the web of secrecy and fear in which they were caught. Some parents would respond that their children 'do not need to know until I am dying', others that they 'knew the children knew'. At best, many parents said they would respond to their children if they began to ask questions, but regularly reported that no such questions were being asked.

So what needs to happen for children to ask questions, and how do we create a context of permission with appropriate time, space, openness and safety? Without parental permission it is not possible to work on issues either with the children, the extended family or the parents themselves. Yet most children were clearly aware that all was not well within the family. Friends and family members died with alarming regularity. Parents attended funerals and then came home and discussed how and why their friends had died. There were regular clinic visits and sudden admissions to hospital. At Milestone it was impossible to escape the conclusion that people died of AIDS, unless you could not read. Parents told me that their children did not know, yet it was not uncommon for a worker to be told 'My daddy is going to die' or 'This is the place where you come to die of AIDS'. Many children found themselves living with a new carer without preparation or acknowledgement of their experience. The new carers, often grandparents, were also unprepared. Bereaved themselves, blaming themselves for their children's lifestyle and premature death, their instinct was to shut the door on the past the moment the funeral was over, to make a 'fresh start' for themselves and their grandchildren.

So what can be done to support the children?

Working in a residential setting

Residential environments are extremely powerful therapeutic resources in their own right. The environment and resources available at Milestone allowed for some creative opportunities to provide support, and to help those families where direct communication between parents and children about the impact of HIV and AIDS in their lives was not possible. The child care facilities, multimedia and arts resources (the latter originally intended for adults) became increasingly important.

The child care facility, supervised by two qualified staff members, offered a safe space in which children could relax and play. For some, it was their only opportunity to 'be children', get support and to develop consistent adult–child relationships on which they could rely during traumatic periods.

The arts facilities were perhaps the most important resource, identified by both parents and children as a means of communicating with each other, and of sharing together, and of building up their relationship. Many parents and children would come to Milestone especially to participate in sculpture workshops. Parents who were unable to communicate verbally with their children about what was happening accepted opportunities to sculpt or paint with their children, write their life-story, or letters to their children, with the help of the Writer in Residence, or make videos about their lives, telling their children those things which were too painful to communicate directly. I often participated in arts activities with the parents and children I was working with.

What makes Milestone unique as a therapeutic environment is its safety, informality and accessibility and the possibility of parents, children, staff and others using the windows of opportunity. If a parent wished to discuss their concerns in the middle of the night, this was possible. If a child was distressed, there was someone to talk to. It was possible for parents, and to a lesser extent, children, to control the pace of the work they wished to undertake.

Creating a memorial page for a dead parent began to be an acceptable way for the surviving parent or new carer, who might be an uncle or aunt, of allowing children to express their grief and openly reminisce. Parents and carers would often be present: this was an opportunity for them to grieve too, and such expression gave children the permission they so often needed. In such sessions the message could be conveyed that it was 'okay to cry'. Parents or new carers might also reminisce and photos be produced, which are an invaluable source of information for the child. Symbolically, such sessions offered the possibility of 'saying goodbye' to one relationship in a ritualised manner, and of beginning the establishment of a new relationship based on shared memories.

This is particularly important if the child has been denied the opportunity to attend the funeral.

By 1994 many more parents were requesting support and assistance to work with their children. The most potent dynamic of a residential environment appeared to be having an effect, namely the shared experience of the peer group. It was Kim who began to encourage other parents to inform the school, borne out of her own experience with Jane, and who was able to reassure some parents that even young children can maintain confidentiality. Another parent showed the life-story book she was creating with her son to a group of mothers. Within an hour I received two requests to begin life-story work.

Most adults have a basic need to protect children from pain and hurt and instinctively believe this can be done by 'hiding' the facts of the adult world. Children and young people have a level of sensitivity to the pain and hurt of the adult world which we all tend to underestimate because it is expressed in a medium we have long forgotten, or not expressed at all.

At Milestone House we had the opportunity to encourage parents, grandparents, aunts, uncles and other workers to see that adults and children do not, in reality, live in two different worlds. Whatever the experience, it is a shared experience, differing only in perception, understanding and interpretation. While the adults found enormous difficulty in sharing this experience in a way which was meaningful for the children, the latter were expressing in numerous ways their need to be involved. Not to share was to deny the children part of their relationship with the most important people in their lives, their parents, in a situation where there would be no second chance.

Children 'protected' from pain were almost certainly enduring pain alone, and would go on doing so following the death of a parent. Pain shared between parent and child left children not just perhaps with less pain, but also with the memory of the sharing.

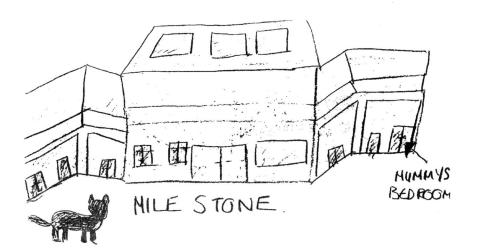

Note

1. Genograms and ecomaps are both diagrammatic constructs. The former depicts a person's family structure through at least three generations, creating a 'family tree'. The latter depicts a person's social network and might include family, friends, GP, school and other relevant agencies. The pictorial nature of these constructions, and the process of discussion and exploration that takes place around their construction, can assist in helping people identify patterns in family behaviour, relationships, traditions and areas of conflict and support which might otherwise remain hidden and confused.

Reference
Stickney, D. (1992), *Waterbugs and Dragonflies*, London: Mowbray.

Chapter 4

◆

BRENDA HOUSE

AN EXPERIENCE OF WORKING WITH DRUG-USING WOMEN AND THEIR CHILDREN IN A RESIDENTIAL SETTING

Joy Barlow
Senior Manager, Brenda House
Isobel Hamilton
Project Leader, Brenda House

Introduction

The Brenda House Project in Edinburgh is one of four Aberlour Child Care Trust Projects in Scotland working specifically with women affected by their own problem drug or alcohol use and their children. The project provides a range of therapeutic interventions including residential rehabilitation, day and outreach provision and supportive aftercare accommodation. Of all our projects, Brenda House has the greatest experience of working with families both infected and affected by HIV and AIDS.

At the heart of our service provision is the belief that drug dependency in women cannot be addressed without an understanding of the fundamental role that gender plays in defining identity, coping style, skills and available opportunities and resources. This approach assumes that the needs and characteristics of drug dependent women are similar to those of all women. It acknowledges that, while financial and emotional dependency in women is given credence by society through the legal system, the health service and social services, only certain forms of dependency are socially frowned upon. Within the project, the strengths and potential which women bring with them are recognised and built upon, thus helping women to develop abilities and capacities that have been limited through past experience and their role in society. We attempt to enable women to establish more adaptive ways of managing situations that have caused conflict and stress and to create more options for them in their own communities.

As a child care organisation, the Trust is obviously concerned about the welfare of the children of drug-using parents and all projects employ specialist playworkers who take responsibility for addressing children's needs. We attempt to ameliorate the damage to children who have been exposed to a chaotic lifestyle, to redress possible damage already done by child-rearing practices, to develop a more positive relationship between mother and child, and thus to help the whole family to develop its ability to care for all its members.

Drug use and mothering

By choosing to use drugs, women are explicitly going against their socially prescribed role as nurturers and servers. Drug use is seen as a highly self-indulgent activity, not compatible with the notion of mothers as guardians of the nation's moral welfare. Women using illegal drugs, particularly opiates, are viewed in a different light from those who use prescribed psycho-tropic drugs or alcohol. They are perceived as being incapable of being good parents, hard workers or socially useful people. In fact they may be all of these. A particularly strong perception current in the drug scene amongst drug-using women is that they cannot be good mothers. This has been instigated and reinforced by some professionals. The Aberlour Child Care Trust Projects grew out of the belief that this is neither a valid nor acceptable way to view chemically dependent women.

Although the majority of drug-using women are mothers, scant attention is being paid to the meaning of the role for them. When the relationship between mothering and drug use is noted, it is usually with the focus on the well-being of the children.

While recognising the need to be mindful of the care of children, the project's programme lays emphasis on seeing the woman as an independent person in her own right. Without that recognition of independence and the perception of women needing special and unique provision we see any attempts to help the children as being in vain (Roulston 1990).

Children affected by drug and alcohol use

Over the years we have begun to understand more fully the needs of children in vulnerable families affected by substance misuse. Children in drug-using families may come from a wide range of backgrounds and display a variety of responses to living in a drug-using family. Nonetheless, for these children, parental problematic drug use can prove to be the central focus of their lives, their feelings and their personalities. Behaviour can be affected more by this reality than by any other. Where there is problematic drug use, the possibilities of creating an imbalance in a family unit due to the unpredictable and often disruptive behaviour of the drug-using member is common. What we often see is that other family members will take on the role to cope with or contain the problematic drug use in order to reduce stress on the family unit and maintain its balance. Problematic drug use in a family can impair or distort the child's development, particularly if external supports are limited or if they are unaware of the extent of the problem.

In families where drug use results in a chaotic lifestyle, a number of characteristics may emerge (Barlow 1993). These have been discussed in Chapter 1.

In summary, problematic drug use not only affects the user but the family as well. Research and clinical experience indicates that a whole system of behaviours and strategies is developed to handle the drug-using family member. As the system develops, individual members may acquire unusual responsibilities that conflict with normal expectations. The conflict over expected behaviour, the lack of a sense of reality, the emotional or physical abuse, and then repression of feelings are major effects of parental problematic drug use on children and adolescents.

The drug-using community is notoriously stigmatised and isolated. Women in this community, or who have previously been problem drug-takers, find asking for help for themselves and their children very difficult. If you have lived with the stigma of apparently being an unfit mother and possibly threatened with the removal of your children, then asking the 'authorities' for help is a frightening experience. The situation is further exacerbated if your views are not given true recognition.

Working at a woman's pace

The Trust has endeavoured to help women to keep the parenting role, with the help of a range of supportive carers, even if eventually most of the caring is in fact performed by someone other than the mother.

Alongside colleagues in both the statutory and non-statutory sectors we have recognised the need to balance support and advice. We have to work at a woman's pace, to enable her to reach decisions and we have to support her decisions. Sometimes that is very difficult when a child is moving at a different pace. There are real dilemmas about when children should learn that their mother is dying, but we cannot intervene arbitrarily and take away this one area of her life that the woman may still be able to control. The best scenario is when a woman either tells her child herself, or asks a member of staff or other carer to help her to tell the child. The worst scenario is when the child should know, wants to know, and may indeed already know, but has never been 'officially' told. Here staff try to support the women in making the best decisions for their children. That is never easy; the child's right to know versus the parent's desire to remain silent is a moral dilemma faced by Brenda House staff on a regular basis, and support for them is very important.

Professional staff working across a variety of disciplines may wish that the situation regarding future planning for children could be more clear cut. It is our experience that this is rarely the case. The desire of most parents in such situations is to keep control and plan the future at their own pace. When a woman is faced by enormous questions about her child's future, coupled with recurring illness and possible problems of drug use, then her pace may inevitably be erratic. Sometimes, when feeling physically and emotionally capable, she may see the reasons for forward planning, though that may be tempered by the fact that when well she sees no need to plan. At other times she may feel tired, ill and increasingly concerned, but emotionally she may want to keep her child close to her, and may not be able to face big questions about the future.

The project's approach to counselling is person-centred and non-directive, which in terms of drug rehabilitation means that a woman's progress in the programme is self-determined. Translating this way of working into counselling on HIV and AIDS issues may be slow and erratic. Advice will be given as to how, when, why and by whom children might be assisted in the better understanding of their situation, but support needs to continue if a woman steadfastly refuses to make decisions. This process is achieved by going over various scenarios: role playing how each one might or might not be dealt with; explaining how a child might react; discussing the possible outcomes and identifying what supports might be necessary.

A useful way of looking at the parenting role is through the various functions of parenting. These can be defined as biological, nurturing, educative and preparation for citizenship. Each of us as parents fulfils these roles more or less well, but usually with the help of others. Women facing the issues of HIV with their children need to know that if one of these functions is taken over by someone else, then they have not failed as parents, but are being supported in the roles they are still capable of undertaking. Most women want to protect both themselves and their children from further pain.

Working with children on HIV issues
Establishing a framework

The Brenda House experience is a unique one because the family will have had the experience of being together in a therapeutic environment. For some it will represent safety and security. Children will already have had the experience of working through some of the issues as to why they are staying at the project and will have talked about fears, anger and so on. Therefore some of the ground work in talking about HIV and AIDS will be laid.

However, the obvious dilemma faced by all professionals and other care givers is continually present, that is the difficulties caused if a family has not given permission for 'the words to be said'. Thus, the partnership between parents and care givers is of vital importance. Brenda House staff have realised the importance of this trust, and therefore permission is sought to answer children's questions honestly, because a child's timetable for asking questions may not coincide with an adult who is carefully preparing the ground.

Our practice experience over time has raised issues which have enabled us to provide a reasonable working framework for working with children affected by HIV. This includes listening to unspoken as well as spoken messages; accepting that responses may not be immediate or obvious; giving permission for hurt and pain to be expressed; helping the child to find constructive outlets for anger, energy and fears; understanding the need for children to continue to address their loss; understanding the need for a bereaved child to establish a new identity; and understanding the need to talk about the parent when the child wishes.

Children require truthful answers which are best given within the context of a trusting therapeutic relationship. It is also important that those speaking to children have at least a basic knowledge and understanding of childhood and child development, for it is important to know the ways in which children differ from adults in their emotional responses.

Communicating with children

From basic information about how people become ill, more emotional responses are drawn upon, using books and poems, not always those written specifically on the issues of loss and bereavement. A great favourite of Brenda House children is the story of *The Velveteen Rabbit*. This children's story book by Marjory Williams (1922) is the story of a toy rabbit in a child's nursery who learns what it is to become real by being loved.

> 'Real is not how you are made', said the skin horse. 'It is a thing that happens to you when a child loves you for a long, long time, not just to play with, but really loves you, then you become real.'

The rabbit is the boy's favourite, until he is thrown away after the boy has had scarlet fever. Abandoned with the other rubbish the rabbit is very sad.

> Of what use is it to be loved and lose one's beauty and become real if it all ended like this? and a tear, a real tear, trickled down his little shabby velvet nose and fell on the ground.

At this point magic takes over in the story and a fairy turns the toy rabbit into a real one.

> 'I am the nursery magic fairy,' she said. 'I take care of all the play things that the children have loved. When they are old and worn out, and the children do not need them any more, then I come and take them away with me and turn them into real.'

The book has been used on a great many occasions to explain the meaning of being loved; how to grow shabby and lose beauty does not mean that this is a reason for abandoning people. Even when people are no longer what they once were, they are still loved and want to be loved.

With the use of the book children are able to explore that how people look is far less important than what they are like as people. The abiding theme of the book is that the power of love is greater than all other powerful emotions, and that there is a kind of existence other than the one we know of now. These themes seem to be important ones which can be communicated both to women and children, through the medium of a child's fairy story.

Staff at the project have always been keen to use the natural world to explain the 'mysteries of the universe', and the children are used to planting flowers, trees, bushes and so forth in order to remember people. One group of children were excited by the idea that the stars in the sky represent those who have died, but who are still with us, and one child always looks for the brightest star in the sky because the person who died was a 'bright, starry person'. This example represents a way of dealing with death, not as a taboo, but as a positive experience, and came from the family of one of the project staff.

What has been recognised is the need of those children directly affected by a death to keep memories alive. Families are particularly keen to hear the stories about mummy before she was ill, what she wore, who her friends were, the music she liked and so forth. This 'oral tradition' is important alongside the preservation of letters, photographs and so on.

Group work with children

In view of the fact that the Brenda House environment encourages openness and honesty, it seems logical that children of all ages will ask questions appropriate to their various levels of emotional and intellectual maturity. Thus, when the process of talking to children in a group developed, it was important to pitch the activities at a level in which all could participate and ask questions.

The group evolved from the discussions about a recent death which all the children knew about, and centred on the question of disease and how our bodies fight off infection, and how people become more ill. Children were encouraged to draw on their own experience of being ill and then explore what happened when the body could not fight off infection any longer. Activities took place using painting and drawing. For example, one boy drew a picture of a castle with the T-cells fighting off the enemy.

In group discussion children have been encouraged to give each other support and reassurance, something which again is encouraged by the philosophy of the project. This peer support becomes an important factor in helping to dispel fears of isolation so often felt by the bereaved.

Other groups have taken place with children, some on particular themes which have elements of HIV and AIDS within them. Other groups have been held specifically in order for children to give support to each other. An example of the latter is the Friday group which met over lunch time. The Friday group would usually involve children aged between 5 and 10 years. These children may deal with their situation by denial, which can cause adults unconsciously to withdraw support. It is at this stage that inner deep feelings need to be acknowledged. In the group children are encouraged to talk about any topic and are not stopped from expressing pain and grief. Stories about shared experiences are told, remembering outings, holidays, good and bad times. Sometimes feelings of guilt may be expressed and it is important to reassure a child that their behaviour did not cause the death. Staff at Brenda House have tried to help children realise that they are not alone, and that they themselves may feel very sad at the death of a child's parent. Explaining their fears may help both child and adult to understand the other's experiences.

Another group, facilitated by one of the playworkers, took the theme of families and family structures, looking at the way people move in and out of relationships and how sibling rivalry develops. Children drew pictures of their own families and talked honestly and openly about things which concerned them regarding the way in which family members behaved or had behaved. Some of the children wanted to explore the issues of 'daddies' and why some of them were not around, and for what reasons.

During the art work children could talk as little or as much as they wanted. This means that the children set their own agenda and sometimes the group might be a 'free play group'.

One of the children in this group had difficulties in the use of his legs, and because of frustration was becoming difficult with the others. The playworker decided to pretend in that particular group that no one could walk properly, and the children spent an hour realising how difficult it was and were able to talk about it and give the little boy in question support.

All the discussion in the group is fed back to the parents and is kept in the children's files. This encourages parents to continue discussion with the children, if they are able.

Conclusion

The aim of working with children on the issues of HIV and AIDS at Brenda House is to prepare children for the future in the knowledge that there are adults who will listen and be available. Children need to understand that they are not alone, and they must be encouraged to be children rather than little adults capable of maturity and responsibilities beyond their years. The project has worked in the belief that the children are children first and affected by HIV second.

The support needs of these children include networks, the chance to talk, the chance to look at the future and talk about it, information at an appropriate age and given in an appropriate manner, the opportunity to grieve and the opportunity to have as normal a childhood as possible (Honigsbaum 1991). Consideration of a child's previous experience of care must be a vital component of any supportive response. Children may have experienced inconsistent and unpredictable relationships, therefore they do not want a constant procession of carers. They do not want separation from their parents. They will have already experienced past separations at either a physical level or because of parental drug-taking behaviour.

Children wish to care, and it is through appropriate supportive adults that care will provide the basis of a future not too disfigured by enormous loss at a very young age.

The following poem is both a tribute to Marley and to her mother. Marley was seven years old when she wrote the poem, on the day she was told that her mother was dying in April 1995. She is one of the children to whom the work described in this book is dedicated.

Marley's Poem
1 April 1995

I love my mum she is beatful
She uset to be nice to me
She made me laugh and uset to give me big cuddles
and kissis and we were happy together but in
this very day she gopt ill and am very sad
everybodys sad and I cry very much and I
still love her very much and I still have my
Dad and aunty Issie I will never forget the happy
days whit my mum in this very day.
She diyd in peace and my aunty Izzy was there
with her. They had pink champagne and strawberries
before she died with Ronnie and Ian and steve and
Lorraine and my dad.

References

Barlow, J. (1993), Speech for 'Issues for Women and Children', Second International Conference on HIV in Children and Mothers, Edinburgh.

Honigsbaum, N. (1991), *Children and HIV: A Cause for Concern*, London: National Children's Bureau.

Roulston, J. (1990), 'Residential services: the example of Brenda House', in S. Henderson (ed.), *Women, HIV, Drug Use Practical Issues*, London: ISDD.

Williams, M. (1922), *The Velveteen Rabbit*, illustrated by W. Nicholson, London: Little Mammoth.

Chapter 5

◆

COMMUNICATING WITH PARENTS AND CHILDREN ABOUT MEDICAL AND NURSING PROCEDURES

Jacqueline Y. O. Mok and Fiona M. Mitchell
Paediatric HIV Service, City Hospital, Edinburgh

Introduction

Paediatric HIV infection is associated with a wide range of complex clinical and psycho-social problems. Like many other chronic childhood conditions, a multi-disciplinary team approach is required. It must be recognised that chronic illnesses are characterised by stable periods which may be interrupted by acute episodes requiring medical attention and hospitalisation. Families usually struggle to establish normality in between episodes of uncertainty and anxiety.

The majority of children are infected through vertical transmission, that is from mother to child during pregnancy, birth or breast feeding. This means that for women infected with HIV, feelings of guilt and blame have to be addressed along with the knowledge that their children require close medical surveillance. This chapter provides information on the medical and nursing procedures involved in the follow-up at the City Hospital in order to help explain why we do the things we do.

The setting

All families are registered with a general practitioner, who is usually the first point of contact. Where referrals are made to the Paediatric HIV Service at the City Hospital, the consultant paediatrician is ultimately responsible for the care of the child, and makes decisions about the medical treatment in conjunction with the family's wishes. Where necessary, other specialists may be involved.

Less than 20 per cent of the families use the out-patient clinic facilities at the hospital. Children are seen wherever it is convenient for the parents, and in the majority of cases the chosen venue is the family home. A familiar environment is usually less distressing for both parent and child. For some families, however, the home is a sanctuary of normality for the child, free from painful interventions and these families may choose a venue outside the home, for example the general practitioner's surgery, health visitor clinic or child's nursery. A breach of confidentiality is the greatest fear of many families and this must always be considered when choosing a suitable venue.

Wherever possible children with HIV will have their care and treatment carried out in the community. If hospitalisation is necessary, admission is to the children's infectious disease ward under the care of the consultant paediatrician who is already known to the family. Parents are encouraged to visit the ward with their child before their illness is apparent, so that they can be introduced to the in-patient nursing staff and become familiar with the surroundings and routines of the ward.

If the child is admitted to the ward, he is usually nursed in a single cubicle to avoid contracting or passing on other infections. Although visiting is unrestricted, this may have to be adapted to circumstances. For example, to protect their immune systems, very young children and babies are not allowed as visitors. A very ill child may require extra rest, and should not be disturbed by constant visitors. The nursing staff will be able to guide parents as to whether their child should have unrestricted visiting.

Parents are encouraged to take an active part in the care of their children. With support and guidance some parents may choose to become involved in certain nursing procedures such as administering medicines, giving nasogastric feeds, filling in fluid balance charts and keeping an eye on monitors and intravenous infusions. It should never be presumed that parents will wish to participate in such care and, as such, parents must not feel compelled to engage in procedures with which they feel uncomfortable.

The children's ward is also used for day cases, for those children who require medications by intravenous (drip) or inhalation (mask) routes regularly, but who are otherwise well and do not need to be admitted to hospital. These out-patient visits last two-six hours depending on the medications, and are timed to suit child and family circumstances. Often parents choose a time when their child has a half day to minimise absences from school. A large room in the ward is used for day cases and the hospital play specialists try to make the children's stay as fun as possible with structured activity and games.

Follow-up of children

It is essential that parents clearly understand the implications of, and reasons for, their child being tested. In accordance with their wishes any information regarding children's HIV status will be discussed with parents. It must be appreciated that all babies born to women with HIV infection will have the mother's antibodies in the first year of life, and are therefore 'HIV antibody positive'. This does not necessarily mean they are infected. Using specialised tests, many infected babies can be diagnosed as early as one week of age, although tests must be repeatedly positive before a definite diagnosis is made. While the importance of close follow-up in the first six months of life is emphasised, it must also be stressed that follow-up is offered on a voluntary basis and as such parents may choose to withdraw their child at any time.

The aims of the follow-up are to:
- detect as early as possible those babies who are infected with HIV;
- offer treatment as soon as possible to improve the quality of life for children infected with HIV;
- reassure most parents that their child has no signs or symptoms of HIV infection;
- support parents and carers through highly anxious times, either before a diagnosis is reached or when children become ill;
- help some parents come to terms with their own illness and plan for the future care of their uninfected child; and
- use the information gained from the follow-up to improve the care of future children born to mothers with HIV.

Nature of follow-up

At each follow-up visit, the doctor takes a medical history to find out if there have been any illnesses or concerns. Questions about child care and development are addressed by the health visitor, who also performs a developmental assessment. Measurement of the child's height (or length), weight and head circumference is done to ensure optimum growth. A physical check on the child allows early signs of HIV infection to be picked up. Finally a sample of blood is taken.

Other screening tests, for example chest x-rays and brain scans are planned annually. Results of these and other tests are usually discussed with parents before the next appointment. Although much has been learnt in the last 10 years about how HIV infection affects children, there are gaps in knowledge about how to treat infected children, whether therapies are effective and when the optimum time is to offer or withdraw treatment. If children require medical care, the options are discussed with parents. This may include enrolling a child into a trial. The parents' and child's wishes are always paramount in any decision made about treatment and follow-up.

Typical visit/consultation

As already stated, parents are given the choice of where they wish their child's follow-up to take place with the majority opting to be seen at home. Each visit typically lasts from around 20 minutes to over an hour, with some initial time being spent on informal conversation to help put parents and children at ease. If not already known, members of the paediatric team are always introduced by name to the family.

Ideally, the family in question will have had adequate preparation and information regarding the impending procedure well in advance of the consultation. This will entail informal discussion between the parents and a member of the paediatric team, usually in the parents' home. Although the first contact is made preferably in the ante-natal period, early contact after the birth will provide an opportunity to meet the parents, establish a relationship and above all admire their baby without the threat of blood tests or other treatment.

At each visit an initial assessment is made of the home situation to gauge any sense of hostility, friction, fear or apprehension. The best approach to examining a child is considered and a decision made as to whether or not the unpleasant procedure of taking blood should be undertaken first.

With babies and small toddlers it is generally the parents who need the greatest explanation and reassurance. Most babies tend to object strongly to having their movement restricted during an examination, particularly while having an arm held still for blood-taking. Consequently, many mothers express immense guilt that their child should undergo these procedures and blame themselves for their child's distress.

In assessing the situation, the following concerns are considered.

Child's concerns

- How has the child reacted to our presence?
- Is the child chatty and inquisitive or frightened and distressed?
- Does the child know why we are here?
- What has the child been told?
- Is the child expecting a blood test?
- What does the child remember from the last time?

Parent's concerns

- Does the parent appear agitated or upset by the impending procedure?
- Does the parent have a clear understanding about the proposed procedure?
- Does the parent seem wary of interruptions, telephone calls or visitors?
- Who else is present in the home?
- Are the other people present in home aware of the HIV issues?
- Is there a danger of inadvertent breach of confidentiality?
- Is the parent looking for an opportunity to discontinue follow-up?

During distressing procedures some mothers will try to soothe their child by rebuking the paediatric staff as 'bad and cruel people' and promising the infant that 'they will not be allowed to do this again'. By directing anger at the paediatric staff, a parent may be helped to cope with their own feelings of guilt and helplessness.

Occasionally a mother will project on to an infant feelings and emotions far in excess of his development capabilities. For example, one such mother insists that her five-month-old baby will only forgive us for taking blood if we bring her chocolate buttons. We comply with this request against our better judgement! Although it is recognised that taking time to discuss the merits or otherwise of certain procedures with a family is desirable, this can be difficult to accomplish and can prove frustrating and complex for the paediatric team. Contact with certain families can be erratic and unpredictable. The desire to have the reassurance of having one's child tested and found to be HIV negative is countered by the fear that testing may reveal children to be HIV positive. Consequently, families who actively avoid contact with paediatric services may suddenly present their child for testing at short notice. This type of situation clearly offers little scope for preparatory work with children.

Concerns of families

Parents worry about disruption to the family's routine by regular visits from the paediatric team or visits to the hospital. Many express fears or reservations regarding prolonged follow-up and their views are taken into account when negotiating intervals between routine check-ups, especially if the child is well. Appointments can be made to suit children's routine, for example after nursery or school hours or during school holidays.

When children have a life-threatening illness parents find it difficult to treat them as they did before their illness. It is important for children to know that the parent or carer is still in control and families are encouraged to maintain the usual level of discipline. By maintaining continuity and stability children are reassured that despite all the confusion and painful treatments the family can be relied on to remain the same. Involving the carers in medical or nursing procedures may help, as well as taking time to explain children's progress by showing parents the growth and development charts. Other siblings in the family may feel left out of all the attention focused on the ill child, and parents need to remain aware that the needs of other children are equally important. In many chronic childhood illnesses support groups exist for siblings but difficulties with confidentiality prevent many siblings living with HIV from using support groups.

Confidentiality

The stigma attached to HIV has led to difficulties in offering a service to many families. One of the greatest fears for families is breach of confidentiality, especially where partners or other family members are unaware of the mother's HIV status. A situation such as this not only poses ethical and moral dilemmas, but also major practical problems when endeavouring to monitor the health of an HIV infected infant whose father may be unaware of his partner or his child's diagnosis. Preparatory work done with such a child will be hampered by the mother's fear of inadvertent disclosure and any communication about procedures will become fraught with difficulty.

The fear of identification and subsequent risk of stigmatisation has meant that some parents have chosen not to have any involvement with paediatric HIV services. Women who have initially chosen to have their child followed up by the paediatric team have found the complexity of arranging suitable venues and maintaining confidentiality too problematic and have subsequently severed contacts with paediatric services for fear of identification.

It is understandable that some parents are reluctant to seek medical care or follow-up and this is especially true when children grow older and start asking questions about the follow-up. Such questions usually demand explanations which may involve disclosing the mother's HIV status or lifestyle and many parents will therefore choose to keep their child in the dark or withdraw them from further follow-up in order to avoid painful explanations.

There is also a worry that children may start telling teachers or friends about family problems. In our experience, where children have been informed of HIV in the family, very few breaches of confidentiality have occurred. Children who are old enough to understand should be involved in discussions which involve future parental illness and plans for their care, at a pace which is comfortable to children and parents.

Parental guilt and anxiety

Many parents living with HIV experience feelings of guilt, blame and powerlessness, which can manifest as aggression towards doctors and nurses. Members of the paediatric team may then be viewed with fear and mistrust and associated with painful procedures. Careful explanation about the necessity of follow-up, as well as an acknowledgement that the medical and nursing profession also get upset about inflicting pain on children, usually allows some working relationship to develop. Parents can be given a choice about the level of their own involvement in a procedure. Some choose to hold their child while blood is being taken, others prefer to leave the room to dissociate themselves from the painful procedures, returning only to comfort the child. Medical interventions should never be used as a threat to children, for example, 'If you don't behave you'll get a jag.'

At one home visit to arrange a subsequent appointment a five-year-old child appeared distressed and agitated by the health visitor's presence. He was reassured by his father who promised that 'he would not get any more jags', while at the same time indicating behind his back that he did wish the child to have further blood tests. This difficult situation was resolved by taking time to talk with the child about his fears and by explaining the proposed treatment in detail. The use of local anaesthetic cream ensured a pain-free procedure a few days later. It was important that this child was offered an honest explanation in order to prevent him losing confidence and trust in his parents.

Parents who choose to administer treatments at home will need training as well as on-going supervision and support. Training must take place at the parents' pace and parental involvement should occur only when the parents feel confident to undertake medical and nursing procedures. Parents should always feel able to seek advice and support from medical and nursing staff even when they are in sole charge of treatments at home.

The early months before a definite diagnosis is made raise many anxieties and feelings of guilt for the parents. Repeated explanations are usually required to reassure them. Some doctors allow parents to record the consultation on to a tape so that the information can be listened to again with other members of the family, if necessary, and important messages reinforced. Parents are also encouraged to write questions down before coming to the clinic.

Children's anxiety and pain relief

Children are often bewildered by the secrecy surrounding family illness and anxious about the nature of medical and nursing interventions. Simple explanations are usually necessary with the level of detail dependent on age and maturity. Medical jargon is best avoided and the same language and terms used by parents should be followed, for example 'jag' or 'jab' for injections, 'check-up' for physical examination. Children are usually given an opportunity to explore the medical kit, trying out instruments such as auriscopes and stethoscopes on themselves. The doctor can also try out the procedure on a teddy bear or doll, allowing children to observe in a non-threatening way. Setting up a hospital corner in the ward or waiting area also allows children to become familiar with medical procedures. A selection of children's hospital books are available in the waiting area and in the children's ward which can be used with children by parents and staff. The use of local anaesthetic cream (often referred to as 'the magic cream') will alleviate the pain involved with injections, although some children are upset by having the cream put on. We try to involve children in decisions such as choosing where they would like the blood taken from, and leave some cream with the parents so that the chosen area can be anaesthetised prior to the next visit. It also helps if parents are provided with some medical equipment, for example syringes, blood tubes and gloves, to enable them to explain procedures to children, through play. Rewards are used to alleviate the anxiety. At the clinic we use customised plasters, gloves, balloons, badges, bravery certificates and sweets.

Children's privacy must be respected at all times. Some children object to being undressed and a compromise can usually be reached, for example listening to the chest or feeling the abdomen through clothes. Parents may worry about the apparently large volumes of blood taken and showing them the size of the blood tubes as well as explaining the variety of tests may help to ease their anxiety. Where possible we may request that stored blood be tested to avoid an unnecessary procedure for children.

It is best that children should be given truthful explanations. It is preferable to say, 'The procedure will only hurt a little and will be finished quickly if you keep nice and still,' rather than, 'It doesn't hurt at all.' Many children accept procedures if given adequate answers and reassurances. Occasionally children may need to assert control and should not be discouraged from crying or refusing a procedure which, on previous occasions, they had not objected to. Each child is an individual. Some prefer to have the painful procedure first before anything else is done, while others like to leave the nasty bits to the end. It is best to respect the child's rights to refuse to have a test, especially if healthy and the test is only in the interest of research. Sometimes we face a dilemma where the carer is agreeable to a blood test but the child is adamant that they are not having blood taken!

Many children will benefit from having an individual to whom they can discuss their fears and anxieties. This trusted adult can be a family friend, play specialist, teacher, counsellor or family support worker.

Terminal care

A child with end-stage HIV disease may have an acute illness which can be treated aggressively and the child returns to a stable period of well-being for weeks or months. This roller coaster in the family's life can go on for several months, and leave the family emotionally and physically drained. During these times there may be conflict between health care professionals and parents as to whether active treatment should be instituted at all costs. When all therapy has failed, parents are involved in the decision to withdraw interventions. They must be reassured that their child will not be in pain and that death will be dignified, but there will be the added pain of the secrecy of AIDS.

The stigma of AIDS in the family prevents many parents from discussing their own or their children's illness. Often parents will not allow any discussion of their illness or impending death with their dying child. Children usually have a greater understanding of their illness than adults believe and feel frightened and bewildered in their isolation. Where parents or carers decide to involve children in discussions, this must be done at a level appropriate to the child's development and with help from a professional counsellor.

Most families wish to care for their terminally ill child at home. Support must be available and on-going to manage the practical aspects of care. The needs of carers as well as other children in the family must not be forgotten.

As HIV infection in children is a relatively new disease, much remains to be learned. Distressing though it may be, parents or carers are usually approached for consent to perform an autopsy examination of children. It is hoped that information gained from that examination may help other children. It is also the responsibility of medical and nursing staff to discuss funeral arrangements including disposal of the

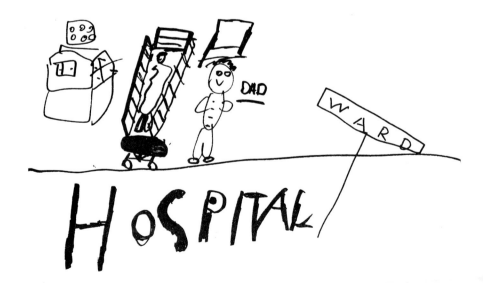

body after death. There never seems to be a right time for such sensitive discussions and many doctors choose to do this early on in the illness to allows carers time to make decisions.

Conclusion

HIV infection in children is a major chronic illness with many complex medical and psycho-social challenges. It is still both a relatively new and rare phenomenon and one where our knowledge base remains inadequate in many areas. However, we have been able to learn from good practice developed in other settings where children with other chronic illnesses are cared for, as well as developing some of our own. It is both possible and desirable to provide a child-friendly environment within clinical settings, where parents and children can feel involved as active participants in their own medical care, where they can be helped to make more informed choices about that care and where basic medical procedures are de-mystified. Such practices will not make all the fears and anxieties associated with HIV disappear, but they will help prevent the medical care itself from adding to those fears.

◆

Chapter 6

Hospital play for children infected and affected by HIV and AIDS

Alison Blair, Rosemary Garrod and Jinty Ramsay
Hospital Play Specialists

Introduction

Play is important for any child's visit or stay in hospital because:
- Play is a normal activity for children.
- Play makes a link with home and the outside world.
- Play helps communication.
- Play reduces stress and anxiety.
- Play provides a way in which children can express emotions, like anger and frustration.
- Play preparation for medical procedures helps a child understand the way treatment is given.
- Play lets a child feel in control.
- Play is *fun*.

Most people feel apprehensive when they or their child have to go to hospital for treatment or tests, so it can be very reassuring to find that children are welcome. Children who have had a previous 'bad experience' of hospital will be apprehensive or scared. This 'bad experience' is often caused by the child having to be rushed to accident and emergency in great pain, with no time for play preparation. Parents, naturally enough, worry; perhaps they have had to leave their child alone overnight in a strange place with strange people; or the child knows of someone who died in hospital. If this is the case, it is hardly surprising that a child associates hospitals with pain, anxiety and negative feelings.

Play specialist team

The role of the hospital play specialist within the ward team is to provide suitable and therapeutic play for all children and teenagers (0–16 years or over) who come to the hospital, taking into account their physical, intellectual, emotional and social needs.

Playing with children affected by HIV and AIDS

In the out-patients' clinic, a few children come to see the doctor or have tests, but many more children accompany parents, relatives or friends. Some of these children may have spent a few days or weeks staying with their family in the hospice, visiting sick parents in hospital wards, or caring for their parents at home. These children are living with HIV and AIDS. Children who need regular treatment, or are ill because they are HIV positive, are treated in the children's ward.

The play which we provide for children affected or infected by HIV and AIDS is in many ways no different from the play we provide for any other children who come to hospital. Most of these children come to the out-patients' clinic, where there is a play area (at one side of a busy corridor), equipped with a home corner, which has a cooker, sink unit, doll's cot and highchair, tea sets and cooking pots. Here the children can imitate scenarios from home, or create their own fantasy home, cafe or hospital. The toy medical set, a white coat and nurse's uniform help them to play out medical situations which may seem very frightening to a young child. There is a low table and chairs used for teaparties; jigsaws, drawings and board games are available for older children. Babies and toddlers are also catered for with rattles, activity centres, shape sorters, inset jigsaws, cars, dumper truck and so on. The rocking horse in the play area is very popular with toddlers and young children, providing movement in a restricted area.

We also provide the opportunity for messy play like painting, play dough and gluing. Nearly all children love to paint. Red and black are often the favoured colours but a full range of colours is provided. Painting is an ideal medium for expressing feelings. It gives the child a sense of control. Some of the affected children who may come from chaotic backgrounds have many fears and worries about their parent's repeated ill health. Sometimes they paint very neat, tidy and precise patterns or pictures. It is as if the paint brush is the only thing they have total control over. Equally, if they need to splash and scribble, draw and block out again, they must be allowed to do so.

Play dough, to thump, squeeze, make models, or roll and cut out, is fun to play with, and at the same time it relieves tension, and provides a satisfying outlet for angry feelings. Children (and adults) relax as they work, gaining satisfaction when they finally produce a simple sausage or wiggly worm, or an elaborate basket of fruit, 'cakes and scones' or nothing in particular. Although help is at hand if needed, there is no pressure on anyone to create a masterpiece or produce something recognisable. Just being able to pick up a piece of dough, to squeeze, roll and feel the texture is as important as making something with it. Older children and teenagers are encouraged to play board games, try puzzle books, word searches, read teenage magazines, draw cartoons, look at diagrams of how our bodies function, listen to someone's heart with a working stethoscope, or put on a Walkman® playing familiar sounds.

While playing with the children, or watching them play in the out-patients' clinic, the biggest influence on how the children play seems to be the condition of the parent they are accompanying. Younger children are often not told about their parent's illness and this can leave them worried and bewildered about unexplained illness. School children may pick up on things they see or hear, and may not know that there is something wrong and are angry at not being told the truth. They share these feelings with the children of those who suffer a chronic illness, but HIV opens up complicated and sensitive issues, such as how the virus was contracted, which parents may feel this is too difficult to explain. The parent may also feel afraid that the child will innocently pass on information to others which could result in a backlash of prejudice. Over a period of time, as we have built up a relationship with the children and their parents when they are visiting the clinic, we have become aware of some of the issues these families face.

One 11-year-old, a regular visitor to the clinic, came one day with a friend. While his parents were seeing the doctor, his friend asked him why his parents were at the hospital. 'Why?' came the further enquiry. 'Just because,' came the abrupt and final reply. He suddenly appeared hostile and angry with his friend. Did he know? If he did not, he knew it was something he should not be talking about. It is true to say these older children can often feel isolated or different from their peers. Some children take a more active role in protecting their parents by actually caring for them.

A parent who frequently visits the clinic often has one of his two daughters with him. Both girls appear immature in their selection of toys or play activities, yet are obviously of great support and practical assistance to their dad. On one visit, dad would not talk to any member of staff without his daughter acting as some kind of mediator. Although she helped willingly, she would always dart back to the play area, taking up an activity which appeared inappropriate to her age. Perhaps the pressure, however willingly taken on, left her with a longing to break back to a period in her life when she had less responsibility to cope with.

It is important for us, in these situations, to let the child choose and direct the play, so they can gain control and comfort from playing.

Working with Zara

On one occasion a three-year-old girl, Zara, refused to leave her mother's side because on a previous visit she had witnessed mum having blood taken for testing. In spite of being comforted and reassured by the nurses at the time, this had distressed Zara greatly, so by staying with her mum it was as if she was trying to protect her. It took longer to build a trusting relationship with Zara because she had been traumatised by her previous experience at the hospital. However, mum and the play specialist both spent time playing with her together. Mum was very forthcoming and used that traumatic experience to explain Zara's extreme clinginess; she then reinforced her behaviour by immediately saying, 'She'll not leave me; she won't stay with you.' This made Zara feel more justified in her action. I decided it was better to change the subject to something other than Zara, but it was important to continue to talk to her mother as it allowed Zara to see there was a comfortable relationship between her mother and myself. By taking the focus away from the child she was allowed to behave in a less self-conscious and more natural way.

It did seem that in some ways Zara's mother subconsciously encouraged this behaviour, partly due to the fact that she herself was quite advanced in her illness and wanted to have as close a relationship with Zara as possible. Although this tired her she was reluctant to pass over the care of Zara to anyone else. Both mother and daughter needed support from the hospital play specialist to enable the mother to relinquish a small amount of the care of her daughter to appropriate people, in order to allow time for herself. By showing the mother that this would not detract from her relationship with Zara, but take some of the intensity away, it helped Zara feel less responsible and protective of her mum.

Mum spent time with me playing with Zara on each visit to the clinic. On the whole, the time needed for Zara to become relaxed and comfortable with me grew shorter on each visit, unless her mother was very ill. I introduced toys and realistic medical equipment, including syringes without needles and a specimen bottle. By using these on a doll first, then by offering them to Zara to try, she was able to act out the procedures she had witnessed. Any misunderstanding shown in her play could be corrected so that doctors, nurses and hospitals became less frightening for her.

On the ward, the children who are infected by HIV come for treatment on a regular basis. Some of these children are very 'hospitalised' as they have been coming for a number of years. Although we provide the same kind of play as in out-patients' clinics, we also have a longer time to assess these children's needs and abilities and so provide a more specialised play programme. Those children who are close in age and in good health come together for their treatment. This lessens their feeling of isolation and offers mutual support.

At these sessions we provide craft work so that the children can each create their own masterpiece to take home, making each visit a positive experience. Recently we decorated plant pots before planting them up. The children look forward to their visits when they can see if their plant has grown or burst into flower yet. We also have pet fish on the ward. If one of the fish dies the children ask endless questions, 'Where is it now?', 'How did it die?', 'Why?' and so on. This allows the children the opportunity to discuss with us the cycle of life and death which affects all living things. The book *Beginnings and Endings and Lifetimes in between* (Mellones and Ingpen 1983) explains this well.

If the health of one of the children deteriorates and they are in hospital more frequently, their play programme may need to be revised. As the child becomes more and more disabled, a stronger input and more help from the play specialist will be required.

Children as patients will have decreasing concentration spans and will easily tire. We have to provide play which stimulates, yet does not exasperate, as well as play to help them deal with their hopes and fears. We often rely on sensory materials, such as finger paint, play dough, sand and water, as these can have great properties for soothing, as well as stimulating, the senses. Many children enjoy using finger paint and it is helpful to let the child choose what colours to use. Very often they choose red, black or brown but a wide variety of colours should be offered to suit any mood. Tell the child, 'That is a good colour to choose.' Later, as they make patterns in the paint with a finger, thumb, or whole hand, it might be helpful to say, 'I wonder why you chose that colour today.' Their answers are revealing, as well as surprising. One child who had chosen red said, 'That's the blood! That's the blood!' When I asked, 'What blood?' he described a horror video most graphically. It sounded like an adult video and he was obviously terrified by it. He swirled his hands in red paint, squeezing it between his fingers, letting it drip off them, and talking all the while about what he had seen. When he was finished he was asked, 'Are you ready to wash your hands yet?' 'Oh yes,' he replied with a huge sigh of relief. He made a very thorough job of washing every last speck of red away but was not satisfied until he had washed the board the paint was on. The cleansing of paint, especially when the colour is chosen because it has negative associations for that child, is as important as the actual finger painting. On the other hand, if a child is reluctant to wash away their design, a piece of paper can be laid on top, pressed down carefully, then lifted to make a print.

Often children are so absorbed in what they are doing that silence reigns and knowing when to speak and when to keep silent is a real skill. Background music may help a depressed child to express themselves more freely. Encouragement, affirmation and the opportunity to express their feelings by making a mess using forbidden 'dirty' or bright colours can be most satisfying for children of all ages.

Adults rarely join in with finger painting but play dough on the other hand, or clay, has its appeal for adults and children alike. Using the sort of home-made play dough described at the end of this chapter means the item can be kept by the child or we can chat to the child about making it as a gift to someone close. This can open up discussion about what the child would like to leave to parents, siblings or friends. This could be a simple form of a will. By doing this with the involvement and support of the child's parents, we can then look at the real possibility of the child's death. This may facilitate more open and helpful discussion about the future. Story telling, too, becomes an important release from their condition, allowing escapism into a fantasy world, as well as a pleasant way of giving factual information.

Conclusion

This chapter has tried to show that the play we provide for children infected or affected by HIV is not unusual or different from other kinds of play. It illustrates well-established, good practice which can be undertaken within residential or day care settings or in the child's own home. It does help to have a good understanding of child development and some knowledge of the social consequences, as well as health issues, relating to HIV. Enjoying children and play oneself are also important prerequisites! The rewards are many. To see children relax and enjoy what they are doing is a small part of it. To know that you have helped a child's understanding, listened to a child's point of view, seen that child grow in self-confidence and affirmed their uniqueness – that's what it's really about.

Some recommended activities and materials

- Painting a large piece of paper, powder paint in assorted colours, mixed with washing-up liquid and a little water, in non-spill pots or ready-mixed paint in non-spill pots, various brushes.
- Palette of paint, finer brushes, water pots for older children (eight years or over) who get to choose which kind of paint to use.
- Play dough

  ### Ingredients

1 cup of plain flour	1 tablespoon cooking oil
1 cup water	1 heaped tea-spoon cream of tartar
1/2 cup salt	a little food colour

  ### Method

  Put a pan over a low heat. Stir all the time till it thickens and forms a ball in the centre of the pan. Cool. Knead. Store in a clean margarine tub with lid or other plastic food box in a cool place. Will last 1–4 weeks depending on storage, how often used and so on. This dough is suitable for modelling, rolling and cutting out.

- Play dough: made with 1 cup flour, 1/2 cup salt and a little water bakes hard and is good for Christmas tree decorations or to decorate a candle holder, edge of a mirror, and so on. Can also be used to make small ornaments.
- 'Newclay' has the advantage over pottery clay as it does not need to be fired in a kiln but dries hard at room temperature.
- Washable PVA adhesive plus spreaders, decant into shallow pot with lid so that unused glue is not wasted.
- Scissors: include one pair of left-handed scissors.
- For collage: provide bits of coloured card or paper, material, sequins, ribbon, tissue paper, anything which will stimulate a child's interest and imagination.
- Junk, cardboard tubes, boxes, and so on, to create objects of their choice.
- Jigsaws for all ages. Not more than 80–100 pieces as concentration span is limited even with older children and teenagers.
- Home corner with full range of equipment to stimulate home play, imaginative play – ages 2–6 years (a toy tea set will do if you are short of cash).
- Medical kit: try to use one with realistic toy instruments, for example, Fisher Price. When an adult is there to supervise safety and encourage medical play, a working stethoscope, spare oxygen mask, cotton wool, bandages and so on.
- Photographs, pictures, books, showing various medical procedures being carried out, or to explain HIV.

- Baby toys: rattles, nesting cups, activity centre, toys which make a noise, squeak, have bells, click and so on.
- Toddler toys: shape sorters, chunky cars, dolls, toys where something disappears then reappears, thick wax crayons, coarse paper, shape boards, and rocking horse.
- Puzzle books, dot-to-dot, felt-tipped washable pens.
- Board games: must be quick to play, robust, easy to learn with not many rules, for example snap, pairs, dominoes, draughts, Frustration, snakes and ladders, Connect 4, Othello, Crossword and so on.
- Story books: use ones which are multi-cultural, non-sexist, non-aggressive. When an adult is there to answer questions and explain, use books about death and bereavement.

Reference

Mellones, B. and Ingpen, R. (1983), *Beginnings and Endings with Lifetimes In Between*, Limpsfield: Dragon's World.

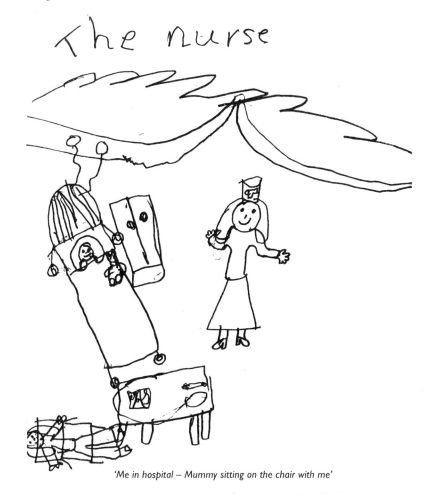

'Me in hospital – Mummy sitting on the chair with me'

Chapter 7

◆

What shall i tell the children?

Group work with women on communicating with their children

Jan McClory
Women and HIV/AIDS Network

Introduction

The principal aims of the Women and HIV/AIDS Network (WHAN) are to provide information relevant to women's lives about HIV, and to encourage and stimulate the mutual support of women affected by HIV and AIDS and workers involved in this field. It was established in 1988, and in 1992, it received funding from the Urban Programme to carry out development work in Lothian Region.

WHAN attempts to work in partnership with agencies and individuals for whom HIV is an issue. We hope to provide a focus for the development of initiatives in this field. Our outreach work is based upon a community development approach, seeking to identify women's needs and, with them, to identify strategies to address these needs. Some of our work has been in the area of HIV prevention, with particular attention to the needs of women from ethnic minorities. Other initiatives have been developed with women whose lives are affected by HIV and AIDS in a major way. This chapter will describe work undertaken by WHAN to support HIV positive mothers.

Women's needs

Talking to children about HIV and AIDS has been an area of much interest over the last few years. For the children of HIV positive parents, the issue has special significance and many workers have expressed concerns about the conflict which can exist between children needing to know about their parents' situation and the reluctance, on some parents' part, to make that disclosure. This issue was one which was also a concern for some of the HIV positive women who were in touch with our agency. They felt under pressure at times to disclose their status to their children. At times they actively wished to be open with their children but drew back from the task, afraid of the possible consequences of their actions.

At a seminar where workers and parents had discussed this issue, one mother commented to me:

> I want to tell my kids, and my social worker keeps on telling me my kids need to know, but nobody tells me how or what to do if it all blows up in my face. Most of the workers seem to talk about needing more training in talking to children about loss and bereavement. What training will I get?

WHAN certainly supported the view that children had needs in these situations which they deserved to have met, including the right to appropriate information, involvement, reassurance and expression of their feelings. On listening to women, it became clear that for many it was fear of rejection by their children, of 'doing it wrong' and causing further pain and damage that held them back from disclosure. For some, fear of disclosing a past history of drug use was enough to compound their silence. Our aim, therefore, was to work with women whose wish to communicate effectively with their children in this sensitive area was undermined by fear and lack of confidence. We believed that, through addressing the needs of parents in this way, we could respect the needs of their children and also support and strengthen the relationship between mothers and their children.

WHAN had already committed itself to the support of women in the HIV epidemic. As a voluntary agency, we had the opportunity and potential to work with women in a manner which might not be possible within the statutory sector. As an adult service, our primary focus was on mothers themselves and on their life experiences. We believed that in order to create a safe environment where women could explore some extremely sensitive issues, the workers involved should be women who possessed an awareness of the issues and life histories which would be the background for this work. We believed that it was essential that facilitators could relate to the experiences women brought with them. However, being female was not sufficient in itself and there were several other essential requirements for the facilitators. Extensive experiences and skills in training were considered a priority, along with practical experience in children and families work. It was also vital to have sound knowledge of child development and both theoretical knowledge and practical experience of loss and bereavement issues.

Both facilitators, in this case, were experienced trainers in a wide variety of settings. One was a clinical psychologist with extensive experience working with families affected by HIV and drug use. The other was a qualified social worker with many years' experience in counselling, particularly with young people in the areas of loss and bereavement.

The consultation process

Our next step was to make contact with agencies who were actively working with women who were HIV positive. This covered a considerable number of organisations from both the voluntary and statutory sectors. We invited representatives from these agencies to a consultation meeting. The primary task on this occasion was to identify the main issues concerning HIV positive mothers as perceived by workers offering support to these women. What emerged clearly was the issue of communicating with children about HIV and its implications for their future. In some cases anxiety had arisen due to increasing ill health and pressure on mothers to make plans for the future care of their children. In other cases, mothers were expressing a clear desire not to wait until their health deteriorated before they talked to their children about their diagnosis.

We then asked what agencies offered in terms of support in this area, in an effort to identify gaps. Some agencies identified a lack of relevant skills available to deal with such a substantial task, while others identified there was not the necessary trust between workers and clients to realise this kind of work. One thing common to most agencies was an awareness that women had a wish for peer support when dealing with the very real challenges HIV presented. Each organisation was aware of individual women voicing very similar concerns, and who were also living in isolation from each other. None of the agencies present felt they were able to progress this area of work.

Following on from this meeting, we decided to use these contacts in an attempt to consult with HIV-positive mothers themselves. It was our wish to bring women together so they might identify their wishes and needs. In addition to our original contacts, we identified key workers in the community. They worked in a variety of settings including children's centres, GP practices, drugs agencies and hospitals. The two facilitators undertook to visit, or contact by telephone, those workers whom we knew were likely to come into close contact with HIV positive mothers. We introduced our idea of the consultation to them, sought their views and support, and enlisted their help in encouraging women to attend such an event. These workers were also able to support women, either by accompanying them or helping with transport to the first meeting.

Seven mothers attended this initial meeting. Most of the mothers were acquainted with each other. What emerged was a request for an event in which women could:

- explore their fears in a safe environment;
- share experiences and learn from each other;
- learn about child development and check out their parenting skills;
- 'rehearse' talking to their children;
- learn about resources;
- learn about children's experiences of loss; and
- plan for the future.

The women involved in this session felt strongly that they would gain much from a group experience, rather than one-to-one support.

The programme

We looked at the requests outlined by the women, and compared them to the content of training courses we had previously delivered to professionals on working with children, loss and HIV. We recognised that our consultation group had requested a skills-based training with much of the programme content common to the work we had already done. We identified key areas and then began to develop a framework which would allow for both exploration of personal experience and learning opportunities. We devised a three-day training which would provide a safe environment for this learning to take place. This included a mixture of individual, small group and large group exercises on an experiential basis with specific inputs on theoretical issues. Over three days, we planned to look at three key areas.

Personal experience of loss and bereavement

Understanding past experience and its impact upon participants. Making connections with their children. Identifying fears and anxieties. Exploring possible outcomes and strategies.

Child development

Understanding developmental tasks and consequent supports or hindrances for children aged 0–16. Giving insight into children facing change and loss.

Support and planning for the future

Identifying goals for participants and their families. Identifying the resources and supports required for the tasks ahead.

There was good initial publicity surrounding this training event. We used key contacts from the consultation process and sent them fliers for the course and application forms. We also used WHAN's mailing list which includes women's organisations. HIV positive mothers, previously unknown to the agency, made enquiries or contacted us to voice support. Some, whilst offering support for the initiative, did not feel this was the time to deal with something which would involve painful explorations of their past, present and future lives. For other women, their own or their partner's health prevented them from participating and, at the last minute, one participant became hospitalised. This is important to mention because a real consideration in doing this kind of work is the unpredictability involved. This work can be demanding and requires flexibility and creativity on the part of facilitators.

I believe that the positive response to the programme was due to effective networking and liaising with women and other agencies. We tried to reach women where they were currently getting some support, that is, via their key workers in children's centres, drugs projects and social work departments. We therefore capitalised on the good support work already in existence and tried to build on its strengths. I think we also listened carefully to the mothers we were in touch with and valued their input to the consultation. This allowed the programme to be owned by them. We also kept the key workers in touch with developments, so they could pass on full and complete information to the women. Frequent communication proved a positive aspect and contributed to trust.

Our aim was to develop a partnership with the women, offering opportunities for exploration of sensitive and sometimes painful areas. However, we believed that it was essential for the women to be empowered in this process, and thus be able to influence and adapt the programme as we worked with it. We negotiated, through the establishment of ground rules within the group, the ways in which we could best support the group to achieve their aims.

For example, we had originally allowed for groups of up to 10 participants. Experience showed that this would have been too large, given the considerable amount of personal work and issues that required to be processed. We realised after the first course that we were trying to pack too much into each day, and, consequently, participants felt over-stretched. Accordingly we shortened the length of each day for our second group and reduced the amount of small-group exercises. We also developed a longer period of time at the start of day two and three for participants to check in with each other and to reflect on the previous day's experience, as this emerged as an important process for participants.

Another important factor was the opportunity for individual support from the facilitator, should any women require this, either during or outside the programme. This was a resource which was used during both courses. Participants commented on the benefits of this in establishing personal safety.

Programme content

The first part of the programme dealt with personal experience. This was painful for most participants and for some was the first opportunity they had to look at the impact of significant changes and losses in their own lives. Connections were readily made with what participants' children might be experiencing. Mutual support was offered in this process and common ground identified which contributed to the cohesion of the group.

We used two experiential exercises with the group. The first, called a Time Line, asked participants to focus on significant changes and issues in their lives. We then focused on how participants understood or dealt with these events and what behaviours they observed in other people at these times. The exercise also enabled us to look at losses, many of which go unacknowledged in our lives, and especially in the lives of children. Participants were able to identify how information, or the lack of it, had affected their ability to deal with the losses they had experienced. For those who underwent particularly significant losses in childhood – through illness, separation from parents, or divorce – the quality of information offered and the opportunity to express feelings and reactions at that time were especially relevant to helping them identify with their children.

The next exercise focused on death and how we come to understand it. We used a questionnaire to reflect on the impact of past experience on current views and feelings (Worden 1991).

Lisa, a 35-year-old single mother with two children, aged 14 and 10, had been struggling with her extended family's reaction to her HIV status. During her marriage to a violent husband, her family had offered some degree of support, but on learning of her diagnosis some of them had withdrawn. She felt isolated and rejected by her family and experienced a powerful sense of loss which overrode the positive support she still received from her brothers. During the Time Line exercise, Lisa identified that she was still very affected by a separation from her parents in early childhood. The third of five siblings, she was placed in care for a year when she was three years old. Her recollections of this period were patchy and she had gained little information from her parents as to why she was the only child in her family to be placed in care. Her parents response was to say she had been a sickly child who needed more attention than they could give. Lisa realised that much of her current experience of her family's behaviour was related to the unresolved issue of separation from her family, or, rather, the loss of her place in the family unit as a child.

The programme went on to consider children's needs and parenting skills. We provided information on child development, focusing on tasks for children at each stage of their physical, social and emotional development. We asked participants to fill in a questionnaire in the form of a grid. This looked at the behaviour one might witness in children affected by change or loss, and what might hinder or help a child deal with their distress. We asked participants to approach each developmental stage separately, looking at age-appropriate reactions in children. Participants discussed their views in pairs and then shared findings with the whole group. In the group exercise, participants were able to demonstrate their ability to understand children's needs and accompanying behaviour, while also considering their responses as parents. Discussion about both helpful and unhelpful responses was extensive, and participants consistently drew on examples from their own experience and considered them in relation to new perspectives.

Some women felt that they were under threat in their role as mothers. Profoundly affected by a sense of having failed in their lives, they withdrew from avenues of support, feeling that any request for help from professional agencies would be interpreted as failure to cope or to provide for their children. They felt this would lead to an examination of their parenting style, from a critical or prejudiced perspective in which they would be seen as inadequate. One woman said she felt she had failed her children by becoming infected with HIV and already felt bad enough about this. Therefore, she felt unable to enter into negotiations around issues such as respite care, without feeling that she might be judged in her role as a mother, and consequently lose her children. We encouraged women to look at how they might feel empowered in negotiations with agencies. Basic assertiveness techniques were explored and role plays or rehearsals of situations were used.

In the next stage, participants were asked to identify their aims in talking to their children and how they would like to achieve them. They were then invited to consider obstacles which prevented them from achieving this. For many women the reasons arose from feeling they could not talk to their children because of a lack of skill. During the three days, this became a more and more relevant issue for all participants. An equally important issue was the stigmatising effect of an HIV diagnosis on the family. Mothers felt that they did not wish to pass the burden of carrying such a secret on to their children. Another important block was the feeling of uncertainty about how much information would be appropriate to share with their children. This task had seemed too difficult for some women to tackle previously but the learning gained during the course of the programme allowed them to explore what they thought their children needed to know, when and how to tell them, and what other support their children needed.

Finally, support and planning for the future were addressed. Setting goals for their families and themselves was where many of the women had started. The range of goals was broad. For some, the immediate goal was to tell their children that their health was deteriorating. For others it was that they had HIV, and for one mother that she and her eight-year-old son were both positive. In some cases, women would be telling their children that other people might be involved in their care.

Joan's story

Joan is 30 and has AIDS. She lives alone with her son, Martin, who is nine years old and she describes their relationship as 'very close'. Joan's parents have offered to care for Martin when she becomes unable to do so. Joan's relationship with her parents has been strained in the past, especially during Joan's marriage to Martin's father.

Joan's health is deteriorating. She feels the need to tell Martin of her diagnosis and future plans. However, her parents are resistant to talking about the future with Joan unless pushed, and they are against disclosing her AIDS diagnosis to Martin.

In the group, Joan was able to focus on Martin's need to understand the changes in his mother and their current circumstances. She was able to explore and articulate the acute pain she felt about the task of talking to Martin about the possibility of her own death. She identified her own needs and wishes and especially what support she needed in order to be able to talk to Martin. Her parents' views and needs were also explored, and Joan could see a role for her social worker in offering support to them. She decided to request help in this area and also to enlist the help of her parents' closest friend.

Joan's immediate task was to set up a support framework for herself and Martin so that she could begin to talk to him about her HIV status. She gained a lot from discussion with another group member who had already told her oldest child of her diagnosis. Joan also received great support from the other women who offered to be available to her in the coming months. This contributed to Joan's feeling of community and self-worth, a sharp contrast to the sense of isolation and fear she had lived with over the previous years. This kind of support continues to be invaluable to Joan, and reflects the experience of many of the women whose lives had been characterised by stigma and isolation. It is a tribute to their strength and compassion that they are now able to reach out to each other across their differences.

Evaluation

At the end of each event, we asked participants for written evaluation. I think that this was a difficult notion to introduce to a group which, although structured throughout, had developed a strong sense of intimacy and did not reflect the formality of professional training courses. We restricted our evaluation to five areas:

- what participants had gained;
- what they had liked most;
- what they had liked least;
- what they would have liked more of; and
- how suitable the venue, child care arrangements, timing and organisation had been for them.

All participants reported that they had gained confidence and a belief in their ability to deal with the difficult task of communicating with their children. Participants were able to anticipate difficulties which might arise in this process and there was a certainty about the importance of finding a way which was right for each mother to meet her children's needs.

Conclusion

These three-day training events were only a small part of a process which is on-going for all women who attended. The challenges facing them will continue to change and take on different aspects as both they and their children learn to live with, and talk to each other about, HIV and AIDS. Hopefully, it might be a process which, though never easy, will be informed and supported by some of the experience gained in these groups. There will still be times when the conflict between parents' and children's needs will present dilemmas. In our experience, many women will put their children's needs first and above their own needs and plans. Their desire to protect their children from the pain and hostility which HIV and AIDS has brought is more than understandable. It is this which is often the driving force behind their reluctance to talk, and their reluctance to accept that the child lives sensitively in the world, capable of deduction, conjecture and fearful imaginings.

Reference

Worden, J. W. (1991), *Grief Counselling and Grief Therapy: A Handbook for the Mental Health Practitioner*, London: Routledge.

Chapter 8

◆

SUPPORTING HIV INFECTED AND AFFECTED CHILDREN IN SCHOOL

Eleanor Carr
Teacher

Liz White
Deputy head teacher

Introduction

The professional role of a teacher has changed considerably in the last 20 years. The emphasis now is much more on building good relationships with children and identifying their individual educational, social and emotional needs. Teachers of younger children in particular have a much closer involvement with students, which, at times, makes being a 'professional only' very difficult. This is especially true when working with HIV infected and affected children in the classroom. Good relationships are often established whereby parents confide in teachers that they or their child are infected or affected by HIV. Teachers then feel an extra responsibility to meet the needs of the individual child and work to support them.

Despite good intentions, there are often limitations to the support a teacher can offer. Teachers are answerable to agendas set by the school, education authority or government and must work within these boundaries. Because of constraints such as staffing, the curriculum and the local environment, support for HIV infected and affected children is not always adequate. For example, HIV and AIDS are not taken into account when compiling the Learning Support Audit for additional resources as schools and individual teachers cannot disclose the HIV status of any child or parent. Therefore, an HIV infected child with health problems or an affected child with behavioural difficulties is unlikely to have one-to-one auxiliary support unless those difficulties are severe. Class teachers must cope with the situation as best they can, but at the same time teachers have the other children in the class and their needs to consider as well. There is also a feeling of working very much alone because of the lack of any real, practical policies on HIV and AIDS issues at both school and regional level. Teachers are advised on how to deal with blood spillage, but not on the issues surrounding the teaching of HIV and AIDS to primary-age children. Even at a curriculum level, HIV and AIDS are only covered under the auspices of the immune system, which is taught at the upper stages of primary school. It is therefore very much at the discretion of individual teachers to discuss HIV and AIDS at earlier stages, and they are in no way required to do so. Added to this are the secrecy and confidentiality aspects of HIV and AIDS, and so teachers wishing to tackle them may find that they lack support.

Two teachers working in suburban Scotland in the early 1990s with infant classes found themselves having to deal with both infected and affected children in their classrooms. This is an account of some of the difficulties they experienced and how they coped. It has to be acknowledged that the situation has changed and improved since this time with more advice, information and help available from a range of sources.

Disclosure and secrecy

Any child in a class could be affected or infected by HIV, but unless a parent chooses to disclose this information directly to the class teacher, the teacher can never be certain. The teacher may often suspect that a child has health problems or difficulties at home through conversations with the child or through their school work. For example, a child may say, 'Mummy is in hospital again,' and does not know why or the child may draw a sad picture. A child could also describe their own hospital visits, blood tests and so on. This does not mean that the teacher automatically assumes that the problem is HIV-related but, nonetheless, he or she becomes aware that the child has particular needs.

Parents who choose to disclose either their own or their child's HIV status to a teacher places a great deal of responsibility and trust upon that teacher. There is always a risk that the teacher will mishandle the disclosure or not be able to cope with it.

> When I first heard that I was having an HIV infected child in my class, my initial reaction was one of shock that something so dreadful could come into my life. I had read reports of the disease's progress in the States and of its spread here, but it had always seemed remote. My understanding was mainly based on in-service training that had been set up by the Region, and at that time we were not particularly well informed. I was told of the situation before the start of term and Joe's family spoke openly and honestly to me about his condition. They did state, however, that they did not want everyone to know about it, only those working with him. As a result, only the head teacher, the nursery nurse attached to the infant classes and I knew.

The initial reaction of shock was replaced with an overwhelming sense of secrecy and not being able to talk about the matter with anyone. In Joe's case, his positive status was almost an open secret in the community, but a teacher could not acknowledge this with other parents. This occasionally posed problems for the teacher as Joe tried to scratch and bite other children in the playground.

After one incident, a parent of another child spoke to me of her concern for other children. She was a neighbour of the family and aware of Joe's condition and family background. She was in no way accusatory and, indeed, very sympathetic to the situation, but did have concerns. (At that time we did not know if biting could transmit the virus.) I could not enter into a discussion with this parent about Joe's condition as I had agreed not to discuss the matter with anyone other than the head teacher and the nursery nurse. I had to be very non-committal and stress that no child was allowed to scratch or bite.

This small incident highlights the importance and difficulty of confidentiality. A teacher cannot share information on a child or parent's HIV status with anyone other than those designated by the parents. The pressure of confidentiality is often most difficult to cope with. As a teacher you are used to sharing ideas, experiences and problems with your colleagues and gaining support from them. However, HIV infection is a problem you cannot discuss unless parental permission is granted. Eventually this was the case with Joe.

In December of Primary Two, Joe's grandmother came back to see me and told me that he had very little time left. She said that I could tell staff at school as she felt it was important that they should know about Joe's situation. I told staff that Joe had AIDS and that this was possibly going to be his last Christmas. I explained that the family had given permission for them to be told, but that it was still not common knowledge and they would prefer that it stayed that way. The staff were very supportive and positive. There was not one hostile or wary response to the information, but it did highlight for them that other infected children could be in their classes. Everyone took their obligation to the family very seriously. Joe was not a subject for open discussion, but when support was needed, it was there.

Support

The issue of support is vital when dealing with HIV infected and affected children. As indicated, teachers can lack support because of confidentiality and the secrecy surrounding HIV and AIDS. The teacher cannot then discuss the issue with the head teacher, unless the teacher has parental permission, and cannot necessarily enlist the support of other agencies, for example, social work departments, as parents do not necessarily involve other agencies. Andrea, whose mother was HIV positive and had shared this information with Andrea's teacher, was a case in point:

As Andrea settled into her new class, she changed from being a quiet, withdrawn child to one who was disruptive and attention seeking. She would deliberately say or do unacceptable things to see how I would react. How far could she push me before I gave up and sent her out of the classroom? For example, she would regularly crawl under desks and make silly noises or throw pencils across the room. She would openly defy me or become physically aggressive towards other children. On a personal level, I could understand this behaviour given her circumstances, but as a teacher I had to prioritise the children's needs. It often felt like Andrea versus the rest of the class.

This brought out great feelings of guilt on my part. I felt I was failing Andrea and she was distraught when she was sent to the head teacher and informally excluded from school. She did not want to be sent home for a few days as school was a lifeline to her. I felt I had failed Andrea's mother. She had confided in me and now I was giving her something else to worry about, having failed to 'contain' Andrea.

Despite these problems, it was very important to let Andrea know that I wanted to support her. This had to be done very subtly. Andrea came to school every day with an overwhelming desire to be 'normal'. She did not want to be seen as 'teacher's pet' nor to get any special, positive attention from me. School was her chance for her life to be like any other child's. Again, when I did talk to Andrea, I had to be careful. Sometimes she would confide in me and tell me how she felt, but at other times she would shout at me and tell me to leave her alone. It was very difficult to predict how she would react.

In time, through communicating with her mother by letter, I realised that Andrea's behaviour was like a barometer for her mother's health. If she was studious and settled, her mother was well, whereas when she was sick, Andrea tended to be more disruptive and volatile. On these latter occasions I tried to be more tolerant and let Andrea know I was there if she needed me. Andrea could also express her feelings through her schoolwork. It was obvious that Andrea had a very good relationship with her mother and loved her deeply, yet at the same time resented her for being ill and tired all the time. I noted a good illustration of this on Mother's Day. The children were asked to draw a picture of their mothers and write a few sentences about her. All of the other children drew happy pictures and said how much they liked their mum as she was kind and bought them sweets and so forth. However, despite making a beautiful card, Andrea's portrait and description of her mum told a different story: 'I hate my mum. She sleeps all day. I guess mum and life don't mix.'

It was very important that I did not dismiss this, nor say that she could not possibly hate her mother. I simply explained that it was possible to love and hate someone at the same time and that this was acceptable. This was difficult for the other children to comprehend when the descriptions were read to the class and I felt the need to protect Andrea from the scorn of her classmates. This feeling of the need to protect ran through the whole year of working with Andrea. On one occasion, when her mother was ill and still asleep when she got up for school, Andrea came to school with her nightdress on under her pinafore. The other children were shocked and began to tease her and asked why her mum had not noticed. I manipulated the situation by saying that Andrea had done this as a joke to see if her classmates would notice. She colluded with this and so the immediate issue was resolved without a fuss.

Strategies

Such events highlight how teachers have to rely very much on their own strategies for supporting HIV infected and affected children. There were no specific HIV-related school policies to refer to when working with both Andrea and Joe. The teachers, quite rightly, treated the children as individuals with individual needs. Behaviour guidelines can be helpful when dealing with the child on a general disciplinary matter but do not take the individual circumstances, like HIV, into account.

In Joe's case, the class teacher, the nursery nurse and the head teacher worked out various strategies to curb his aggressive play, with rewards for good behaviour and setting targets for him to achieve in the playground. For example, if he did not get into a fight at playtime, he was allowed to go to lunch first. The other children were involved in helping with his behaviour modification and were very encouraging. They allowed him to join in their games which they had originally stopped doing in the first few days of the term. The staff concerned found that a combination of approaches worked and by the end of the first term Joe's behaviour had improved.

It was good that the other children participated in supporting Joe, but, at the same time, it was very important that their needs were not forgotten. Teachers must try to treat everyone as fairly as possible. In Joe's case though, this proved difficult.

> As his health declined, Joe could no longer take part in PE lessons and this distressed him as it had been one of his favourite activities. In order to lessen the blow I made him the 'Gym Assistant' and he became my helper. He was given a whistle and would give signals to the rest of the class during games and activities. The others were not upset by him having a special job as they knew that he was not well enough to take part in the lessons, but I always tried to ensure that when others could not do gym, they also got a 'job' to do.
>
> Joe found it difficult to concentrate on work without a great deal of adult support and his progress was slow. The nursery nurse who worked with the class was invaluable as she worked with Joe on a one-to-one basis, as well as working with his group. This gave him the support he needed and the others in the group also got the benefit of extra adult input.
>
> I limited the amount of class written work as Joe found it very tiring. If he was required to copy from a board or a work card, he became very frustrated as he would lose the place or forget what he was working on. It was simpler to ask Joe to find and write the answers only.

Attendance

Children infected and affected by HIV and AIDS can often have frequent absences due to their own or their parent's ill health. This makes continuity of education difficult. A class teacher will try to compensate for this without compromising the needs of other children.

Joe's attendance from the first was not perfect as there were regular visits to hospital, but there were also days here and there when he just did not come to school. This was mainly because his family wanted him at home and they kept him away for the slightest reason. This made consistent teaching impossible and, as a result, he was difficult to motivate. Like most children, he found it hard to return to school and fit in when everyone else was doing new things which he had missed the beginning of.

When he returned to school after being absent he lacked concentration and was more aggressive than usual. He also found it hard to re-establish friendships. His family quite understandably spoiled him but realised that his absences were becoming a problem. They were invited to school for an informal meeting with me and we discussed the negative effects of unnecessary absence, for example, changed special groupings in class and groups having moved on to new reading books and so forth. As a result of our discussions, Joe's attendance improved, and so did his general attitude to his work and his classmates.

Health

Health is obviously a relevant issue in the classroom when an HIV-infected or affected child is in the class and teachers have to respond to questions which arise from the child or classmates. For example, Joe's visits to hospital were regular throughout the year and the children often asked why he had to go. He did not know what was wrong with him, but he always told us what had happened to him. The hospital staff explained processes to him and the other children enjoyed listening to how they took his blood, weighed him and so on. He had been told that these visits to the hospital were to check up on his health and to keep him healthy. The doctors had to do tests on him to see that there were no germs in his blood that would make him ill.

These conversations were potentially stressful for the teacher, but were managed by normalising the issue through general health talks. It was found that most of the children in the class had been to hospital or the doctor's and so could share their experiences, too. Children, at the infant stage of school, accept many explanations at face value and are not interested in exact diagnosis. Therefore, when Joe was told that his heart was sick, that is what he told the class. They accepted it and asked questions about why that made him feel tired and puffed out.

I explained that your heart was what gave you energy as it pumped the blood around your body. They already knew that the blood is full of good things to keep you healthy. Therefore, if your heart was tired your body did not get all the good things it needed and you got tired or ill. Then, as a class we talked about germs and how our white blood cells captured them and stopped them from making us ill. If the germs were too strong for our blood cells to fight or if our white blood cells were not working properly, then we could get ill. Although very young, the class seemed to understand the explanation.

In this case, HIV and AIDS was not directly discussed, although some of the issues were dealt with. Talking specifically about HIV and AIDS in an infant class is a more difficult thing to do and at the moment teachers are not required to do so. Individual teachers, when teaching a general health topic, may choose to discuss HIV and AIDS, although many are prohibited through their own lack of knowledge or discomfort. Therefore, young children at present will only learn about HIV and AIDS at school if their teacher wishes to discuss the subject.

HIV in the classroom

Children are likely to be at various stages of knowledge about HIV and AIDS and, therefore, will require different inputs. Some children will not have heard of HIV and AIDS, whereas, at the other end of the spectrum, there will be some whose family members have died or are dying of AIDS. They may also be familiar with some of the HIV- and AIDS-related agencies. Thus, when approaching the issue, class teachers have to be very sensitive to individual needs. It is important to teach children about HIV and AIDS, but at the same time, teachers do not want to frighten them, particularly affected children. Thus, when a child asks, 'Can you die of AIDS?', the response has to be very carefully worded. Teachers in this situation should try to answer honestly, but positively, by saying that people with HIV and AIDS can be healthy and live for a long time, but one day may get sick and die. A simple response of 'Yes, you die of AIDS' will terrify the affected child. Younger children in particular are concerned with the here-and-now and accept explanations at face value. There is always a danger that affected children will expect their parent to be dead by the time they get home from school if they hear such a response.

Questions and answers

Questions relating to HIV and AIDS are often very difficult to answer, particularly at the lower end of a primary school. The term Human Immunodeficiency Virus is not exactly child-friendly. When asked what HIV is, it is better to relate it to something children will understand:

> I start by discussing the children's favourite cartoon characters and ask them who the 'goodies' and the 'baddies' are. From this point I move on to a general health topic and we discuss all the times the children themselves have been ill and what it feels like. I ask them to tell me the name of all the illnesses or diseases they know about. This allows me to gauge the different stages individual children are working at. I then move back to the cartoon imagery by equating white blood cells with 'goodies' who move round the body helping us to stay healthy. A 'baddie' might come along, for example Mr Tummy Bug, and have a fight with the 'goodies'. He is strong to start with and makes the person feel ill, but then the 'goodies' fight back and win. Mr Tummy Bug goes away and

the person feels better. The problem with HIV, I tell the children, is that he does not go away. He hides for a long time then comes out for a fight. He zaps a few 'goodies' and sneaks back to his hiding place. He does this for a long time and one day there are not enough 'goodies' left in the body to fight him and so the person gets sick and may die. HIV is such a clever 'baddie' that doctors do not know how to make him go away yet, but they are trying very hard.

The most obvious questions which follow this explanation are, 'Have I got HIV?' and 'How do you get HIV?' The first question can be answered by saying that it is unlikely, as not many children are HIV positive, but the latter question is more difficult. The nature of HIV transmission is not comprehensible to young children, nor would it be welcomed as suitable teaching material since it mostly relates to sexual relationships or intravenous drug use. As a teacher of infants, it is more appropriate to answer the question by highlighting all the ways that you cannot get HIV. *Come sit by me* by Margaret Merrifield (1990) illustrates this well and is a good starting point for discussions. This is one of the few available books which is appropriate for use with a younger audience. In general, there is a lack of both fiction and non-fiction in this subject area. The lack of suitable teaching material leaves most teachers in the dark. Obviously, HIV and AIDS are only some of many issues which a teacher deals with in the classroom but, nevertheless, teachers need information for both themselves and their class if they are to communicate such complex issues successfully.

Practical problems and dilemmas teaching an HIV infected child

Teaching an infected, asymptomatic child throws up many practical issues which can be stressful for the class teacher. In Joe's case, his health declined quite rapidly and the teacher was faced with many problems and dilemmas.

> As the first year progressed it became obvious that Joe was not a risk to other children's health as had first been feared, but rather that they were a risk to him. Every small infection that went round the class caused Joe great problems. A minor ailment for the rest of the class caused him to have a severe infection and days off school. In June of Primary One, he caught a cold. He could not fight the infection and was absent for the rest of term. During the summer the infection spread to his heart and he was very seriously ill. When he returned after the holidays, the change in his appearance was striking.
>
> Joe had been quite a plump little boy, but now he was very thin with dark rings around his eyes. The infection had damaged his heart. Other children commented on his weight loss but thought that he had been on a diet. They did not see it as something to worry about, although I found it very distressing. Joe's general health was no longer good and he had to be given medication in school. He suffered from loss of appetite which made lunch times very difficult.

The dining supervisors were concerned about his not eating and there was a danger of this being made into a daily drama. I started eating with the children and would sit near Joe. However, this only worked for a short time. I also tried a reward system for everything he ate. This consisted of Joe being taken swimming, but gradually the rewards had to be more passive activities.

By the end of the autumn term Joe's health had deteriorated so much that people were commenting on his appearance. Further weight loss and lack of energy were noticed by the rest of the class, although they were very matter-of-fact about it. They played games that Joe could join in and stayed in with him on cold days. The level of discomfort Joe was suffering increased quickly and was more difficult to deal with. For example, the practicalities of keeping drugs locked safely away, while having them accessible when needed, were all but impossible when I was teaching a class. I was very lucky to have a nursery nurse there to help facilitate this. She also took Joe away when he was having spasms of pain. These did not last long, but we did not want the others to be upset by seeing him in discomfort. There were other times when all Joe needed or wanted was a cuddle. I thought the class would be jealous of this, but they accepted it and asked him themselves if he needed a cuddle.

It was very difficult to remain professional as Joe's health declined because I was so emotionally involved. Although we had agreed to keep him in school for as long as possible, by the end of May it was obvious that Joe was not coping. He became too ill to attend and was absent for the rest of the term. I moved schools after the summer and during the first week of the new term I received a phone call at work telling me that Joe had died.

When a child dies of AIDS, or indeed of any illness, support is available for the bereaved family, yet teachers can be forgotten. There is a feeling that they are 'only a teacher' and do not matter as much. As professionals, we are supposed to remain more distanced and detached. This is also true when working with affected children and their families. In Andrea's case, the teacher worked very closely with Andrea and her mother, but felt at times she was going beyond the parameters of her professional role as a teacher. She felt that she became too involved practically and emotionally and began to need support herself, but because of confidentiality issues and the feeling of having gone beyond her remit, she felt she had to remain silent and did not request help and support for herself.

Conclusion

The change in role of teachers needs to be acknowledged if HIV infected and affected children are to be supported in schools. Teachers now work very closely with children, catering for their individual educational, social, emotional and physical needs wherever possible. HIV and AIDS will not go away in the foreseeable future, so if children and teachers are to be supported in HIV- and AIDS-related issues then perhaps a more unified inter-agency response is required. Added to this would be clearer educational guidelines and support systems so that teachers do not have to take individual approaches only. This, at least, would make them feel less isolated. However, this will only be achieved if we can find a way through some of the constraints imposed by the stigma and secrecy which surround this illness.

Reference

Merrifield, Dr M. (1990), *Come sit by me*, illustrated by H. Collins, Toronto: Women's Press.

Chapter 9

◆

GOOD PRACTICE IS GOOD PRACTICE IS GOOD PRACTICE

HIV AS A FACTOR IN REFERRALS TO CHILDREN'S HEARINGS

Jean Raeburn, MBE, MSC, NNEB

Introduction

The children's hearings system is unique to Scotland and is part of a welfare-based system of juvenile justice. Children from the first day of birth until they are 17½ years old may be referred to a hearing if their situation satisfies any one ground of referral, and the reporter considers that they may be in need of compulsory measures of care.

The Kilbrandon Report (Scottish Home and Health Department 1964), which introduced the system, reinforced the principle that the test for public intervention in families and the use of compulsion must always be 'the best interests of the child'. The differences between children it stated, whether they were in need of care and protection, beyond parental control, truanting or offending, were far outweighed by their similarities.

> Common to all such children is that the normal upbringing processes have for whatever reason fallen short or been disrupted and that the primary focus of intervention must always be, wherever possible to strengthen and supplement and further these natural influences for good which will assist the child's development into a mature adult.
>
> (Kilbrandon Report 1964)

HIV and AIDS and the hearings system

Almost certainly the vast majority of children involved in some way with HIV and AIDS will not be referred to a children's hearing. HIV and AIDS are not in themselves grounds for referral. Such families will quite appropriately be receiving help and support from a number of sources entirely on a voluntary basis.

A small number of children, who may have been referred to a children's hearing on a variety of grounds, will have HIV as an additional factor in their lives. It may be quite unconnected with the reason that a compulsory order is considered necessary and is therefore unlikely to figure at all in the discussion of the hearing. This is appropriate in such cases.

For some children, however, the presence of the virus within the family may contribute to difficulties which result in grounds of truanting, beyond parental control or offending behaviour. For others, the virus may be related to the parent's lifestyle, which has already resulted in lack of parental care grounds with regard to the children.

Since on their own HIV and AIDS are not reasons for referral to the reporter, figures are not available which would indicate the numbers of cases involved. In one urban area in the central belt, it is estimated that those who are referred make up less than 1 per cent of the hearings' workload. That this is so is entirely in keeping with the principles as well as the legislation governing the system. The hearings system offers support and access to services. It does so, however, from a basis of compulsory supervision, the hearing is the point of compulsory intervention in the lives of families and should be necessary only in a minority of cases.

This means that panel members' responsibilities are likely to be different from those of others who work with families in these situations. In a 45-minute hearing, informal only by comparison to court, panel members must explore the issues and engage the families' co-operation in a search for resolution. The decision about whether or not to make a compulsory order, and if so, what conditions must be applied, is taken by the panel members whether or not the family agrees with it.

It also means that the numbers of cases involving HIV referred to hearings will be small and the opportunity for panel members to build up expertise in this area is likely to be limited. Clearly it is important therefore to identify good practice in order to reinforce it and to provide guidance for panel members who may be called upon only rarely to deal with such issues.

Developing good practice

This is best attempted, in the first instance, by trying wherever possible to link good practice dealing with HIV and AIDS situations to more familiar principles underpinning everyday practice in the hearing room. In other words, to what extent and in what ways will the usual behaviour and response of a children's hearing be appropriate when dealing with a case involving HIV? Are there any situations which will require a departure from usual practice? This is not to deny the impact of HIV and AIDS, but is instead an attempt to re-evaluate the principles of the children's hearings system, measuring them against the needs of this particular group of children and young people.

The Kilbrandon Report (written in 1964, long before AIDS became an issue) made a number of points illustrating the complexities of family relationships and drew conclusions from these about helpful methods of intervention. These have been incorporated into both legislation and into practice.

- Children were to be seen as 'individual' in terms of their need, yet not to be assessed in isolation from their parents, family and community.
- Good, or good-enough, parenting was recognised as an extremely powerful and direct influence on young people. Yet the limitations of ordering, forcing

or coercing mothers and fathers to be better parents was acknowledged and accepted.

- Helpful intervention, which the report described as a process of social education, would best be achieved through forms of partnership, working in closest co-operation; parents, children, carers, social work and other agencies would all contribute to the resolution of difficulties.
- Early identification of problems and comprehensive assessment would allow intervention to encourage and support parents to resolve the difficulties and to provide adequate care, or to provide good-enough parenting.
- A fundamental aim of the system therefore must be to engage families co-operation in both identifying and resolving problems.
- In a 'hearing', three lay members of the community, using informal language, should involve the family in a full and frank discussion, before deciding 'in the best interests of the individual child'.

Despite such grand intentions, that many decisions will involve pain and anger is not at all surprising. It is a cosy idea to assume that the needs of the child will coincide with the needs and wishes of the parent. Frequently they do not. Indeed that is the whole premise on which children's hearings operate – compulsory care.

Core principles

The basic principles of the system which apply in all cases, not simply those where HIV is a factor, may be summarised as follows:

- **The welfare of the individual child is paramount.** Need, the assessment of needs and meeting these, is the lynch pin of the children's hearing system.
- **Children and parents have rights.** There are limitations and constraints on the powers of panel members, reporters and on professionals who interact with the system. Checks and balances are a necessity in a welfare-based system of justice.
- **Communication is a crucial factor** in the seeking and the gathering of valid information, in the exploration of options, and in the search for consensus which is a part of the decision-making process. It necessarily involves family, professionals and panel members.

It follows therefore that preparation, openness, confidentiality and sensitivity are important general features of the children's hearings system which are likely to have particular relevance for families facing HIV and AIDS.

Current practice

The description of current practice which follows draws on interviews with reporters and panel members in busy city panels.

There is a general feeling, confirmed by those interviewed, that the system is working well with regard to this small group of children and families. These are very definitely a small minority of cases, most relating to children whose parents are HIV positive, and perhaps because numbers are small, practice is considered to be good; that is, professionals prepare well, resources are generally available as required and panel members address the issues appropriately.

Referral to the reporter

Good practice begins at the point of referral to the reporter and preparation is an important aspect of that. Reporters, in deciding whether or not a case is referred to a hearing, will seek information from the usual range of sources. To this extent these cases are dealt with on an individual basis, no differently from any other. HIV status may be a contributing factor but is not in itself sufficient reason to justify a referral to a hearing. As part of the exploratory role, the reporter will also try to discover what the specific agenda is, in any particular situation.

- There is an important role for the statutory social worker in co-ordination but how do the links between child, parent and social work seem to be operating in practice?
- Are there up-to-date medical reports?
- Who knows what, and what are the parents' wishes about this?
- The child may or may not know about the HIV status. Should they attend the hearing?
- What does the child's age and stage of development suggest in this particular case?
- What are the social workers' views?

Once investigations are complete, if the child is to be referred to a hearing, the reporter is likely to prepare a briefing note for panel members alerting the hearing to these kind of issues.

The panel member's role (preparation)

Legislation requires that panel members receive reports three days in advance of the hearing to allow them to prepare appropriately. Clearly it is crucial therefore that important reports from professionals arrive in good time, otherwise panel members can find themselves ill-prepared for difficult situations.

As part of their preparation, panel members may well be asked to consider whether or not the child should attend the hearing. Whatever position individuals adopt in advance in relation to this, the decision to dispense with the child's attendance can only be taken in a hearing. The basis for any such decision is likely to be information from the social worker.

- It is assumed that children will attend their own hearing unless there is good reason that they should not.
- Any request that the hearing dispense with the child's attendance should give reasons why that is believed to be in the child's interest and should be sent out in good time to allow panel members to advise the reporter whether or not the child is to be brought to the hearing.
- The hearing may decide that children should be present for all/part/or none of their hearing.

For some children, those whose parents are HIV positive, it may be the wish of the parents that the children are not told, particularly if very young. In many of these situations the child does not attend the hearing and that is seen as appropriate by panel members and reporters.

In other cases, similar to other instances of undisclosed information, panel members may well wish to consider and pass comment, without the presence of the child, on whether or not the child should in fact be informed.

- It would not be appropriate, however, for children to learn about a parent's HIV status in the setting of a hearing and panel members would consider it detrimental to disclose such information themselves.
- Where children are to attend the hearing, and do not know about the virus, it is not appropriate for panel members to refer to it in their presence.

If, nonetheless, the health of the parent is an issue for the hearing, they may, depending on what is most appropriate for the child, refer to the parent's illness in the same way they would any other health problem; for example it is not unusual to have a conversation with a cancer patient about how they are and how the illness is progressing without using the word 'cancer'. Alternatively, panel members may ask the child to leave for part of the hearing. This does not, however, automatically 'protect' the child, who is, after all, living daily with the illness and may simply feel excluded, and become more anxious about what is being discussed in their absence.

Where the child knows their parent is ill but not what the illness is, it will be important for panel members to satisfy themselves, at successive hearings, without direct reference to HIV and AIDS, that the child at each stage has access to the necessary information about his or her care and the care of the sick parent and, where appropriate, that issues of loss will be addressed. The needs of a child in this situation will be similar in many ways to those of the child who has been fully informed about the illness.

Panel members are likely also to find themselves facing a number of different situations involving HIV positive parents where the young person does know the nature and name of the illness. The consensus from both panel members and reporters is that these situations are often dealt with better in hearings than are some other parental problems, for example alcoholism, which can sometimes attract moral judgements. Panel members are a group of people who are likely to be concerned with social issues and there has been a great deal of education about AIDS. That may explain, to some extent, why there is rarely any condemnation of the family. Panel members see, appropriately, HIV and AIDS as health problems, like any other serious long-term or terminal illness. Frequently, for hearing families, this is simply another problem among multiple problems.

Openness and sensitivity

The task for panel members in hearings involves openness and sensitivity and in this respect is not unlike other extremely difficult family circumstances, for example cases involving sexual abuse. Hearings are frequently highly charged, emotions running high for parents and children. While there will be a need to address the parents' feelings and the difficulties they face, any such discussion should turn on how these feelings and difficulties will impact on the child. Hard as it may seem, the hearing must not allow the parent's dying, their needs and wishes in relation to dying, to submerge the needs of the child.

Parents facing death, who have initially been referred for lack of parental care, frequently become painfully aware of their earlier failures. They are suddenly in touch with the needs of their child, may feel guilty and want desperately to meet these needs. One positive result from that is this they may become more co-operative in the hearing than at any time previously. It becomes urgent, pressing, for them to have a coherent plan for the future of their child. However, while workers and panel members are concerned with providing support to allow the child and parents to be together as much and as often as possible, the ill parent's main aim may be to see the child settled with permanent carers. Although this may be the eventual plan for the child, they may be unable to consider such a situation while they have yet to face and come to terms with the loss of a parent. Despite their concern for the parent, panel members must retain their focus on the needs of the child.

In a different situation, a young person, referred to a hearing because of their own acting-out behaviour, may be angry with the ill parent, whose lifestyle has created this problem. As the parent wishes to be close and caring, the young person is rejecting and angry. The parent can be very vocal about their illness, yet the young person's knowledge about the illness comes out in anger towards the parent. They are 'beyond parental control' or aggressive. The parent sees only that the young person is getting their own way.

Alternately, the demands created by the parent's illness may have placed an unfair burden on the young person or resulted in lack of supervision. Such absence of parenting at an extremely difficult time for the child can sometimes lead to truancy or offending.

It would be wrong to suggest that all parents become co-operative as the illness progresses. Some who have been aggressive and violent remain so, demanding that situations are resolved taking account of their needs and using the hearing as a platform to that end, rather than to address the needs of their child.

Despite the presence of such competing demands and powerful emotions, which can both de-skill and divert panel members from their task, the hearing has a limited time in which to reach a reasoned decision.

- The hearing must not shy away from the important issue of the health of the parent and its impact on the child.
- Panel members must speak the unspeakable in clear simple language in an unemotive way.
- They should acknowledge the pain and difficulty involved in talking about such issues.
- Without being patronising they should attempt to use the language of the young person.
- They are unlikely to find it helpful to go straight into painful issues without some attempt to make the family feel comfortable and to build some sense of rapport.
- Since these situations are rarely resolved in single hearings, it will be important to make good use of continuity among the panel members.
- Panel members will want to maintain the focus on the changing needs of the young person as the situation worsens or improves.
- These are likely to include the need for information: about the course of the illness; about care of and contact with the ill parent; about the future care of the young person.
- Each of these will involve the need for some preparation, preparation for loss as well as preparation for the future.
- Panel members will seek a flexibility of response from the social work department, in providing the appropriate resource as it is required whether to maintain a child and parent together or to provide respite care, where the health of the parent has worsened.
- Despite the obvious needs of the ill parent, panel members will seek to maintain clarity about their role and focus on the child as the client whose needs will be addressed by the hearing.
- The hearing, as in all other situations, will clarify these needs, whether for information, preparation, care or bereavement counselling, and identify how they will be met. The hearing will not see it as its role to meet the young person's need, but will instead seek to determine that appropriate arrangements have been made.

Creating the culture

Despite encouragement, panel members were reluctant to offer formulae for ways of talking to young people in hearings: 'We do what we always try to do, what we've learned in training, sometimes more successfully than others.' That is not difficult to understand.

Clearly panel members must set a scene which facilitates communication, while at the same time acknowledging blocks which are unavoidable. The purpose of the interaction of the hearing is different from most other situations. Power, authority and responsibility are involved. There are different pressures at play for the adults, and the previous experiences of the children will also contribute to the way in which they experience this situation.

In speaking with children of different ages and levels of ability, panel members must take account of the very different means by which these ages, stages and experiences are reflected in, and affect, the young person's behaviour and speech. Panel members must try to tune into the individual child and to find the appropriate vocabulary for each situation.

It will also be important to reflect upon the various feelings and assumptions which influence the ways one communicates: that is, whether the young person is male or female; young child or adolescent. To some extent panel members' own experiences of childhood and adolescence will also influence the way they relate to children and families.

In short these are considerations which exist for panel members in all cases of extreme difficulty. The task of the hearing is to engage the family in meaningful discussion about the difficulties, to learn what the young person thinks, feels and would like to happen. This information will not only inform their decision-making but should also begin to involve the family in a search for consensus, if that is at all possible. An appropriate response from panel members to each individual situation is likely to be more constructive than any specific routine approach, no matter how well phrased.

Having said that, clearly it is important to reinforce good practice by highlighting some of the straightforward communication skills on which panel members might usefully draw.

Communicating

Active listening is likely to be particularly helpful; allowing the family to define the problem; reinforcing the speaking of the child; the use of non-verbal encouragement – or discouragement where the parent speaks to the exclusion of the young person.

Mirror and echo statements can usefully extend or continue the contribution from the child without further complicating the conversation, like bouncing a ball back. They can also serve to check out you are understanding correctly. 'You didn't like that?', 'He was cross with you?'

Extending statements more directly seek further information, 'Could you say a bit more about what happened when …?', 'Do you think that maybe …?'

Understanding statements can be helpful. 'It does seem to me that there has been a lot for you to cope with …', 'Sometimes young people in your position …'

Response

The way panel members respond is likely to be crucial to whether or not the family remain open and involved in the discussion. Judgemental statements are rarely helpful, yet sometimes the information offered has been damning. 'I know I shouldn't allow anyone to use drugs in front of the children, but sometimes ...' The problem for panel members here is to reinforce the speaking, the honesty, without endorsing the message. Echo statements are useful to keep the lines of communication open. If the nature of the disclosure has been very negative, it is sometimes more helpful to simply acknowledge how difficult it must have been to share that information.

Panel members' opinion

It is appropriate for panel members to introduce their own thinking in the process of moving towards a decision. Helpful ways of offering that view include:

- I wonder if maybe ...?
- Would it be fair to say ...?
- Do you think possibly ...?
- Are you suggesting that ...?

All of these can be accepted, denied or modified by the family with less risk of confrontation.

Here and now

It can also be particularly helpful to use what is going on in the hearing room, to deal with the here and now.

- You looked upset when he said ...?
- You seem angry ...?
- Is John always as quiet as this?
- Are you surprised to hear how worried mum is about what will happen?

This can also be useful with regard to panel members themselves.

- I'm not sure I understand?
- It's difficult to know what would be most helpful.
- I think we've gone as far with these arrangements as we can at the moment.

None of these phrases refer specifically to HIV and AIDS, but that is not inappropriate. Panel members are never likely to be required to either introduce the subject to the young person for the first time or to delve into painful examination of the details of the illness. As in all cases before them, they are charged with identifying and deciding in the best interests of the individual child.

There is little doubt that consistent exercising of such skills in stressful hearings is not easy. Panel members require a degree of confidence (not false bravado) based on experience of hearings, if they are to relax sufficiently in their role, to allow these skills and their human concern to come to the fore.

Conclusion

When addressing HIV and AIDS issues in hearings, panel members will most helpfully bear in mind the general principles of the hearings system and draw on their usual range of communication skills. They should prepare thoroughly in advance giving consideration also to whether the child should attend all, part, or none of the hearing. Families should be treated with dignity and respect in all contacts and their rights to confidentiality also respected. In the hearing, panel members should speak openly, yet sensitively, with the child and their parents addressing important issues about current care, loss and the future care of the young person. In the often highly charged atmosphere of these painful hearings, the hearing will seek to maintain the focus of the discussion on the child and their needs. Although seeking agreement with the family about the best course of action, the hearing is charged with reaching a reasoned decision based on the best interests of the child.

Such behaviour would be recognised as good practice in any hearing, no matter the specific ground of referral or underlying family problems. Good practice may at times be more difficult to achieve in a hearing involving HIV and AIDS. It is nonetheless what is required. To do otherwise, to single such cases out for some kind of special treatment, might be counter-productive.

Reference

Scottish Home and Health Department (1964), Children and young persons Scotland: Report by the committee appointed by the Secretary of State for Scotland (The 'Kilbrandon Report'), Edinburgh: HMSO.

Chapter 10

◆

WHEN A PARENT DIES

SUPPORTING BEREAVED CHILDREN THROUGH INDIVIDUAL WORK

Judith Morkis
Barnardo's Riverside Project Leader

Introduction

The Lothian Planning Service is part of Barnardo's Riverside Project, which was set up in conjunction with Lothian Regional Council to work with children and families affected by HIV and AIDS. The project is a voluntary agency and works in partnership with parents who wish to engage in the vital task of making plans for the time when they may be unable to care for their children themselves. Our aim is to help families retain control of their lives and be together for as long as possible. The welfare of the children is our priority, and their wishes and feelings are always taken into account when plans are being made so that much of our work goes on 'face to face' with children, trying to help them make sense of what is happening in their lives.

All of the children who come to the project are likely to lose, or will have already lost, at least one significant person through HIV-related illness. In many cases that person will be the child's parent. In this chapter, I shall attempt to describe the underpinning philosophy and my practical approach to working with children who have experienced a bereavement.

Children and bereavement

The normal development of a child's understanding of death has been described by Nagy (1948) and Anthony (1971). For very young children under the age of around 3–5 years, death is a temporary state synonymous with absence or going away. For example, a three-year-old who has been told about the death of a Grandparent may ask, days later, 'Is grandpa still dead?' By the age of five years, children start to be able to differentiate between death and absence, and develop an interest in animate and inanimate objects. Between the ages of 5–8 years they begin to adopt rituals and superstitions around the topic which are evident in their play, 'Step on a crack, break your mother's back', and they are uncertain about whether death is funny or frightening. By the time most children are 9 or 10 years old, they know that death is final and inevitable.

In the normal course of life, children's understanding of separation and death is gradually acquired through experiences in which they learn to cope with the loss of familiar objects, people, routines and how to adapt to the changes these losses necessarily entail. For most children the first experience of death within the family will be that of a grandparent and, while this makes them sad, they usually recover very quickly, understanding that when people get old their bodies get worn out and death seems natural. In addition, children usually know at least one or two others in their peer group who have lost a grandparent and are clearly surviving. There is no need to feel less 'safe' and less 'normal'. When a dependent child experiences the death of a parent, the loss of the person who loved and cared for them whom the child expected to be always there, the world seems to collapse. The child, quite correctly, knows and fears that nothing is, nor can ever be, as it was.

Children whose parent has died of an HIV-related illness have all this to contend with and more, because of the fear, stigma and discrimination, which still clouds the lives of those affected. They may not know why mum or dad has died, or be aware of the circumstances but have been told that 'it needs to be kept secret'. They feel ashamed, guilty and afraid without really understanding why, and the secrecy creates a sense of isolation. They may want to ask questions and to talk about how they feel. They need to do that essential piece of work, but they fear the consequences. Will the other important people in their life be angry? Will they be rejected or abandoned if the secret gets out? For some children too, where parental drug use has been a feature of their life with resultant chaos and little in the way of security and stability, there is a huge need to grieve for something that never was and never can be, which often goes unrecognised or ignored.

Helping these children is an immense challenge. In the literature on bereavement and its effects on children, Dr Kubler-Ross (1969) has identified five stages of grieving. In the first 'shock and denial' phase children may show little emotion early on, seeming nearly mechanical and easily conforming in their behaviour. Gradually they may develop attention problems and become forgetful, and appetite and sleep disturbances are common. During the next 'angry' stage the child's feelings are frequently projected on to current care givers and anger may be demonstrated actively or passively, with minor frustrations precipitating intense outbursts of furious rage. The next phase is 'bargaining' and may be characterised by the child making promises about future behaviours before moving into stage four, disorganisation and despair. During this phase the child may experience a variety of emotions – yearning and pining for the dead person, anger, anxiety and guilt. Tears appear more easily. The child may seem sad and withdrawn and regression is common. In the last 'resolution' stage, children accept their loss, and anger and despair have been dealt with.

Working with bereaved children

As workers we can feel quite alarmed by the task of undertaking grief work with children and I think there are four basic and inter-related reasons for this. First, such work is often described as 'therapeutic', a word which implies a certain amount of mystique and a high level of 'professional expertise'. Second, we are terrified of making mistakes during this 'therapeutic' intervention, especially when our clients are children. The third reason, I feel, is to do with the need for us, as adults, to retain control in situations we share with children. We are frankly terrified that the children, or ourselves, will become overwhelmed by the emotion of it all. Finally, we have probably all experienced times when we have patently failed in our communication with children and we are loathe to repeat an experience in which we and the child have felt awkward and miserable. So before starting, we need to put these issues into perspective.

First of all, let's debunk the mystique around the word 'therapeutic', defined in the *Collins English Dictionary* as 'an adjective, pertinent to the art of healing'. I believe this is exactly what our work with children is about. We cannot cure the source of their sadness. Nothing we do will bring back the person whose loss they mourn, but we can help in the healing process by helping children to get in touch with, and express, their feelings about their loss.

The second issue is our fear of making mistakes. I have to accept that I will occasionally say or do 'the wrong thing', but I know I'll learn from it and will not make the same mistake again. There are also, however, some basic methods of avoiding major blunders. For example, if you don't know the answer to a question a child asks, say so, don't try to bluff it out, and even more importantly, take time to discover the child's story and you'll spot the booby-traps when they arise. I remember working with a 15-year-old boy, 'Bob', who had been in 'the system' for several years because of his 'anti-social' behaviour. Bob's mum had died of a heart attack when he was 4 years old, and when Bob was 10, he asked a trusted well-meaning adult, 'So what happens when you have a heart attack?' and the adult replied, 'Well if you get help quickly enough you'll be okay'. Bob was devastated. He'd been the only one in the house when his mum died, and from that point he shouldered a burden of guilt and self-blame which turned his life upside down. I also want to say on this point, that if children express anger with you for your mistake, welcome that as a sign of the trust they have in you. Remember that you are there, reducing their isolation and loneliness, and responding to them in a way which lets children know that you are concerned, are trying to understand, and are willing to give comfort and support.

The fear of becoming overwhelmed is a real one and yes, there will be times when that will be how it feels, but if you know the child's story and you've been moving at the child's pace, you will be aware most of the time that you are getting close and can prepare yourself. In my experience, the most alarming times arise when children become 'stuck' in their grief work. It can feel pretty risky when we, as adults, have to then take full control of the situation and intervene in a directive way. I feel very strongly that we must be prepared to take the risks, for if we ignore the child's pain or try to seduce them away from the reality of their feelings, the child will be the one left with an emotional burden which may last a lifetime.

We cannot avoid talking about death and dying when we are helping a child with grief work, and we are very aware that we are dealing with a taboo subject for many people. Avoiding euphemisms and saying words like 'dead', 'died' and 'dying' to a child can make us feel uncomfortable and brings us right back to our own fear of making mistakes as a child struggles to come to terms with the reality of their loss, and may want to ask questions about what happens to people after they've died. The truth is that none of us have the answer to that one, do we? We may have strongly held beliefs of our own, but that is as far as it goes. My rule of thumb is that if children have a concept of death which gives them comfort, explore it with them and then accept it. During the exploration process you'll become familiar with the child's terminology and understanding which opens up the space to talk about the physical and spiritual aspects of death. You can also explore any ideas which might be causing anxiety, for example a child who likens death to going to sleep and is suffering sleep disturbance. The child's concepts may be new and unfamiliar to you. Let the child and their family help you to understand. I remember sitting with a child looking at photographs of his mother on holiday. This child had told me that his mum had died and gone to heaven and I wondered if there were sunbeds there. He replied, 'Don't be silly, Judith, they've got the clouds!'

There are times when it will be apparent that the child's understanding of death gives no comfort at all, and I think on these occasions it is appropriate to challenge their thinking. Bob, for example, talked about his belief in 'nothingness', but also about seeing his mum as a ghost, two conflicting statements which warned me that he was struggling with something. I discussed various beliefs with him, like the Christian understanding of the afterlife, and reincarnation, and agreed that yes, there were a lot of people who thought 'death was the end'. I admitted that I didn't know who was right, and wouldn't know until the day I died, but I liked the idea of an afterlife as I would get to see people I had known and loved and say sorry for one or two things I had done. Bob was intrigued, and I explained that lots of people who lost some one they loved had guilty feelings about something because we were none of us perfect. This gave Bob the space to talk about his 'unfinished business'. In my opinion, it's important to question the use of negative concepts and terminology, the fire and brimstone notions of sin, hell, purgatory and limbo, which cause untold fear and distress. I would strongly suggest that it is especially important to do so in our work with children and families affected by HIV and AIDS, who can experience the rejection, guilt and blame attached to these conditions every day of their lives.

I find Bion's (1962) concept of 'a container', a person able to accept and hold in a chaotic input of largely painful feelings, and D. W. Winnicott's (1964) notion of the 'Holding Environment', in which he describes the relationship between a stable adult who accepts and contains a child's negative feelings, really useful in understanding what we should be doing in our work with children. It is a natural adult response to try to protect them from pain. Often our communication with them gets blocked because either 'They're too young to understand' or 'They're far too sensitive to cope.' I question whether either approach actually serves the best interests of the child. It seems to me that both are defence mechanisms adopted by adults to avoid dealing with a child's pain.

I cannot emphasis too strongly, that we, as adults, must be prepared to put our adult methods of communication aside when we work with children and get back in touch with the child within ourselves and recognise play as communication. Adult interview situations do not work with children. As adults we are all too familiar with interview situations in which we anticipate disaster at every turn, but know that we have to impress if we are going to get that new job or overdraft. We try to give the answers we think the interviewer wants to hear so that we can avoid rejection and disappointment, and escape with our self-esteem still intact. Remember those feelings of anxiety and powerlessness, and imagine how a child would feel, and you will be able to recognise the potential for feelings being denied and minimised.

For example, a child may say, 'I loved my mummy, but I'm doing okay. I don't need anybody to help me so you can go now'. While thinking, 'I can't tell this grown-up [powerful you] that I used to get angry with my mummy sometimes. Now she's died and I can't tell her I'm sorry and I feel horrible. This person will think I didn't love mummy and she'll think I'm horrible too. I'm scared and I want *out* of here.'

On meeting children for the first time and explaining why you have arrived in their life, and what you can and cannot do, the opportunity is there to explain that children often have thoughts/feelings which scare and worry them and which they think they should not have. This begins the process of creating the 'Holding Environment' and giving the child permission to express themselves out loud.

I always get down on the floor with a child and the work takes place around both of us being involved in play activity. You will be amazed at how adept the children are communicating reality this way! The use of play materials also serves another important function as a 'defuser of tension'. For example, think about yourself in a situation where you are talking to someone about a subject which is giving you distress. As the tears come, you want to look away, or down, and your shoulders droop. A child whose gaze can fall on to their game, drawing or whatever will feel safer and more able to accept a comforting arm around their shoulders (which they can shrug off more easily too!). A word of caution here: in these situations do follow through, saying something like, 'I guess this bit is really hard for you.' The child will let you know by their response whether they want to stop or go on.

Working with Jane

When I met Jane she already knew that her mum was HIV positive and very ill, and she had been told that her mum was going to die. Her dad had asked for help because there were some important practical considerations and legal issues to resolve if he was to be able to give Jane the security and stability he wanted for her. He was also concerned that Jane might need help in coping with a situation which he knew was causing her great anxiety and distress.

My first task with Jane was to establish the basis of my contact with her and use some time to learn her story and allow her to check me out as a person whom she might trust. The fact that I was introduced to Jane and her family by Zoe, a volunteer from an organisation called Positive Help, was of immense value. Zoe had given consistent practical and emotional support to Jane and her mum and dad for several years, and because of their trust in her, my arrival on the scene was more readily and quickly accepted.

I explained that dad and Zoe had asked me to help because they understood how hard it must be for her right now. Jane readily accepted this agenda and having been given permission to talk about mum, set about putting a 'memory store' together with great enthusiasm. As we looked at old photographs and momentoes, Zoe's assistance was invaluable. She helped Jane to share her good and bad memories, and helped me to learn about Jane and her family's story and her understanding of what happens when someone dies. Jane's family held strong spiritual beliefs and she told me that her mummy would go up in the sky to heaven, where she would become an angel, an understanding which she illustrated in several drawings.

Jane was eight years old when her mum died, and Zoe and I had been working with Jane for around three months. Given her age, we could be reasonably sure that Jane would have an understanding of the reality of death, but may not have fully accepted its finality. This was apparent immediately. When I visited her the day afterwards, Jane confided that she felt really frightened and I asked if she wanted to tell me why. Jane told me that she was frightened of ghosts, and I tried to explain that, although I knew many people who have died, I had never seen a ghost, so I didn't think there were any. I explained that maybe when you went to heaven it was like a moving staircase that only went one way, so no matter how much you loved the people still on the earth, you couldn't go back, and heaven was such a great place you didn't feel sad. I went on to say, sometimes we think so hard about the person who has died, our mind might seem to flash a photograph of them in front of our eyes and we think we see them sitting in their favourite chair or standing at the kitchen sink like we often saw them. Jane became really angry, shouting, 'I don't care what I have to do, I will see my mummy again, I will, I will.' At this point I was thinking what a really clumsy explanation I had given Jane, but as I comforted her, I remembered that Jane was experiencing her first shock and denial, and had expressed it out loud! When Jane calmed down, her first question was, 'Will you be at the funeral?' I promised I would be. I wondered if Jane knew what would happen there, and we talked about all the people who had cared about mummy being there to say goodbye before she went to heaven. The importance of children attending funerals does not need to be repeated here. Jane drew a picture of how mummy would look as an angel for her memory box.

An understanding of the grief process in children helped to alert me to Jane's difficulties as they arose. She had expressed her initial denial of her mother's death, and had seemed to move quite rapidly to the 'angry' stage when someone, usually her father, had to withstand her frequent expressions of frustration and rage. She had shed few tears for her mum, although it was clear that her thoughts were very much focused on her. She talked about her mother freely and openly and often added items to her box.

Over the next few weeks, Jane gained great comfort from her memory box and various items were added, including her mum's favourite earrings and her make-up, which had strong, happy memories for Jane. Whenever Jane brought her memory box out, people knew she wanted to talk about her mum, although her father admitted this was very painful at times. Jane created some beautiful images of her mother. On an outing one day she pointed to a rainbow saying, 'Look at that, I bet my mummy's playing on it.'

About two months later Jane became sad, withdrawn and, at times, angry. She did not want to look at her memory box or share her feelings, and during our sessions, would do anything to divert my efforts; plastering me in shampoo and talcum powder proved extremely effective! After two sessions like this, I suspected that Jane was back into denial and struggling with feelings she was scared to share, but needed to express. It was time to take a risk and I used a grief story from the book *Once Upon a Time* by Nancy Davis (1990), to try to help Jane become unstuck. I read the story to her and she asked me to read it again and again. Jane then read the story to me, and carefully coloured in the accompanying picture. As she did so, she began to cry softly and whispered that she'd had two dreams about mummy, both the same. In the dream, mummy came to her room and said to Jane that she wanted her to go with her but she would have to hurry. Jane couldn't move fast enough and mummy went away without her. By the time Jane got to this part she was furiously putting a red border round her picture, and she said, 'I can't go with her because I didn't get the virus. If only I had, I could have gone.' While I cuddled her, I told Jane that I guessed one of mummy's happiest days was when the doctor told her Jane hadn't got the virus, because mummies love their children and want them to live for a long, long time and be happy. By this time Jane was sobbing bitterly, and I was wondering if I should really be making her suffer like this. But again I remembered that Jane was suffering like this already, but keeping all the pain of loss and self-blame to herself. Jane's dad joined us now and took Jane from me, rocking her in his arms until her sobs subsided, crying with her. Jane had become stuck in her grieving process, unable to deal with her feelings of despair, and had needed help.

Conclusion

To sum up, we as helping adults have an important role to fulfil in the lives of children whose parents have died, but helping the child come to terms with a new, very different reality can seem like a daunting prospect.

The ideas contained in this chapter are not new, they have been tried and tested by generations of adults who, personally and professionally, have in common a willingness to understand, and a commitment to and compassion for, the children in their care. In essence, our task is to create an environment within which the child feels safe enough to explore the experience of loss. It is important to understand children's comprehension of death, and how children react to loss, and vital to take the time to learn their story and get down alongside them as they control the pace and communicate with you the way they know best. Be honest about what you know and what you do not know; about what you can and cannot do, and the child will trust you as a person strong enough to share their pain as much and as often as they need. It can feel hard at times, but it is most definitely not all doom and gloom. Children experience pleasure as well as pain in the work, and will share this with you too. As adults we will learn, grow and change with the child and the rewards for both are immense. I left Jane's story at the point where the pain of her loss had seemed to become almost too much to bear but I would like, with her permission, to offer as a conclusion to this chapter, something which she had added to her memory box when I saw her again. It is a beautiful and moving piece of work. She is still sad, but her good memories are uppermost and her guilt and self-blame have gone.

> *-My Favourite Memories-*
> *Of You*
>
> My favorit memories of my mum is when she lookt at the miror and put on hir macup on. and I liykt it wen she gaveus cudels and cisses and gave me all the atenchin and sed that she luved me and I liykt wen she was happy and I got upset wen she was criyin I luve my mumy so wmuch.

References

Anthony, S. (1971), *The Discovery of Death in Childhood*, London: Penguin.

Bion, W. R. (1962), *Learning from Experience*, London: Heinemann.

Davis, N. (1990), *Once Upon a Time – Therapeutic Stories*, Psychological Associates of Oxon Hall.

Kubler-Ross, E. (1969), *On Death and Dying*, New York: Macmillan.

Nagy, M. (1948), in the *Journal of Genetic Psychology* 45.406.

Winnicott, D. W. (1964), *The Child, the Family and the Outside World*, London: Penguin.

Chapter 11

◆

MY DAD'S IN HEAVEN, TOO

SUPPORTING BEREAVED CHILDREN THROUGH GROUP WORK

Daryl Cuthbert
St Matthew's Family Centre, City of Dundee Council

Introduction

St Matthew's Family Centre is based in Dundee and part of City of Dundee Council Social Work Department's child and family services. We have a remit to support families with children under 12 within the local community who are experiencing difficulty or crisis. The staff group come from a multi-disciplinary background. The Family Centre was initially an urban aid project for families of very young children in the immediate locality. It has since developed into providing a range of family support services for families with a variety of difficulties.

Over the summer of 1993 the Centre received a number of requests for support to vulnerable children. One issue children brought to our attention was bereavement, specifically the isolation and loneliness they felt. One girl stated that meeting other children like her, who had lost a dad, would help her. At that time no other specific child-centred services for bereaved children existed in Dundee. Surveys across both voluntary and statutory agencies confirmed the lack of services, but also the need for support to children experiencing crisis due to bereavement. A group work experience for bereaved children aged from 7 to 11 years was devised by the staff group at St Matthew's. The children all came from the Dundee area and the groups were co-worked by a centre worker, a centre manager and social work students.

A death in the family

Grant was five years old when his dad died. He hadn't known him that long, only five years, but that was all Grant's life. His dad had been in the armed services and often wasn't around, but to Grant his dad was really important and didn't have to be around all the time, although Grant would have liked that.

Although Grant was only five, he could tell mum and dad didn't get on. He had heard them fighting and arguing a lot. Dad might not live with them now; he moved to Grant's granny's, but Grant could still see him.

Grant wanted mum and dad to live together as a family again and for all of them to be happy again. But it was scary when they argued and even scarier when dad hit mum. It was scary the night when dad was drunk and came to the house. Mum wouldn't let him in to see Grant or his sisters. Mum and dad argued; they shouted a lot in the street. It was really scary when dad fell and mum wouldn't help him. Dad said really horrible things to mum and he went away. Grant was upset at that and also because mum would not let Grant help dad, to see if he was all right.

The next day mum was really angry at dad; she shouted and cried a lot. This frightened Grant, seeing her like this, because he didn't know why she was upset. Grant couldn't remember who told him dad was dead, but it felt really strange. His dad couldn't be dead. Grant felt angry; angry at mum for not letting him help dad when he fell. When he asked what made dad die, his questions weren't answered and all the grown-ups wouldn't talk about it. Mum and granny had fallen out and aunts and uncles didn't visit.

One day mum was angry at the children asking about dad. She said he took pills and died. Grant and his sisters felt that they couldn't talk about dad after that.

Grant's dad had not died from a fall as Grant believed. His dad had returned to granny's house where he had taken an overdose of painkillers. His body was found the next day by his mother.

When Grant was eight he was referred to a bereavement support group at St Matthew's. He was still struggling to come to terms with the losses his father's death had caused in his life. His behaviour towards his mum was extremely challenging and their relationship almost in crisis. His school and peer relationships were very difficult and causing concern to the support worker who referred him to the attention of the group.

Grant's losses

To Grant, his dad was dead and could never return. Loss of this kind is overwhelming enough, but the other losses it created meant that Grant lost a great deal more. He lost the mother he knew. His mum, now a widow, was left with guilt and blame for her partner's actions. Tortured by the 'what if' or the 'if only' questions in her mind, while still being angry and traumatised by what she saw as her partner's actions and selfishness, Grant's mum coped by denying the effects on her and by shutting out much of what had happened. Grant had not only lost the physical presence of his father, he had lost:

- his future with his father;
- his opportunity to relate to his dad in the context of the past, present and future;
- his father's family, who blamed his mum for his dad's death;
- his granny, who also blamed mum, but was also blamed by mum for not finding dad sooner;

- his right to be 'proud' of his father and proud of the things they shared together; and
- his right to develop an unbiased view of his father's memory.

These losses went on and on for Grant, impinging on his everyday life, setting his experiences apart from other children. His father's death involved Grant in becoming the victim of silences, secrets, taboos and confusion.

Difficult deaths

Suicide, murder, traumatic deaths, disaster, stigmatised deaths, like AIDS, are often referred to as 'difficult' deaths, increasing the probability of the bereaved not coming to terms with their loss.

Grant's circumstances highlight the need to offer support to children who experience 'difficult' deaths. It may be argued that all children who experience death should be offered support, but in doing so, we may intervene too quickly, infringing on the family's ability to support each other.

The workers in the bereavement group recognised that the pain of grief cannot be taken away. One has to experience and work through the grief, coming to terms with the loss, possibly having grown and changed because of it. Not being able to work through the grief, becoming stuck in the process can make children, as well as adults, vulnerable. Authors on bereavement indicate that unresolved grief issues can impair one's ability to cope with later bereavements, loss or crisis (Wertheimer 1992). Worden (1992) recognises that children in particular are vulnerable to issues around unresolved grief which can impair their ability to cope.

Intervention via a group work experience was thought to be an appropriate method to allow bereaved children space to acknowledge, and begin to address, any issues relating to their loss. Models of issue-based group work were looked at, including bereavement groups, and a 10-week time limited group decided upon which would give clearer focus and purpose to the group (Cruse 1993).

The group was to be facilitated by adults experienced in bereavement work, group work and supporting vulnerable children. We wanted to offer children a space to reflect upon their experiences and to be supported by peers who could acknowledge their right to be 'normal' and not alone. Worker philosophy placed clear emphasis on the rights of the family and the child.

The referral

The referral to the group recognised behaviour which was being described as 'bad' or 'difficult' as a child's expression of just how difficult it was for them to cope with the changes in their lives. Every child referred was part of a family or community, and recognition was given to these and their roles in supporting the child. Children were not bereaved in isolation. Parents, carers, siblings and other significant people needed to be included in discussing the issues for the child attending the group, and how that in turn might affect them.

A leaflet in simple children's language, 'When Someone Special Dies' (Cuthbert 1993), was produced and given to families by referrers or ourselves on our first visit to the child's home. Our intention was to leave families with information which would help them talk about pain and the emotions around bereavement, with their children. We found ourselves in contact with families, wary of trusting our motives, wary of trusting our purpose, wary of letting these 'well-intentioned adults' become involved in asking their children to share their pain, suffering and confusion around their bereavements. But they did, and our respect for those families' strengths grew after every contact. Their stories, their pain and their suffering seemed almost unbearable to us but they survived and were still surviving.

Stories unfolded before us where we were allowed to hear families' darkest secrets, and asked to collude with those secrets; 'Don't tell the children, they don't know it was suicide, they think it was an accident.' It transpired that 70 per cent of the bereavements in the group were through suicide.

Wertheimer (1992), in her book *A Special Scar*, describes suicide as, 'The most difficult bereavement crisis for any family to face and resolve in an effective manner.' We recognised her words in the families struggling to regain control in their lives, having been bereaved by suicide. In the same way the experience of HIV in families can lead to secrets and taboos within the family. Children can feel responsible for 'keeping secrets' for their parents, unable to talk about their fears lest they let the secret slip.

The other children's bereavements were sudden, unexpected deaths. Each bereavement was unique and its impact on each individual unique. What each child had in common was that his or her bereavement was getting in the way of him or her coping with life. They were being seen as unable to resolve their grief and regain some sense of control over their lives.

Aim of the group

The aim of the group was to give children permission to talk about their bereavement in a safe, supportive environment. We told them what had brought them to our attention. 'Someone special had died, and that had changed things.' Children were invited to join a group 'bringing together other children who also knew a special person that had died'. Through activities, games and new experiences we aimed to talk about how things had changed for them and what was making things hard. This simple, clear language was developed from our working aims of providing:

- a safe, secure setting which encouraged relationship-building, trust, sharing, honesty, confidence, self-esteem and self-worth;
- opportunities for new and positive experiences;

- a safe outlet for reflecting on, and sharing, the experience of loss and developing an understanding of one's own feelings and behaviour; and
- consistent adult support to the group.

Some bereavements opened up secrets of parenthood, of extra-marital relationships, previous losses and accidental deaths, but all the children, no matter the circumstances, recognised the loss of their significant person as the issue. To them, the nature of the death made no difference, be the death through suicide, accident or ill health. The children saw themselves as children whose 'fathers' had died, as children whose 'mothers' had died, as children whose 'brothers' had died, as children whose 'friend' had died.

It may be that some deaths can cause a shift in the child's view of significant adults where an illness has been kept 'secret' from them. A breach of trust, as it may be perceived by the child, can lead to a reinterpretation of past events and damage their ability to 'believe' adults again. With highly stigmatised illnesses, like AIDS, there is always the danger of this happening because of the potential secrecy and taboos surrounding them.

Group work

The group met over three months on 10 consecutive evenings. Much of the work in the group took place in a large, comfortable room, with the workers often sitting on the floor at children's eye level. Talking with the children in this kind of environment allowed them to tell their stories through planned activities, often using art materials and exercises. For example, when discussing memories, we asked each child to bring the group a special belonging which reminded them of the dead person. Having a material, concrete object in their hands seemed to help them both remember and share memories.

A 'question box' was introduced to the group, a small box placed in the room we worked in, with pencils and paper to hand. We suggested to the children that if they wanted to ask a question, but the evening was finishing, they could write it down and post it in the box, knowing that next week we would work on it in the group. If a child put their name on it we would do the work individually and privately. If the question was anonymous, then the whole group would be involved. Snack time was an appropriate time to have these discussions. The children worked through the usual jokes and statements, but within these they began to express thoughts on rules and boundaries in the group. One question tested the safety in the group, 'Is it all right to get really angry?' Others told us the extent of the children's pain, 'It's hard to talk about mum, do I have to?'

The accumulated information contained within the weekly recordings proved valuable, not only as a means of assessing whether needs had been met, but also as a learning tool that helped the adult workers gain a deeper understanding of bereavement and a child's capacity to deal with the facts of death. Even with our knowledge, thought and planning, we probably still took the typically adult approach of being too cautious and tentative in judging the pace at which we introduced discussions, games or activities designed to encourage expression of feelings. What our collected recordings started to demonstrate was that, given the right conditions in an atmosphere of trust and support, bereaved children will talk about the person they have lost, what that person meant to them and how they experience a whole range of feelings. Many exercises were designed specifically to build up confidence, esteem and self-worth, supporting the children in taking risks and trusting in new experiences.

The children tended to see only simple choices in their coping skills. As individual children, this is what we expected, but even within the group context their peers shared similar, limited coping mechanisms. All the children at sometime in the group's life stated they were victims of bullies. Some of the experiences they discussed were real, some imaginary. We concluded from this that the children saw themselves individually as 'victims', even in situations where this was not the case.

My dad's in heaven, too

All the children in the group were white, all from Dundee families and from either Roman Catholic or Protestant backgrounds. At the time of the home visits to the adults, we asked them what they believed the children's interpretation to be of where their deceased parents were. This way we were able to ascertain each child's knowledge base. The group workers encouraged the children to explore their individual views. All the children had a perspective of a heaven and were able to discuss age-appropriate understandings of their beliefs. With the children's permission, we fed their understandings back to their carers during the home visits, in order to allow families and carers to continue working with their children.

During one exercise, Dorothy, the only girl in any of the groups, spoke of her dad. 'My dad's a mechanic, but he can't fix cars anymore because he's in heaven.' 'My dad's there, too,' put in Robert, aged eight. 'Where's heaven?' I asked. The children explained their view of heaven, helping each other in their explanations: 'It's beyond the clouds,' 'No you can't fly to it on a plane or rocket,' 'You can't see it, but in heaven they can watch over you.' I wanted to explore their thoughts fully. Robert's mum was worried that he hadn't accepted that his dad could not return. She told us that Robert claimed to still be able to see his dad in the house. This gave me an opportunity to check out Robert's understanding. 'So how do you get to heaven?' I asked. 'You have to die first,' stated Dorothy. Robert agreed, 'That's right and then you get buried.' 'Buried, what's buried?' I began to doodle a picture alongside the children who were also drawing. 'When you die you get put in a box and get put in the ground,' said Robert. At that, he presented Dorothy and me with a picture he had been working on. 'That's Jesus; he came and got my dad when he was buried and took him to heaven with him.' 'Did he take the coffin and your dad too?' I asked tentatively. 'No!' exclaimed Robert, *Jesus Leaves The Skin*'. Dorothy nodded in agreement, both children looking at me as if I was clueless. Robert and Dorothy had shown me age-appropriate understandings of concepts such as heaven not being a two-way process; a 'soul' or spirit leaving the body, and a sense that Jesus, for them, is a safe, caring being, looking after their fathers. Clearly, in a multi-faith group, we would have to pay attention to all perspectives.

Listening to children

The children who attended the groups seemed to recognise that they only had 10 Wednesdays to attend to business. We weren't their friends, or even befrienders. We were people who ran a group for bereaved children, children who, like them, had known someone special who had died. Their parents had introduced us to them as people whom they would want them to trust; as adults who listened to children. Only one child, Alec's brother Kenny, withdrew without reason after six weeks. His right to do so was respected.

Alec, up until Kenny's departure, was hesitant in becoming involved in activities. After Kenny's departure he began to take on a different role. Alec began to ask questions about his mum's death in ways he had not before. He began to use the group to meet his own individual needs, perhaps freed up by Kenny's absence, but perhaps because we were able to view him as an individual, rather than as a part of a sibling group.

Every appropriate opportunity was taken to explore issues in the 10 weeks. 'Snack time', 'group time', 'activity time' and 'home time' all allowed opportunities for exploring themes of memories, events, questions and so forth. This didn't happen by accident. Two-hour group time on Wednesdays was preceded and followed by approximately five hours of planning and review, recording details of conversations with each individual and evaluating activities and group process. The implications for our individual workloads should not to be underestimated.

The value of listening to children, taking note of what they said, sharing it with co-workers at reviews, checking it out with our consultants in the child and family psychiatry service, all enabled us to really hear the children and their stories.

Home visiting was an integral part of the group work. Adult-to-adult contact was vital in making links and discussing issues. Elements of knowledge and understanding had to be discussed without the children being present. One father told me that he didn't think his children knew that their mother had killed herself, but at a group session one of his sons said that he believed his mum had meant to die.

A case in point

Grant's dad, you will remember, had died three years earlier. Grant brought his dad's army belt to the 'shared memories' session. In fact, he wore it to hold up his trousers. This adult parade belt, with it's engraved buckle, holding up an eight-year-old's trousers, was a sight to behold. Grant was oblivious to the mismatch. He walked into the room 10 feet tall, bursting with silent pride, continuously looking for ways in which to draw attention to his belt. 'I've brought in this,' he said. 'It's my dad's army belt,' he proudly proclaimed. 'It was my dad's; he was in the army'... and Grant talked and talked about his dad. This was the beginning of a child talking about his father and how he missed him and grieved for him, using words which had not been available to him before.

This exercise marked a turning point in Grant's attendance at the group. The group was important to him but Grant's mother also played an integral part in allowing her son's need to recognise his father's memory. It was she who allowed him to choose one of his father's possessions. We were witnessing her being able to separate out her pain as a partner, from her child's pain as a bereaved son, and allow him the right to be proud of the things he and his father shared.

Grant's confidence grew from this point on and he played a more active role in the group. Each week he brought to the group something else of his dad's, negotiating with his mum to carry on wearing his belt to hold up his own combat trousers and wearing his dad's shoulder braids over his own jacket. The group had its own Action Man! Grant's need to explore the facts of his dad's life overrode the workers' interest in not encouraging stereotypical roles for children. Although concerned at the emphasis Grant placed on the 'GI Joe' image and its possibly violent connotations, it was an important vehicle for his grieving and, in fact, his mother reported that Grant's general behaviour had improved.

Grant was a private child, often spending time in his room playing with his action figures. Initially, he and his mother choose to stay out of each other's way because of the friction between them. During the life of the group, Grant began to leave his door open, allowing his mother the opportunity to quietly observe his play and also overhear the conversations he was having with his teddy. Grant had many action toys, but when there was something on his mind he would ask questions out loud to his teddy. His mum had overheard some and spoke to us about what she should do. We felt that Grant had engineered the situation so that his mum would overhear, and was sharing his thoughts out loud in a safer and less threatening way than by asking his mum directly. However, we did feel it appropriate to check Grant's behaviour, and we asked him about talking to his dad through his teddy. We asked him if he ever heard dad answer his questions through his teddy. His answer was the simplest of 'no's', presented with the kind of gaze which clearly indicated how stupid he thought we were!

Grant's teddy didn't talk back to him; that wasn't the point. Grant had found a way to talk about dad in the house. Mum was allowing this to happen and supporting him in doing so. It was a safe start to a different kind of relationship between the two of them.

Protecting children from pain

Our starting point with children was to work with them from where they were in their bereavement, not where we felt they 'should' be. We agreed with the children's carers that 'adult business' was separate from 'family business'. In 'family business', we encouraged each member of the family to be involved. 'Adult business', on the other hand, was for adults only.

Like HIV, many of the issues facing the families who had been bereaved placed the worker in the centre of a complex web of knowledge, at times knowing facts that the children were unaware of. The issues for us were difficult to come to terms with, and we tried to strike a balance of encouraging the adults to inform the children of the truth at a level appropriate to the child's age, and the ability of the parent to cope with supporting the child through any subsequent distress. We could not offer adults the support we were giving their children during the group. Our focus was the child's best interests, although this often meant respecting the adult's wish not to share knowledge that they had trusted to us. Parents did draw strength from each other, however, and through the group. Phone numbers were exchanged, visits and contacts arranged, new networks of mutual support opened up.

As workers, we were probably quite cautious in our questioning, fearing that we would cause distress to the children. They soon showed us that our manoeuvring around emotive subjects was not what they wanted. Their special person had died. They didn't want that to happen, but it did. Our gentle exploration was often superseded by the children asking us to be more direct with our use of language. There is a natural tendency in workers to want to minimise children's hurt; but what right have we to do that? Who might we be doing that for? We had gained the children's trust, asked their permission to discuss their pain and now found ourselves initially avoiding it.

Children need honesty from us as workers which we have to be prepared to give. We have to be strong enough to engage with the pain. For example, we also asked the children if they ever felt like hurting themselves in the kinds of ways their parents had. This felt an important question as some of the pain and confusion the children exhibited stemmed from feelings of guilt, blame and the hurt of wanting to be with a dead parent. These feelings might be particularly prevalent where HIV features.

Feed back

With the children's permission we fed back to their families, the thoughts, questions and confusion they had shared with us. In family meetings we supported the children in asking questions they had about the changes they had experienced. For some questions there were no answers, but families could generally be more open and honest about their inability to provide answers to everything.

The group work experience ended as it had begun, with the involvement of all the families in a shared exercise. A picnic and day trip was organised.

After the group ended, each family, child, referrer and school was invited to a review where we could feedback issues and any thoughts for future support. We recognised that because we had made a decision to put the family in the centre of decision-making, we may not have gained the widest possible picture of the children. Schools and teachers were informed by some of the carers as this put them in control of the discussions and sharing of information. It did limit our ability to gain a balanced perspective of how the child was using the time at the group to address issues in other, wider settings. In future, clearer expectations could be built into the referral process which would allow us contact with school, clubs and so forth, although we recognise the philosophical tensions which arise. As a service which places the family at the centre of the process, there are many things we might like to know about people's lives, but we focused only on the area that we 'needed' to know, in order to respect the families' rights to retain control and ownership of the work.

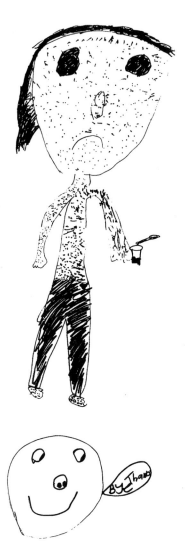

Conclusion

The issues and vulnerabilities of families bereaved by suicide, and other 'difficult deaths', are complex and often demanding. The rights of the child to know the truth and the rights of parents to protect children from the 'pain' of the truth is a critical tightrope. We found that workers offering support to children were also faced with the adult's needs, which we were unable to meet, although we did pass on information about adult support agencies.

Parents also supported each other. One mother was extremely vulnerable at the time of the group, but her child's involvement did force her to face issues in her life about suicide and secrets in the family and she received support from another mum to stay with the group.

Throughout the 10-week programme all the children, at different stages, expressed and demonstrated a range of emotions and behaviours. The strength and effectiveness of the group lay in the realisation that they had all felt the pain of bereavement but that they were not alone. Given that attendance was voluntary, the fact that there were 95 out of a possible 100 attendances indicates how much the children themselves valued the group. One child felt particularly strongly that other boys and girls who had lost someone should come to groups like this because it would 'help them'.

When the children first came into the group they had all felt the pain of bereavement. They all left with the prospect of more pain and upset ahead of them, because that is 'normal'. What the group experience had hopefully done was to help normalise the grieving process by giving the children permission to grieve.

To mark the final goodbye to the group, each child was given a 'thank-you card'. Each card, individually made, reflected the child's interests, making it unique to them. Inside was an acknowledgement of their strengths, their bravery at sharing their pain, their stories and the workers' thanks for trusting them. With a 10-pence piece, permission was given to the children of each group to phone us if they got sad and had no one to talk to about their 'special' person who had died. Referring to the 10 pence in the card, one child said, 'My mum's got a phone, so I don't need to use a call box. Can I spend it on sweets instead?' This seemed a healthy ending!

References

Cruse (1993), *Supporting Bereaved Children and their Families: A Training Manual*, Cruse Bereavement Care.

Cuthbert, D. (1993), *When Someone Special Dies*, St Matthew's Family Centre.

Wertheimer, A. (1992), *A Special Scar: The Experience of those Bereaved by Suicide*, London: Routledge.

Worden, W. (1992), *Grief Counselling and Grief Therapy: A Handbook for the Mental Health Practitioner*, London: Tavistock.

FURTHER READING

Available from Children in Scotland

Alexander, H. (1995), *Young Carers and HIV*, Children in Scotland.
Marshall et al. (1995), *Children's Rights and HIV*, Children in Scotland.
Children and HIV Resource Lists – A comprehensive guide to publications for children, young people, parents and professionals.
From Children in Scotland, Princes House, 5 Shandwick Place, Edinburgh EH2 4RG.

HIV and children

Barlow, J. (1996), *HIV and Children – A Training Manual*, Edinburgh: HMSO.
Batty, D. (ed.) (1993), *HIV infection and Children in Need*, London: BAAF.
Honigsbaum, N. (1991), *Children and HIV: A Cause for Concern*, London: National Children's Bureau.
Imrie, J. and Coombes, Y. (eds) (1995), *No Time To Waste: The Scale and Dimensions of the Problem of Children affected by HIV/AIDS in the United Kingdom*, London: Barnardo's.
The Scottish Office (1993), *Children and HIV: Guidance for Local Authorities and Voluntary Organisations*, Social Work Services Group.

Bereavement

Cruse (1993), *Supporting Bereaved Children and the Families: A Training Manual*, Cruse Bereavement Care.
Jewett, C. (1982), *Helping Children Cope with Separation and Loss*, Harvard: Common Press.
Worden, J. W. (1991), *Grief Counselling and Grief Therapy: A Handbook for the Mental Health Practitioner*, London: Routledge.

HIV/General

Gaitley, R. and Seed, P. (1989), *HIV and AIDS: A Social Network Approach*, London: Jessica Kinglsey.

Gaitley, R., Mallinson, W. and Taylor, D. (1993), *HIV and AIDS: A Social Work Perspective*, London: BASW.

Books for Children

AVERT, 'HIV/AIDS and Sex: Information for young people', leaflet, Horsham: AVERT.

Baker, Dr L. S. (1991), *You and HIV*, London: Harcourt Bruce Jovanovich.

Fassler, Dr D. and McQueen, l. (1990), *What's a Virus Anyway?,* Buringlington: Waterfront.

Jordan, M. (1989), *Losing Uncle Tim*, illustrated by J. Freidman, Morton Grove: Whitmand & Co.

Merrifield, Dr M. (1990), *Come sit by me*, illustrated by H. Collins, Toronto Women's Press.

Mystrom, C. (1990), *Emma says Goodbye*, illustrated by A. Large, Oxford: Lions.

Perkins, G. and Morris, L. (1991), *Remembering Mum*, London: A & C Black.

Stevens, R. (1992), *It's Clinic Day*, illustrated by F. McKenzie, Edinburgh: Edinburgh District Council Women's Committee. Available from Lothian Health Board.

Varley, S. (1985), *Badger's Parting Gifts*, Oxford: Lions.

Williams, M. (1922), *The Velveteen Rabbit*, iIllustrated by W. Nicholson, London: Little Mammoth.

Useful Contacts

Aberlour Child Care Trust
36 Park Terrace
Stirling FK8 2JR
Tel. 01786 450335

AVERT
11 Denne Parade
Horsham
West Sussex RH12 1JD
Tel. 01403 210 202

Barnardo's Riverside Project
235 Corstorphine Road
Edinburgh EH12 7AR
Tel. 0131 334 9893

Brenda House
7 Hay Road
Edinburgh EH16 4QE
Tel. 0131 669 6676

Children's Panel Training
Centre for Continuing Education
University of Edinburgh
11 Buccleuch Place
Edinburgh EH8 9LW
Tel. 0131 650 4400

Children in Scotland
Princes House
5 Shandwick Place
Edinburgh EH2 4RG
Tel. 0131 228 8484

Dundee Royal Infirmary
Social Work Department
Barrack Road
Dundee DD1 9ND
Tel. 01382 346659

Health Education Board of Scotland
The Priory
Cannan Lane
Edinburgh EH10 4SG
Tel. 0131 447 8044

Milestone House
113 Oxgrands Road North
Edinburgh EH14 1EB
Tel. 0131 441 6989

National AIDS Trust
6th Floor
Eileen House
80 Newington Causeway
London SE1 6EF
Tel. 0171 972 2845

PARC (Paediatric AIDS Resource Centre)
20 Sylvan Place
Edinburgh EH9 1UW
Tel. 0131 536 0806

Paediatric HIV Service
City Hospital, Ward 17a
51 Greenbank Drive
Edinburgh EH10 5SB
Tel. 0131 536 6000

Positive Help
64a Broughton Street
Edinburgh EH1 3SA
Tel. 0131 558 1122

St Matthew's Family Centre
  Tranent Grove
  Whitfield
  Dundee DD4 4DW
  Tel. 01382 501966

Scottish Adoption Association
  34 Bernard Street
  Edinburgh EH6 6PR
  Tel. 0131 553 5060

SOLAS
  2–4 Abbeymount
  Edinburgh EH8 8EJ
  Tel. 0131 661 0982

Waverley Care Trust
  4a Royal Terrace
  Edinburgh EH7 5AB
  Tel. 0131 556 3958

Women and HIV/AIDS Network
  13a Great King Street
  Edinburgh EH3 6QW
  Tel. 0131 557 5199

ABOUT THE CONTRIBUTORS

Joy Barlow

Joy Barlow, Senior Manager with the Aberlour Child Care Trust, responsible for the management and development of projects in Edinburgh and Glasgow in the alcohol/ drug dependency sector. These projects provide residential and day support, outreach, follow-on and respite services for women who are affected by their own problem drug or alcohol use, and their children. Since the early 1980s, she has been involved at both policy and practice levels with regard to drug misuse and parenting, and the affects of HIV and AIDS on children. Joy has been a member of the Scottish Task Force on HIV and AIDS (1992) and on drugs (1994). She is currently a member of a variety of national and international committees.

Alison Blair

Alison Blair became involved with children affected by HIV and AIDS as a volunteer in providing play for children in hospital. In 1994 she qualified as a Hospital Play Specialist by which time she had already begun working in the Out-patients' Department at the City Hospital in Edinburgh. At present she is working at Rachel House, Scotland's first children's hospice.

Eleanor Carr

Elanor Carr graduated from Edinburgh University with MA(Hons) in French/ European Institutions. She has a Postgraduate Certificate in Education from Moray House College of Education and has been a class teacher for four years. She has worked as a volunteer at Milestone House for three years.

Daryl Cuthbert

Daryl Cuthbert is a centre worker at St Matthew's Family Centre, City of Dundee Council Social Work Department, which provides direct service in supporting vunerable children and families across Dundee. Trained as a youth and community worker, he has worked as a volunteer for the Scottish Society for Mentally Handicapped, running a social club for adults with learning disabilities and promoting the Tay Award Scheme, a community award scheme similar to the Duke of Edinburgh Award, for adolescents and adults with learning disabilities.

He has trained and worked as bereavement counsellor for Cruse Breavement Care, counselling both adults and children. Within his role as centre worker, he has facilitated a number of groups with adults, parents and children, specifically supporting bereaved children in both groups and individually. He is currently involved in planning for a group to support children affected by HIV issues in partnership with Barnardo's.

Rosemary Garrod

Rosemary Garrod has been providing appropriate play for children for over twenty years, first in playgroups, then as a childminder for children with special needs, and finally as a hospital play specialist. In 1985 she cared for one of the first babies diagnosed as being HIV positive in Lothian and has continued to work with children (and adults) affected by HIV since then. Through community education classes, study days and working with students on placement, she has been able to share her knowledge and practical experience of play with a wide range of adults.

Isobel Hamilton

Isobel Hamilton has been Project Leader at the Brenda House Project since November 1988, and was responsible for the implementation of the service and development of its policy and practice. Prior to her appointment with Aberlour she has worked extensively in drug-related fields, having a particular interest in the issues for women and children. She has been involved in the issues of HIV and AIDS since the beginning of the epidemic in Scotland in the early 1980s and is currently a management committee member of Body Positive Lothian.

Jan McClory

Jan McClory qualified as a social worker in 1979 and worked with families in Lothian and the Borders. Since 1984 she has worked with Brook Advisory Centre counselling on matters related to pregnancy, sexual and psychosexual behaviour. For three years from 1989 Jan was employed as Training Officer with specific responsibility for HIV/AIDS within the Social Work Department in Lothian Region undertaking training for all staff groups. Since 1992 she has worked for the Women HIV/AIDS Network as Project Co-ordinator.

Fiona Mitchell

Fiona Mitchell is a Specialist Health Visitor HIV/AIDS at the City Hospital in Edinburgh and is involved the follow-up and care of children born to HIV positive mothers and includes counselling, support and liaison. Previous to this, she was a health advisor in the Department of Genito-Urinary Medicine, Edinburgh (1989–90); and a health visitor in Edinburgh and West Lothian (1985–8). She completed her midwifery and health visitor training in Glasgow and general nurse training in Edinburgh.

Dr Jacqueline Mok

Jacqueline Mok is a consultant paediatrician with the Edinburgh Sick Children's NHS Trust. She has responsibility for the integration and care of children with chronic diseases and handicap in the community, liaising with the social work and the education departments. Since January 1986 her special remit has been the follow-up of all infants born to women with HIV infection in and around Edinburgh. Dr Mok is responsible for the care of a cohort of infants born to HIV infected women in the Lothians.

Dr Mok has sat on various working parties: the Royal College of Physicians Committee to consider ethical aspects of HIV infection (May 1987); British Paediatric Association working party in AIDS in Infancy and Childhood (November 1987); Technical Working Group from WHO on the Clinical Treatment Issues of HIV Infected Children (November 1989); Technical Working Group from WHO on Prevention of the Prenatal Transmission of HIV by Pharmacological and Immunological Means (October 1992); and Steering Committee from WHO on Clinical Research and Drug Development (February 1993).

Judith Morkis

Judith Morkis is a qualified social worker and has worked with children and families in clinical and community settings. She was seconded to Barnardo's Riverside Project by Lothian Health Board from October 1994 until February 1996. She has a particular interest in bereavement work with children. Judith now works at Rachel House, Scotland's first children's hospice.

Jean Raeburn

Jean Raeburn MBE, MSc, NNEB University of Edinburgh had worked with children and families in health, education and social work settings. She was a children's panel member in Edinburgh for a number of years, sitting at approximately 1000 hearings in that time. Based in the Centre for Continuing Education, she developed and continues to present the programme of training for panel members on Lothian, Borders and the Western Isles. She received the MBE in the New Year's Honours List 1993 for her services to children and to child care.

Jinty Ramsay

Jinty Ramsay is a state-enrolled nurse, nursery nurse and a hospital play specialist. She has experience of working in schools, nurseries and special schools. For the last two years she has worked in the infectious disease ward of the City Hospital in Edinburgh and has worked with children infected and affected by HIV.

Hazel Robertson

Hazel Robertson qualified as a social worker in 1986 and has worked specifically with people with HIV infection since February 1990. She is Senior Social Worker/ Senior Care Manager of the HIV team in Tayside Regional Council Social Work

Department and has also been involved in practice-based research, HIV training and in the publication of information in relation to HIV both locally and nationally.

Ann Sutton

Ann Sutton has worked in the field of substitute family care since the mid-1960s. From 1987 until 1992 she was a member of Lothian Region's Family Finding Unit and had a special responsibility for developing substitute family services in relation to families affected by HIV and AIDS. She is currently Director of Scottish Adoption.

Ingrid von Arnim

Ingrid von Arnim has worked with children and young people since 1984. Following four years with Berkshire Social Services as a residential and field social worker, she set up a generic social work service at Milestone House in Edinburgh when it opened in February 1990. Over a period of four and a half years she increasingly focused on the provision of pre- and post-bereavement support for children affected by HIV and AIDS in the family. In 1995 she took up the post of Senior Practitioner with Barnardo's Riverside Project in Dundee, continuing to offer a therapeutic support service to children and families affected by HIV and AIDS. Training social workers and other disciplines in ways of offering the same service is an important aspect of her work.

Liz White

Liz White has been a teacher for more than 20 years. She gained a Teaching Diploma from Callander Park College of Education in Falkirk and also has an Infant and Nursery Special Qualification from Moray House College of Education. She has taught at all stages of primary school in Central, Lothian and Fife regions. She is currently deputy head teacher.

INDEX

SCOTLAND

Published by The Stationery Office Limited and available from:

The Stationery Office Bookshops
71 Lothian Road, Edinburgh EH3 9AZ
(counter service only)
South Gyle Crescent, Edinburgh EH12 9EB
(mail, fax and telephone orders only)
0131-479 3141 Fax 0131-479 3142
49 High Holborn, London WC1V 6HB
(counter service and fax orders only)
Fax 0171-831 1326
68-69 Bull Street, Birmingham B4 6AD
0121-236 9696 Fax 0121-236 9699
33 Wine Street, Bristol BS1 2BQ
0117-926 4306 Fax 0117-929 4515
9-21 Princess Street, Manchester M60 8AS
0161-834 7201 Fax 0161-833 0634
16 Arthur Street, Belfast BT1 4GD
01232 238451 Fax 01232 235401
The Stationery Office Oriel Bookshop
The Friary, Cardiff CF1 4AA
01222 395548 Fax 01222 384347

The Stationery Office publications are also available from:

The Publications Centre
(mail, telephone and fax orders only)
PO Box 276, London SW8 5DT
General enquiries 0171-873 0011
Telephone orders 0171-873 9090
Fax orders 0171-873 8200

Accredited Agents
(see Yellow Pages)
and through good booksellers

Printed in Scotland for The Stationery Office Limited by CC No. 13129 15C 11/96

LA CINQUIÈME MONTAGNE

Marie, conçue sans péché, Priez pour nous
qui faisons appel à vous, Amen.

PAULO COELHO

La Cinquième Montagne

TRADUIT DU PORTUGAIS (BRÉSIL)
PAR FRANÇOISE MARCHAND-SAUVAGNARGUES

ÉDITIONS ANNE CARRIÈRE

Titre original :

A QUINTA MONTANHA

Cette édition a été publiée avec l'accord de
Sant Jordi Asociados, Barcelone, Espagne.

À A. M., guerrier de la lumière

Note de l'auteur

La thèse centrale de mon livre *L'Alchimiste* réside dans une phrase que le roi Melchisédech adresse au berger Santiago : « Quand tu veux quelque chose, tout l'univers conspire à te permettre de réaliser ton désir. »

Je crois entièrement à cette affirmation. Cependant, l'acte de vivre son destin comporte une série d'étapes, bien au-delà de notre compréhension, dont l'objectif est de nous ramener sans cesse sur le chemin de notre Légende Personnelle — ou de nous enseigner les leçons nécessaires à l'accomplissement de ce destin. J'illustrerais mieux ce propos, me semble-t-il, en racontant un épisode de ma propre vie.

Le 12 août 1979, j'allai me coucher avec une seule certitude : à trente ans, j'atteignais le sommet de ma carrière de producteur de disques. Directeur artistique de CBS au Brésil, je venais d'être invité à me rendre aux Etats-Unis pour y rencontrer les patrons de la maison de disques et, assurément, ils allaient m'offrir les meilleures conditions pour réaliser tout ce que je désirais dans ce domaine. Bien sûr, mon grand rêve — être écrivain — avait été mis de côté, mais quelle importance ? En fin de compte, la vie réelle était très différente de celle que j'avais imaginée ; il n'y avait aucun espace pour vivre de littérature au Brésil.

Cette nuit-là, je pris une décision, et j'abandonnai mon rêve : je devais m'adapter aux circonstances et saisir les occasions. Si mon cœur protestait, je pourrais toujours le tromper en composant des textes de chansons chaque fois que je le désirerais et, de temps à autre, en signant un article dans un journal. Du reste, j'étais convaincu que ma vie avait pris une voie différente, mais non moins excitante : un avenir brillant m'attendait dans les multinationales de musique.

A mon réveil, je reçus un appel téléphonique du président : j'étais remercié, sans autre explication. J'eus beau frapper à toutes les portes au cours des deux années qui suivirent, je n'ai jamais retrouvé d'emploi dans ce domaine.

En achevant la rédaction de *La Cinquième Montagne*, je me suis souvenu de cet épisode — et d'autres manifestations de l'inévitable dans ma vie. Chaque fois que je me sentais absolument maître de la situation, un événement se produisait, et me faisait échouer. Je me suis demandé pourquoi. Etais-je condamné à toujours approcher de la ligne d'arrivée, sans jamais la franchir ? Dieu serait-il cruel au point de me faire entrevoir les palmiers à l'horizon uniquement pour me laisser mourir de soif au milieu du désert ?

J'ai mis longtemps à comprendre que l'explication était tout autre. Certains événements sont placés dans nos existences pour nous reconduire vers l'authentique chemin de notre Légende Personnelle. D'autres surgissent pour nous permettre d'appliquer tout ce que nous avons appris. Enfin, quelques-uns se produisent pour nous *enseigner* quelque chose.

Dans *Le Pèlerin de Compostelle*, j'ai tenté de montrer que ces enseignements ne sont pas nécessairement liés à la douleur et à la souffrance ; la discipline et l'attention suffisent. Bien que cette compréhension soit devenue une importante bénédiction dans ma vie, malgré toute ma discipline et toute mon attention, je n'ai pas réussi à comprendre certains moments difficiles par lesquels je suis passé.

L'anecdote que j'ai relatée en est un exemple : j'étais un bon professionnel alors, je m'efforçais de donner ce qu'il y avait de meilleur en moi, et j'avais des idées qu'aujourd'hui encore je considère bonnes. Mais l'inévitable a surgi, au moment précis où je me sentais le plus sûr et le plus confiant. Je pense que cette expérience n'est pas unique ; l'inévitable a frappé la vie de tous les êtres humains à la surface de la Terre. Certains se sont rétablis, d'autres ont cédé — mais nous avons tous été effleurés par l'aile de la tragédie.

Pourquoi ? Pour trouver une réponse à cette question, j'ai laissé Elie me conduire par les jours et les nuits d'Akbar.

PAULO COELHO

« Et il ajouta : "Oui, je vous le déclare, aucun prophète ne trouve accueil dans sa patrie. En toute vérité, je vous le déclare, il y avait beaucoup de veuves en Israël aux jours d'Elie, quand le ciel fut fermé trois ans et six mois et que survint une grande famine sur tout le pays ; pourtant ce ne fut à aucune d'elles qu'Elie fut envoyé, mais bien dans le pays de Sidon, à une veuve de Sarepta." »

Luc, 4, 24-26

Prologue

Au commencement de l'année 870 avant Jésus-Christ, une nation connue sous le nom de Phénicie, que les Israélites appelaient Liban, commémorait presque trois siècles de paix. Ses habitants avaient de bonnes raisons de s'enorgueillir : comme ils n'étaient pas très puissants sur le plan politique, ils avaient dû mettre au point une force de négociation qui faisait des envieux, seul moyen de garantir leur survie dans un monde constamment dévasté par la guerre. Une alliance contractée aux environs de l'an 1000 avant J.-C. avec Salomon, roi d'Israël, avait favorisé la modernisation de la flotte marchande et l'expansion du commerce. Depuis lors, la Phénicie n'avait cessé de se développer.

Ses navigateurs avaient déjà atteint des régions lointaines, comme l'Espagne et les rivages baignés par l'océan Atlantique. Selon certaines théories — qui ne sont pas confirmées —, ils auraient même laissé des inscriptions dans le Nordeste et dans le sud du Brésil. Ils faisaient le négoce du verre, du bois de cèdre, des armes, du fer et de l'ivoire. Les habitants des grandes cités de Sidon, Tyr et Byblos connaissaient les nombres, les calculs astronomiques, la vinification, et ils utilisaient depuis presque deux cents ans un ensemble de caractères pour écrire, que les Grecs dénommaient *alphabet*.

Au commencement de l'année 870 avant J.-C., un conseil de guerre était réuni dans la cité lointaine de Ninive. Un groupe de généraux assyriens avait en effet décidé d'envoyer des troupes conquérir les nations bordant la mer Méditerranée et, en premier lieu, la Phénicie.

Au commencement de l'année 870 avant J.-C., deux hommes, cachés dans une étable de Galaad, en Israël, s'attendaient à mourir dans les prochaines heures.

Première partie

« J'ai servi un Seigneur qui maintenant m'abandonne aux mains de mes ennemis, dit Elie.

— Dieu est Dieu, répondit le lévite. Il n'a pas expliqué à Moïse s'Il était bon ou mauvais, Il a seulement affirmé : *Je suis*. Il est tout ce qui existe sous le soleil — le tonnerre qui détruit la maison, et la main de l'homme qui la reconstruit. »

La conversation était la seule manière d'éloigner la peur ; d'un moment à l'autre, les soldats allaient ouvrir la porte de l'étable, les découvrir et leur proposer le seul choix possible : adorer Baal, le dieu phénicien, ou être exécutés. Ils fouillaient maison après maison, convertissant ou exécutant les prophètes.

Le lévite se convertirait peut-être, échappant ainsi à la mort. Mais Elie n'avait pas le choix : tout arrivait par sa faute, et Jézabel voulait sa tête de toute façon.

« C'est un ange du Seigneur qui m'a envoyé parler au roi Achab et l'avertir qu'il ne pleuvrait pas tant que Baal serait adoré en Israël », expliqua-t-il, en demandant presque pardon pour avoir écouté les paroles de l'ange. « Mais Dieu agit avec lenteur ; quand la sécheresse commencera à produire son effet, la princesse Jézabel aura détruit tous ceux qui sont restés fidèles au Seigneur. »

Le lévite resta silencieux. Il se demandait s'il devait se convertir à Baal ou mourir au nom du Seigneur.

« Qui est Dieu ? poursuivit Elie. Est-ce Lui qui tient l'épée du soldat exécutant les hommes fidèles à la foi de nos patriarches ? Est-ce Lui qui a mis une princesse étrangère sur le trône de notre pays, afin que tous ces malheurs s'abattent sur notre génération ? Est-ce Dieu qui tue les fidèles, les innocents, ceux qui suivent la loi de Moïse ? »

Le lévite prit une décision : il préférait mourir. Alors il se mit à rire, parce que l'idée de la mort ne l'effrayait plus. Il se tourna vers le jeune prophète et s'efforça de le tranquilliser :

« Demande à Dieu qui Il est, puisque tu doutes de Ses décisions. Pour ma part, j'ai déjà accepté mon destin.

— Le Seigneur ne peut pas désirer que nous soyons impitoyablement massacrés, insista Elie.

— Dieu peut tout. S'Il se limitait à faire ce que nous appelons le Bien, nous ne pourrions pas le nommer Tout-Puissant ; Il dominerait seulement une partie de l'univers, et il y aurait quelqu'un de plus puissant que Lui qui surveillerait et jugerait Ses actions. En ce cas, j'adorerais ce quelqu'un plus puissant.

— S'Il peut tout, pourquoi n'épargne-t-Il pas la souffrance à ceux qui L'aiment ? Pourquoi ne nous sauve-t-Il pas, au lieu de donner gloire et pouvoir à Ses ennemis ?

— Je l'ignore, répondit le lévite. Mais il y a à cela une raison, et j'espère la connaître bientôt.

— Tu n'as pas de réponse à cette question.

— Non. »

Ils restèrent tous deux silencieux. Elie avait des sueurs froides.

« Tu as peur, mais moi j'ai accepté mon destin, commenta le lévite. Je vais sortir et mettre fin à cette agonie. Chaque fois que j'entends un cri là-dehors, je souffre en imaginant ce qui se passera lorsque mon heure viendra. Depuis que nous sommes enfermés ici, je suis mort une bonne centaine de fois, et j'aurais pu mourir une seule fois. Puisque je vais être égorgé, que ce soit le plus vite possible. »

Il avait raison. Elie avait entendu les mêmes cris et il avait déjà souffert au-delà de sa capacité de résistance.

18

« Je t'accompagne. Je suis fatigué de lutter pour quelques heures de vie supplémentaires. »

Il se leva et ouvrit la porte de l'étable, laissant la lumière du soleil révéler la présence des deux hommes qui y étaient cachés.

*

Le lévite le prit par le bras et ils se mirent en marche. A l'exception de quelques cris, on aurait dit un jour normal dans une cité pareille à n'importe quelle autre — un soleil pas trop brûlant, la brise venant de l'océan au loin, rendant la température agréable, les rues poussiéreuses, les maisons faites d'argile mélangée à de la paille.

« Nos âmes sont prisonnières de la terreur de la mort, et c'est une belle journée, dit le lévite. Bien souvent, alors que je me sentais en paix avec Dieu et avec le monde, la chaleur était insupportable, le vent du désert emplissait mes yeux de sable et ne me laissait pas voir à deux pas. Le plan de Dieu ne correspond pas toujours à ce que nous sommes ou sentons ; mais je suis certain qu'Il a une raison pour tout cela.

— J'admire ta foi. »

Le lévite regarda vers le ciel, comme s'il réfléchissait. Puis il se tourna vers Elie :

« N'admire pas, et ne crois pas autant : c'est un pari que j'ai fait avec moi-même. J'ai parié que Dieu existe.

— Tu es un prophète, répliqua Elie. Tu as aussi entendu des voix, et tu sais qu'il existe un monde au-delà de ce monde.

— C'est peut-être le fruit de mon imagination.

— Tu as vu les signes de Dieu », insista Elie, que les commentaires de son compagnon commençaient à rendre anxieux.

« C'est peut-être le fruit de mon imagination, lui fut-il répété. En fait, je n'ai de concret que mon pari : je me suis dit que tout cela venait du Très-Haut. »

*

La rue était déserte. Les gens, dans leurs maisons, attendaient que les soldats d'Achab accomplissent la tâche exigée par la princesse étrangère : l'exécution des prophètes d'Israël. Elie cheminait avec le lévite, et il avait la sensation que, derrière chacune des fenêtres et des portes, quelqu'un l'observait et l'accusait de ce qui était en train de se passer.

« Je n'ai pas demandé à être prophète. Tout cela est peut-être aussi le fruit de mon imagination », se disait Elie.

Mais après ce qui était arrivé dans la charpenterie, il savait qu'il n'en était rien.

*

Depuis son enfance, il entendait des voix et conversait avec les anges. Aussi ses parents insistèrent-ils pour qu'il consultât un prêtre d'Israël. Ce dernier, après nombre de questions, reconnut en lui un *nabi*, un prophète, un « homme de l'esprit », qui « s'exalte à la voix de Dieu ».

Après plusieurs heures d'entretien ininterrompu avec lui, le prêtre expliqua à ses parents que tout ce que cet enfant viendrait à dire devait être pris au sérieux.

Sur le chemin du retour, les parents exigèrent qu'Elie ne racontât jamais à personne ce qu'il voyait ou entendait ; être un prophète impliquait des liens avec le gouvernement, et c'était toujours dangereux.

De toute façon, Elie n'avait jamais rien entendu qui pût intéresser les prêtres ou les rois. Il ne conversait qu'avec son ange gardien et écoutait des conseils concernant sa propre vie. De temps à autre, il avait des visions qu'il ne parvenait pas à comprendre — des océans lointains, des montagnes peuplées d'êtres étranges, des roues avec des ailes et des yeux. Lorsque les visions avaient disparu, obéissant à ses parents, il s'efforçait de les oublier le plus vite possible.

Ainsi les voix et les visions s'étaient-elles faites de

plus en plus rares. Ses parents, satisfaits, n'avaient plus abordé le sujet. Lorsqu'il fut en âge d'assurer sa subsistance, ils lui prêtèrent de l'argent pour qu'il ouvrît une petite charpenterie.

*

Fréquemment, il regardait avec respect les autres prophètes dans les rues de Galaad : ils portaient des manteaux de peau et des ceintures de cuir, et affirmaient que le Seigneur les avait choisis pour guider le peuple élu. Mais en vérité, ce n'était pas son destin. Jamais il ne serait capable de connaître une transe lors d'une danse ou d'une séance d'autoflagellation, une pratique normale chez les « exaltés par la voix de Dieu », parce qu'il avait peur de la douleur. Jamais il ne marcherait dans les rues de Galaad, exhibant fièrement les cicatrices des blessures obtenues au cours de l'extase, parce qu'il était trop timide pour cela.

Elie se considérait comme une personne ordinaire, qui s'habillait comme tout le monde et dont l'âme était torturée des mêmes craintes et tentations que celle des autres mortels. A mesure que progressait son travail dans la charpenterie, les voix cessèrent complètement parce que les adultes et les travailleurs n'ont pas de temps pour cela. Ses parents étaient contents de leur fils, et la vie s'écoulait dans l'harmonie et la paix.

La conversation qu'il avait eue avec le prêtre lorsqu'il était petit devint peu à peu un lointain souvenir. Elie ne pouvait croire que Dieu tout-puissant eût besoin de converser avec les hommes pour faire valoir ses ordres. Ce qui s'était passé dans son enfance n'était que la fantaisie d'un gamin oisif. A Galaad, sa cité natale, il y avait des gens que les habitants considéraient comme fous. Incapables de tenir des propos cohérents, ils ne distinguaient pas la voix du Seigneur des délires de la démence. Ils erraient dans les rues, annonçant la fin du monde et vivant de la charité d'autrui. Pourtant, aucun prêtre ne les considérait comme « exaltés par la voix de Dieu ».

Elie en vint à penser que les prêtres n'avaient jamais la certitude de ce qu'ils affirmaient. Il y avait des « exaltés de Dieu » parce que le pays ne savait pas où il allait, que les frères se querellaient et que le gouvernement était instable. Il n'y avait aucune différence entre les prophètes et les fous.

*

Quand il apprit le mariage de son roi et de Jézabel, princesse de Tyr, Elie n'y accorda pas grande importance. D'autres rois d'Israël avaient agi de même. Il en avait résulté une paix durable dans la région, et le commerce avec le Liban s'était développé. Peu importait à Elie que les habitants du pays voisin croient en des dieux qui n'existaient pas ou se consacrent à des cultes étranges, comme l'adoration des animaux et des montagnes ; ils étaient honnêtes dans les négociations, voilà l'essentiel. Elie continua donc à acheter leur bois de cèdre et à leur vendre les produits de sa charpenterie. Même s'ils se montraient un peu orgueilleux, aucun des commerçants du Liban n'avait jamais cherché à tirer parti de la confusion qui régnait en Israël. Ils payaient les marchandises à leur juste prix et n'émettaient aucun commentaire sur les constantes guerres intestines, ni sur les problèmes politiques auxquels les Israélites étaient sans cesse confrontés.

*

Après son accession au trône, Jézabel avait demandé à Achab de remplacer le culte du Seigneur par celui des dieux du Liban.

Cela aussi était déjà arrivé auparavant. Elie, bien qu'il fût indigné par le consentement d'Achab, continua d'adorer le Dieu d'Israël et d'obéir aux lois de Moïse. « Cela ne durera pas, pensait-il. Jézabel a séduit Achab, mais elle ne parviendra pas à persuader le peuple. »

Mais Jézabel n'était pas une femme comme les autres ; elle avait la conviction que Baal l'avait fait venir au monde pour convertir les peuples et les nations. Subtilement et patiemment, elle se mit à récompenser tous ceux qui se détournaient du Seigneur et acceptaient les nouvelles divinités. Achab ordonna la construction d'un temple pour Baal à Samarie, à l'intérieur duquel il fit bâtir un autel. Les pèlerinages commencèrent, et le culte aux dieux du Liban se répandit de toutes parts.

« Cela passera. Cela durera peut-être une génération, mais ensuite cela passera », pensait toujours Elie.

Alors survint un événement auquel il ne s'attendait pas. Un après-midi, tandis qu'il finissait de fabriquer une table dans sa charpenterie, tout s'obscurcit autour de lui et des milliers de points blancs se mirent à scintiller. Sa tête lui faisait mal comme jamais ; il voulut s'asseoir, mais constata qu'il n'arrivait pas à bouger un seul muscle.

Ce n'était pas le fruit de son imagination.

« Je suis mort, pensa-t-il sur-le-champ. Maintenant, je découvre l'endroit où Dieu nous envoie après notre mort : le milieu du firmament. »

Une des lumières brilla plus fort et soudain, comme si elle venait de partout en même temps, « *la parole du Seigneur lui fut adressée : "Dis à Achab que, par la vie du Seigneur, le Dieu d'Israël au service duquel je suis, il n'y aura ces années-ci ni rosée ni pluie sinon à ma parole."* »

L'instant suivant, tout redevint normal, la charpenterie, la lumière du crépuscule, les voix des enfants jouant dans la rue.

*

Elie ne dormit pas cette nuit-là. Pour la première fois depuis des années, les sensations de son enfance étaient de retour ; et ce n'était pas son ange gardien qui lui parlait, mais « *quelque chose* » de plus puissant. Il redouta, s'il n'obéissait pas à cet ordre, que toutes ses activités ne fussent maudites.

Le lendemain matin, il décida de faire ce qu'on lui avait demandé. En fin de compte, il se contenterait de délivrer un message qui ne le concernait pas ; une fois cette tâche terminée, les voix ne reviendraient plus le déranger.

Il n'eut aucune difficulté à obtenir une audience auprès du roi Achab. Des générations plus tôt, lorsque le roi Saül était monté sur le trône, les prophètes avaient acquis de l'importance dans les affaires et le gouvernement de son pays. Ils pouvaient se marier, avoir des enfants, mais ils devaient rester en permanence à la disposition du Seigneur, afin que les gouvernants ne s'écartent jamais trop du droit chemin. La tradition affirmait que, grâce à ces « exaltés de Dieu », on avait gagné de nombreuses batailles et qu'Israël survivait parce que, quand ses gouvernants se fourvoyaient, il y avait toujours un prophète pour leur faire regagner la voie du Seigneur.

En arrivant, Elie avertit le roi que la sécheresse allait dévaster la région jusqu'à ce que le culte des dieux phéniciens fût abandonné.

Le souverain n'accorda guère d'importance à ces paroles, mais Jézabel, qui se tenait à côté d'Achab et écoutait attentivement, se mit à l'interroger. Elie lui parla alors de la vision, du mal de tête, de la sensation que le temps s'était arrêté quand il écoutait l'ange. Pendant qu'il décrivait ce qui lui était arrivé, il put regarder de près la princesse dont tout le monde parlait. C'était l'une des plus belles femmes qu'il eût jamais vues, avec de longs cheveux noirs descendant jusqu'à sa taille parfaitement tournée. Ses yeux verts, qui brillaient dans son visage brun, restaient fixés sur ceux d'Elie. Il ne parvenait pas à déchiffrer la signification de ce regard, et il ne pouvait pas savoir quel effet lui causaient ses propos.

Il sortit de cette entrevue convaincu qu'il avait accompli sa mission et pouvait désormais retourner à son travail dans la charpenterie. Sur le chemin du retour, il désira Jézabel de toute l'ardeur de ses vingt-trois ans. Et il pria Dieu qu'il lui fût permis de rencontrer plus tard une femme du Liban, parce qu'elles étaient belles, avec leur peau sombre et leurs yeux verts emplis de mystère.

*

Il travailla le reste de la journée et dormit en paix. Le lendemain, il fut réveillé avant l'aurore par le lévite. Jézabel avait persuadé le roi que les prophètes étaient une menace pour la croissance et l'expansion d'Israël. Les soldats d'Achab avaient reçu l'ordre d'exécuter tous ceux qui refuseraient d'abandonner la tâche sacrée que Dieu leur avait confiée. Mais à Elie ils n'avaient pas donné la possibilité de choisir : lui devait être mis à mort.

Elie et le lévite passèrent deux jours cachés dans l'étable au sud de Galaad, tandis que quatre cent cinquante *nabis* étaient exécutés. Cependant, la plupart des prophètes, qui vagabondaient d'ordinaire dans les rues en s'autoflagellant et en prédisant la fin du monde à cause de la corruption et de l'absence de foi, avaient accepté de se convertir à la nouvelle religion.

*

Un bruit sec, suivi d'un cri, interrompit les pensées d'Elie. Alarmé, il se tourna vers son compagnon :

« Que se passe-t-il ? »

Mais il n'obtint pas de réponse : le corps du lévite s'écroula sur le sol, une flèche plantée au milieu de la poitrine.

Devant lui, un soldat mit une nouvelle flèche dans son arc. Elie regarda autour de lui : la rue, les portes et fenêtres fermées, le soleil éblouissant dans le ciel, la brise qui venait d'un océan dont il avait tant entendu parler mais qu'il n'avait jamais vu. Il songea à courir, mais il savait qu'il serait rattrapé avant d'atteindre le coin de la rue.

« Si je dois mourir, que ce ne soit pas d'un coup dans le dos. »

Le soldat banda de nouveau son arc. A sa grande surprise, Elie ne ressentait pas la peur, ni l'instinct de survie, ni rien. C'était comme si toute la scène avait déjà été définie voilà très longtemps, et que l'un et l'autre — lui aussi bien que le soldat — tenaient un rôle dans un drame qui n'avait pas été écrit par eux. Il se rappela son enfance, les matins et les après-midi à Galaad, les ouvrages inachevés qu'il allait laisser dans sa charpenterie. Il songea à sa mère et à son père, qui n'avaient jamais désiré avoir un fils prophète. Il pensa aux yeux de Jézabel et au sourire du roi Achab.

Il pensa qu'il était stupide de mourir à vingt-trois ans, sans avoir jamais connu l'amour d'une femme.

La main lâcha la corde, la flèche fendit l'air, passa en sifflant près de son oreille droite, et se planta derrière lui dans le sol poussiéreux.

Le soldat, encore une fois, arma son arc et le visa. Pourtant, au lieu de tirer, il fixa Elie dans les yeux.

« Je suis le meilleur des archers de toutes les armées d'Achab, dit-il. Cela fait sept ans que je n'ai pas manqué un seul tir. »

Elie se tourna vers le corps du lévite.

« Cette flèche était pour toi. » Le soldat gardait son arc bandé, et ses mains tremblaient. « Elie était le seul prophète qui devait être mis à mort ; les autres pouvaient choisir la foi en Baal.

— Alors, termine ton travail. »

Il était surpris de sa propre tranquillité. Il avait imaginé la mort tant de fois durant les nuits passées dans l'étable, et maintenant il comprenait qu'il avait souffert plus que nécessaire. En quelques secondes, tout serait fini.

« Je n'y arrive pas », dit le soldat, les mains encore tremblantes, et l'arc changeant à chaque instant de direction. « Va-t'en ! Hors de ma présence ! Je pense

26

que Dieu a dévié mes flèches, et qu'il va me maudire si je réussis à te tuer. »

Ce fut alors — à mesure qu'Elie découvrait qu'il avait une chance de survivre — que la peur de mourir afflua de nouveau. Il était encore possible de connaître l'océan, de rencontrer une femme, d'avoir des enfants et d'achever ses ouvrages dans la charpenterie.

« Finis-en vite, dit-il. En ce moment, je suis calme. Si tu attends trop, je vais souffrir pour tout ce que je serai sur le point de perdre. »

Le soldat regarda alentour pour s'assurer que personne n'avait assisté à la scène. Puis il abaissa son arc, remit la flèche dans son carquois, et disparut.

Elie sentit que ses jambes flanchaient ; la terreur revenait dans toute son intensité. Il devait fuir immédiatement, disparaître de Galaad, ne plus jamais avoir à se trouver face à face avec un soldat, l'arc tendu, pointé sur son cœur. Il n'avait pas choisi son destin, et il n'était pas allé voir Achab pour se vanter auprès de ses voisins d'avoir conversé avec le roi. Il n'était pas responsable du massacre des prophètes. Il n'était pas non plus responsable d'avoir vu, un après-midi, le temps s'arrêter et la charpenterie se transformer en un trou noir, empli de points lumineux.

Imitant le soldat, il regarda autour de lui. La rue était déserte. Il songea à vérifier s'il pouvait encore sauver la vie du lévite mais bientôt la terreur revint et, avant que quelqu'un n'apparût, Elie s'enfuit.

Il marcha pendant des heures, s'engageant dans des chemins qui n'étaient plus fréquentés depuis longtemps, et arriva enfin au bord du ruisseau du Kerith. Il avait honte de sa lâcheté, mais il se réjouissait d'être en vie.

Il but un peu d'eau, s'assit, et alors seulement se

rendit compte de la situation dans laquelle il se trouvait : demain, il lui faudrait se nourrir, et il ne trouverait pas de nourriture dans le désert.

Il se rappela la charpenterie, le travail de tant d'années, qu'il avait été contraint de laisser derrière lui. Certains de ses voisins étaient ses amis, mais il ne pouvait pas compter sur eux. L'histoire de sa fuite s'était déjà sans doute répandue dans la cité, et tous le haïraient de s'être échappé, pendant qu'il envoyait au martyre les véritables hommes de foi.

Tout ce qu'il avait fait jusque-là était ruiné uniquement parce qu'il avait cru accomplir la volonté du Seigneur. Demain, et dans les prochains jours, semaines et mois, les commerçants du Liban frapperaient à sa porte, et on les avertirait que le propriétaire s'était enfui, semant derrière lui la mort de prophètes innocents. On ajouterait peut-être qu'il avait tenté de détruire les dieux qui protégeaient la terre et les cieux. L'histoire franchirait bientôt les frontières d'Israël, et il pouvait renoncer pour toujours au mariage avec une femme aussi belle que celles qui vivaient au Liban.

*

« Il y a les navires. »

Oui, il y avait les navires. On avait coutume d'accepter pour marins les criminels, les prisonniers de guerre, les fugitifs, parce que c'était un métier plus dangereux que l'armée. A la guerre, un soldat avait toujours une chance de rester en vie ; mais les mers étaient un territoire inconnu, peuplé de monstres, et, lorsqu'une tragédie survenait, il n'y avait pas de survivant pour raconter ce qui s'était passé.

Certes, il y avait les navires, mais ils étaient contrôlés par les commerçants phéniciens. Elie n'était pas un criminel, un prisonnier ou un fugitif, c'était un homme qui avait osé élever la voix contre le dieu Baal. Lorsqu'on le découvrirait, il serait mis à mort et jeté à la mer, car les marins croyaient fermement que Baal et ses dieux étaient maîtres des tempêtes.

Il ne pouvait pas se diriger vers la mer. Ni continuer vers le nord, car là se trouvait le Liban. Il ne pouvait pas non plus aller vers l'orient, où des tribus israélites menaient une guerre depuis deux générations.

*

Il se souvint de la tranquillité qu'il avait ressentie devant le soldat. En fin de compte, qu'était la mort ? Un instant, rien de plus. Même s'il éprouvait de la douleur, elle passerait rapidement, et le Seigneur des Armées le recevrait en son sein.

Il se coucha sur le sol et resta très longtemps à contempler le ciel. Comme le lévite, il tenta de parier, non sur l'existence de Dieu — il n'avait pas de doutes sur ce point —, mais sur la raison de sa propre vie.

Il vit les montagnes, la terre qu'allait dévaster une longue sécheresse — ainsi l'avait annoncé l'ange du Seigneur — mais qui conservait encore la fraîcheur de nombreuses années de pluies généreuses. Il aperçut le ruisseau du Kerith, dont les eaux se tariraient bientôt. Il fit ses adieux au monde avec ferveur et respect, et pria le Seigneur de l'accueillir quand viendrait son heure.

Il se demanda quel était le motif de son existence, et n'obtint pas de réponse.

Il se demanda où il devait se rendre, et comprit qu'il était cerné.

Le lendemain, il ferait demi-tour et se livrerait, bien que la peur de la mort fût revenue.

Il tenta de se réjouir puisqu'il lui restait quelques heures à vivre. En vain. Il venait de découvrir que l'homme a rarement le pouvoir de prendre une décision.

Lorsque Elie se réveilla le lendemain, il regarda de nouveau le Kerith. Demain, ou dans un an, ce ne serait plus qu'un chemin de sable fin et de galets polis. Les habitants continueraient de le nommer Kerith, et peut-être indiqueraient-ils leur route aux voyageurs en disant : « Tel village se trouve au bord de la rivière qui passe près d'ici. » Les voyageurs marcheraient jusque-là, verraient les galets et le sable fin, et se feraient cette réflexion : « Là, sur cette terre, il y avait une rivière. » Mais la seule chose importante concernant une rivière — son torrent d'eau — ne serait plus là pour étancher leur soif.

Comme les ruisseaux et les plantes, les âmes avaient besoin de la pluie, mais d'une autre sorte : l'espoir, la foi, la raison de vivre. Sinon, même si le corps continuait à vivre, l'âme dépérissait ; et les gens pouvaient dire que « là, dans ce corps, il y avait eu un homme ».

Ce n'était pas le moment de songer à tout cela. Encore une fois il se rappela sa conversation avec le lévite, un peu avant qu'ils ne sortent de l'étable : à quoi bon mourir de tant de morts, s'il suffisait d'une seule ? Tout ce qu'il devait faire, c'était attendre les gardes de Jézabel. Ils arriveraient, sans aucun doute, car les itinéraires n'étaient pas nombreux pour fuir de Galaad. Les malfaiteurs se dirigeaient toujours vers le désert — où on les retrouvait morts au bout de quelques jours —, ou vers le Kerith où ils finissaient par être capturés. Bientôt, donc, les gardes seraient là. Et il se réjouirait en les voyant.

*

Il but un peu de l'eau cristalline, se lava le visage, et chercha un endroit ombragé où attendre ses poursuivants. Un homme ne peut lutter contre son destin — il avait déjà tenté de lutter, et il avait perdu.

Bien qu'il fût considéré par les prêtres comme un prophète, Elie avait décidé de travailler dans une charpenterie, mais le Seigneur l'avait reconduit vers son chemin.

Il n'était pas le seul à avoir essayé d'abandonner la vie que Dieu avait écrite pour chacun sur terre. Il avait eu un ami, doté d'une voix remarquable, dont les parents n'avaient pas non plus accepté qu'il fût chanteur — car c'était un métier qui déshonorait la famille. Une de ses amies d'enfance savait danser comme personne, mais sa famille le lui avait interdit — pour la bonne raison que le roi aurait pu la faire appeler et que nul ne savait combien de temps durerait son règne. En outre, l'atmosphère du palais était dépravée, hostile, écartant à tout jamais l'opportunité d'un bon mariage.

« L'homme est né pour trahir son destin. » Dieu ne mettait dans nos cœurs que des tâches impossibles.

« Pourquoi ? »

Peut-être parce que la tradition devait être maintenue.

Mais ce n'était pas une bonne réponse. « Les habitants du Liban sont plus avancés que nous parce qu'ils n'ont pas suivi la tradition des navigateurs. Alors que tout le monde utilisait le même type de bateau, ils ont décidé de construire un instrument différent. Beaucoup ont perdu la vie en mer, mais leurs navires ont été perfectionnés, et maintenant ils dominent le commerce dans le monde. Ils ont payé un prix élevé pour s'adapter, mais cela en valait la peine. »

L'homme trahissait peut-être son destin parce que Dieu s'était éloigné de lui. Après avoir placé dans les cœurs le rêve d'une époque où tout était possible, Il était allé s'occuper d'autres nouveautés. Le monde s'était transformé, la vie était devenue plus difficile, mais le Seigneur n'était jamais revenu pour modifier les rêves des hommes.

Dieu était loin. Pourtant, s'Il envoyait encore les anges parler aux prophètes, c'est qu'il restait quelque chose à faire ici-bas. Alors, quelle pouvait être la réponse ?

« Peut-être nos parents se sont-ils trompés et ont-ils peur que nous commettions les mêmes erreurs. Ou peut-être qu'ils ne se sont jamais trompés et ne sauront pas comment nous aider si nous avons un problème. »

Il sentait qu'il approchait.

Le ruisseau coulait près de lui, quelques corbeaux tournoyaient dans le ciel, les plantes s'obstinaient à pousser sur le terrain sableux et stérile. S'ils avaient écouté les propos de leurs ancêtres, qu'auraient-ils entendu ?

« Ruisseau, cherche un meilleur endroit pour que tes eaux limpides réfléchissent la clarté du soleil, puisque le désert a fini par t'assécher », aurait dit un dieu des eaux, si par hasard il existait. « Corbeaux, la nourriture est plus abondante en forêt qu'au milieu des rochers et du sable », aurait dit un dieu des oiseaux. « Plantes, jetez vos semences loin d'ici, car le monde est plein de terre fertile et humide, et vous pousserez plus belles », aurait dit un dieu des fleurs.

Mais ni le Kerith, ni les plantes, ni les corbeaux — l'un d'eux s'était posé tout près — n'avaient le courage de faire ce que les autres rivières, oiseaux ou fleurs jugeaient impossible.

Elie fixa le corbeau du regard.

« J'apprends, dit-il à l'oiseau. Même si c'est un apprentissage inutile, parce que je suis condamné à mort.

— Tu as découvert comme tout est simple, sembla répondre le corbeau. Il suffit d'avoir du courage. »

Elie rit, car il plaçait des mots dans la bouche d'un oiseau. C'était un jeu amusant — qu'il avait appris avec une femme qui confectionnait du pain — et il décida de continuer. Il poserait les questions et se donnerait à lui-même une réponse, comme s'il était un véritable sage.

Mais le corbeau s'envola. Elie attendait toujours l'arrivée des soldats de Jézabel, parce qu'il suffisait de mourir une fois.

*

Le jour passa, et rien de nouveau ne se produisit. Avaient-ils oublié que le principal ennemi du dieu Baal était encore en vie ? Pourquoi Jézabel ne le poursuivait-elle pas, puisqu'elle savait probablement où il se trouvait ?

« Parce que j'ai vu ses yeux, et c'est une femme

sage, se dit-il. Si je mourais, je deviendrais un martyr du Seigneur. Considéré comme un fugitif, je ne serai qu'un lâche qui ne croyait pas en ce qu'il disait. »

Oui, c'était cela la stratégie de la princesse.

*

Peu avant la tombée de la nuit, un corbeau — était-ce le même ? — vint se poser sur la branche sur laquelle il l'avait vu ce matin-là. Il tenait dans son bec un petit morceau de viande que par inadvertance il laissa tomber.

Pour Elie, ce fut un miracle. Il courut jusque sous l'arbre, saisit le morceau et le mangea. Il ignorait sa provenance et ne cherchait pas non plus à la connaître ; l'important était d'apaiser sa faim.

Malgré le mouvement brusque, le corbeau ne s'éloigna pas.

« Cet oiseau sait que je vais mourir de faim ici, pensa Elie. Il alimente sa proie pour avoir un meilleur festin. »

Jézabel aussi alimentait la foi en Baal par l'histoire de la fuite d'Elie.

Pendant quelque temps, ils restèrent — l'homme et l'oiseau — à se contempler mutuellement. Elie se rappela son jeu du matin.

« J'aimerais converser avec toi, corbeau. Ce matin, je pensais que les âmes avaient besoin de nourriture. Si mon âme n'est pas encore morte de faim, elle a encore quelque chose à dire. »

L'oiseau restait immobile.

« Et si elle a quelque chose à dire, je dois l'écouter. Puisque je n'ai plus personne à qui parler », continua Elie.

Faisant appel à son imagination, Elie se transforma en corbeau.

« Qu'est-ce que Dieu attend de toi ? se demanda-t-il à lui-même, comme s'il était le corbeau.

— Il attend que je sois un prophète.

— C'est ce qu'ont dit les prêtres. Mais ce n'est peut-être pas ce que désire le Seigneur.

— Si, c'est cela qu'Il veut. Car un ange est apparu dans la charpenterie, et il m'a demandé de parler à Achab. Les voix que j'entendais dans l'enfance...

— ... que tout le monde a entendues dans l'enfance, interrompit le corbeau.

— Mais tout le monde n'a pas vu un ange », remarqua Elie.

Cette fois, le corbeau ne répliqua pas. Au bout d'un moment, l'oiseau — ou, mieux, son âme elle-même, qui délirait sous l'effet du soleil et de la solitude du désert — rompit le silence.

« Te souviens-tu de la femme qui faisait du pain ? » se demanda-t-il à lui-même.

Elie se souvenait. Elle était venue lui demander de fabriquer quelques plateaux. Tandis qu'il s'exécutait, il l'avait entendue dire que son travail était une façon d'exprimer la présence de Dieu.

« A la manière dont tu fabriques ces plateaux, je vois que tu éprouves la même sensation, avait-elle ajouté. Tu souris pendant que tu travailles. »

La femme classait les êtres humains en deux groupes : ceux qui étaient heureux et ceux qui se plaignaient de ce qu'ils faisaient. Ces derniers affirmaient que la malédiction que Dieu lança à Adam : *« Le sol sera maudit à cause de toi. C'est dans la peine que tu t'en nourriras tous les jours de ta vie »* était l'unique vérité. Ils n'avaient pas plaisir à travailler et s'ennuyaient les jours de fête, lorsqu'ils étaient obligés de se reposer. Ils se servaient des paroles du Seigneur comme d'une excuse pour leurs vies inutiles, oubliant qu'Il avait aussi dit à Moïse : *« Le Seigneur ton Dieu te bénira abondamment sur la terre qu'Il te donne en héritage, pour la posséder. »*

« Oui, je me souviens de cette femme, répondit Elie au corbeau. Elle avait raison, j'aimais mon travail dans la charpenterie. » Chaque table qu'il montait, chaque chaise qu'il taillait lui permettaient de comprendre et d'aimer la vie, même s'il ne s'en rendait compte que maintenant. « Elle m'a expliqué que, si je parlais aux objets que je fabriquais, je serais surpris de constater que les tables et les chaises me répondraient, parce que j'y mettrais le meilleur de mon âme, et recevrais en échange la sagesse.

— Si tu n'avais pas été charpentier, tu n'aurais pas su non plus mettre ton âme hors de toi-même, faire semblant d'être un corbeau qui parle, et comprendre que tu es meilleur et plus sage que tu ne le penses. C'est dans la charpenterie que tu as découvert que le sacré est partout.

— J'ai toujours aimé faire semblant de parler aux tables et aux chaises que je fabriquais. N'était-ce pas suffisant ? La femme avait raison. Lorsque je conversais ainsi, il me venait souvent des pensées qui ne m'étaient jamais passées par la tête. Mais au moment où je commençais à comprendre que je pouvais servir Dieu de cette manière, l'ange est apparu et... Eh bien ! tu connais la suite de l'histoire.

— L'ange est apparu parce que tu étais prêt, repartit le corbeau.

— J'étais un bon charpentier.

— Cela faisait partie de ton apprentissage. Quand un homme marche vers son destin, il est bien souvent forcé de changer de direction. Parfois, les circonstances extérieures sont les plus fortes, et il est obligé de se montrer lâche et de céder. Tout cela fait partie de l'apprentissage. »

Elie écoutait avec attention ce que disait son âme.

« Mais personne ne peut perdre de vue ce qu'il désire. Même si, à certains moments, on croit que le monde et les autres sont les plus forts. Le secret est le suivant : ne pas renoncer.

— Je n'ai jamais pensé être un prophète, dit Elie.

— Tu l'as pensé. Mais tu as été convaincu que c'était impossible. Ou que c'était dangereux. Ou que c'était impensable. »

Elie se leva.

« Pourquoi me dis-je des choses que je ne veux pas entendre ? » s'écria-t-il.

Effrayé par ce mouvement, l'oiseau s'enfuit.

*

Le corbeau revint le lendemain matin. Plutôt que de reprendre la conversation, Elie l'observa, car l'animal parvenait toujours à se nourrir et lui apportait même quelques restes.

Une mystérieuse amitié se développa entre eux, et Elie commença à apprendre grâce à l'oiseau. Il vit comment il trouvait sa nourriture dans le désert et découvrit qu'il pourrait survivre quelques jours de plus s'il réussissait à en faire autant. Quand le vol du corbeau devenait circulaire, Elie savait qu'il y avait une proie à proximité ; il courait alors jusqu'à l'endroit et tentait de la capturer. Au début, beaucoup des petits animaux parvenaient à lui échapper, mais peu à peu, à force d'entraînement, il acquit une certaine habileté. Il se servait de branches en guise de lances et creusait des pièges qu'il dissimulait sous une fine couche de cailloux et de sable. Lorsque la proie tombait, Elie partageait sa nourriture avec le corbeau et en gardait une partie pour servir d'appât.

Mais la solitude dans laquelle il se trouvait était terriblement oppressante, si bien qu'il décida de converser de nouveau avec l'oiseau.

« Qui es-tu ? demanda le corbeau.

— Je suis un homme qui a découvert la paix, répondit Elie. Je peux vivre dans le désert, subvenir à mes besoins, et contempler l'infinie beauté de la création divine. J'ai découvert que j'avais en moi une âme meilleure que je ne pensais. »

Ils continuèrent à chasser ensemble au clair de lune. Alors, une nuit que son âme était possédée par la tristesse, il décida de se demander de nouveau :

« Qui es-tu ?

— Je ne sais pas. »

*

Un autre clair de lune mourut et renaquit dans le ciel. Elie sentait que son corps était plus fort, et son esprit plus clair. Cette nuit-là, il se tourna vers le corbeau, toujours posé sur la même branche, et répondit à la question qu'il avait lancée quelque temps auparavant :

« Je suis un prophète. J'ai vu un ange pendant que je travaillais, et je ne peux pas douter de ce dont je suis capable, même si tous les hommes du monde m'affirment le contraire. J'ai provoqué un massacre dans mon pays parce que j'ai défié la bien-aimée de mon roi. Je suis dans le désert — comme j'ai été avant dans une charpenterie — parce que mon âme m'a dit qu'un homme devait passer par différentes étapes avant d'accomplir son destin.

— Oui, maintenant tu sais qui tu es », commenta le corbeau.

Cette nuit-là, lorsque Elie rentra de la chasse, il voulut boire un peu d'eau mais le Kerith était asséché. Il était tellement fatigué qu'il décida de dormir.

Dans son rêve, apparut l'ange gardien qu'il ne voyait pas depuis longtemps.

« L'ange du Seigneur a parlé à ton âme, dit celui-ci. Et il a ordonné : *"Va-t'en d'ici, dirige-toi vers l'Orient et cache-toi dans le ravin du Kerith, qui est à l'est du Jourdain. Tu boiras au torrent ; et j'ai ordonné aux corbeaux de te ravitailler là-bas."*

— Mon âme a écouté, dit Elie dans son rêve.

— Alors réveille-toi. L'ange du Seigneur me prie de m'éloigner, et il veut parler avec toi. »

Elie se leva d'un bond, effrayé. Que s'était-il passé ?

Malgré la nuit, l'endroit se remplit de lumière, et l'ange du Seigneur apparut.

« Qu'est-ce qui t'a mené ici ? demanda l'ange.

— C'est toi qui m'as mené ici.

— Non. Jézabel et ses soldats t'ont poussé à fuir. Ne l'oublie jamais, car ta mission est de venger le Seigneur ton Dieu.

— Je suis prophète, puisque tu es devant moi et que j'écoute ta voix, dit Elie. J'ai changé maintes fois de direction, tous les hommes font cela. Mais je suis prêt à aller jusqu'à Samarie et à détruire Jézabel.

— Tu as trouvé ton chemin, mais tu ne peux pas détruire sans apprendre à reconstruire. Je t'ordonne : *"Lève-toi, et va à Sarepta qui appartient à Sidon, tu y habiteras ; j'ai ordonné là-bas à une femme, une veuve, de te ravitailler."* »

Le lendemain matin, Elie chercha le corbeau pour lui faire ses adieux. Pour la première fois depuis qu'il était arrivé au bord du Kerith, l'oiseau n'apparut pas.

Elie voyagea pendant des jours et atteignit enfin la vallée où se trouvait la cité de Sarepta, à laquelle ses habitants donnaient le nom d'Akbar. Alors qu'il était à bout de forces, il aperçut une femme, vêtue de noir, qui ramassait du bois. La végétation de la vallée était rase, de sorte qu'elle devait se contenter de menu bois sec.

« Qui es-tu ? » demanda-t-il.

La femme regarda l'étranger, sans comprendre ses paroles.

« Donne-moi de l'eau, dit Elie. Je suis seul, j'ai faim et soif, et je n'ai plus assez de forces pour menacer personne.

— Tu n'es pas d'ici, dit-elle enfin. A ta façon de parler, tu viens sans doute du royaume d'Israël. Si tu me connaissais mieux, tu saurais que je n'ai rien.

— Tu es veuve, m'a dit le Seigneur. Et j'ai moins que toi. Si tu ne me donnes pas maintenant de quoi manger et boire, je vais mourir. »

La femme eut peur. Comment cet étranger pouvait-il connaître sa vie ?

« Un homme devrait avoir honte de réclamer de la nourriture à une femme, répliqua-t-elle en se ressaisissant.

— Fais ce que je te demande, je t'en prie », insista Elie, sentant que les forces commençaient à lui manquer. « Dès que j'irai mieux, je travaillerai pour toi. »

La femme rit.

« Il y a un instant, tu m'as dit une vérité : je suis veuve, j'ai perdu mon mari sur l'un des navires de mon pays. Je n'ai jamais vu l'océan, mais je sais que, comme le désert, il tue celui qui le brave. »

Et elle poursuivit :

« Maintenant, tu me dis un mensonge. Aussi vrai que Baal vit en haut de la Cinquième Montagne, je n'ai rien à manger. Il y a tout juste une poignée de farine dans une cruche et un peu d'huile dans une jarre. »

Elie sentit que l'horizon vacillait et il comprit qu'il allait bientôt s'évanouir. Rassemblant le peu d'énergie qui lui restait, il implora pour la dernière fois :

« Je ne sais pas si tu crois aux songes, ni si j'y crois moi-même. Pourtant le Seigneur m'a annoncé qu'en arrivant ici, je te rencontrerais. Il a déjà fait des choses qui m'ont fait douter de Sa sagesse, mais jamais de Son existence. Et ainsi, le Dieu d'Israël m'a prié de dire à la femme que je rencontrerais à Sarepta :

> Cruche de farine ne se videra,
> jarre d'huile ne se désemplira
> jusqu'au jour où le Seigneur
> donnera la pluie à la surface du sol. »

Sans expliquer comment un tel miracle pouvait se produire, Elie s'évanouit.

La femme demeura immobile à regarder l'homme tombé à ses pieds. Elle savait que le Dieu d'Israël n'était qu'une superstition. Les dieux phéniciens étaient bien plus puissants et ils avaient fait de son pays une des nations les plus respectées du monde. Mais elle était contente ; elle vivait en général en demandant l'aumône, et aujourd'hui, pour la première fois depuis très longtemps, un homme avait besoin d'elle. Elle se sentit plus forte. En fin de compte, il y avait des gens dans une situation pire que la sienne.

« Si quelqu'un me réclame une faveur, c'est que j'ai encore une certaine valeur sur cette terre, pensa-t-elle. Je ferai ce qu'il demande, simplement pour soulager sa souffrance. Moi aussi j'ai connu la faim, et je sais comme elle détruit l'âme. »

Elle retourna jusque chez elle et revint avec un morceau de pain et une cruche d'eau. Elle s'agenouilla, posa contre elle la tête de l'étranger et mouilla ses lèvres. Au bout de quelques minutes, il recouvra les sens.

Elle lui tendit le pain, et Elie mangea en silence, tout en regardant la vallée, les défilés, les montagnes qui pointaient silencieusement vers le ciel. Il apercevait les murailles rouges de la cité de Sarepta, dominant le passage par la vallée.

« Donne-moi l'hospitalité, je suis poursuivi dans mon pays, dit-il.

— Quel crime as-tu commis ?

— Je suis un prophète du Seigneur. Jézabel a ordonné la mort de tous ceux qui refusaient d'adorer les dieux phéniciens.

— Quel âge as-tu ?

— Vingt-trois ans. »

Elle regarda avec compassion le jeune homme qui se tenait devant elle. Il avait les cheveux longs et sales. Il portait la barbe, une barbe encore clairsemée, comme s'il désirait paraître plus vieux qu'il ne l'était réellement. Comment un malheureux pareil pouvait-il braver la princesse la plus puissante du monde ?

« Si tu es ennemi de Jézabel, tu es aussi mon ennemi. Elle est princesse de Tyr et, en épousant son roi, elle a reçu pour mission de convertir son peuple à la foi authentique. C'est ce qu'affirment ceux qui l'ont connue. »

Elle indiqua l'un des pics qui encadraient la vallée.

« Nos dieux habitent au sommet de la Cinquième Montagne depuis des générations. Ils parviennent à maintenir la paix dans notre pays. Mais Israël vit dans la guerre et la souffrance. Comment peut-on continuer à croire au Dieu unique ? Qu'on donne à Jézabel le temps d'accomplir sa tâche et tu verras la paix régner aussi dans vos cités.

— J'ai entendu la voix du Seigneur, répondit Elie. Quant à vous, vous n'êtes jamais montés au sommet de la Cinquième Montagne pour savoir ce qu'il y a là-haut.

40

— Celui qui gravira ce mont mourra par le feu des cieux. Les dieux n'aiment pas les inconnus. »

Elle se tut. Elle s'était souvenue que, la nuit dernière, elle avait vu en rêve une lumière vive, d'où sortait une voix disant : « Reçois l'étranger qui viendra à ta recherche. »

« Donne-moi l'hospitalité, je n'ai nulle part où dormir, insista Elie.

— Je te l'ai déjà dit, je suis pauvre. J'ai à peine assez pour moi et pour mon fils.

— Le Seigneur t'a priée de me permettre de rester, jamais Il n'abandonne quelqu'un qui aime. Je t'en prie. Je serai ton employé. Je suis charpentier, je sais travailler le cèdre, et j'aurai de quoi faire. Ainsi, le Seigneur se servira de mes mains pour tenir Sa promesse : *"Cruche de farine ne se videra, jarre d'huile ne se désemplira jusqu'au jour où le Seigneur donnera la pluie à la surface du sol."*

— Même si je le voulais, je n'aurais pas de quoi te payer.

— C'est inutile. Le Seigneur y pourvoira. »

Déconcertée par son rêve de la nuit, et bien qu'elle sût que l'étranger était un ennemi de la princesse de Sidon, la femme décida d'obéir.

Les voisins découvrirent bientôt la présence d'Elie. Les gens racontèrent que la veuve avait installé un étranger dans sa demeure, sans respecter la mémoire de son mari — un héros qui avait trouvé la mort alors qu'il cherchait à étendre les routes commerciales de son pays.

Dès qu'elle eut connaissance de ces rumeurs, la veuve expliqua qu'il s'agissait d'un prophète israélite affamé et assoiffé. Et la nouvelle se répandit qu'un prophète israélite, fuyant Jézabel, était caché dans la cité. Une commission alla consulter le grand prêtre.

« Qu'on amène l'étranger devant moi », ordonna-t-il.

Ainsi fut fait. Cet après-midi-là, Elie fut conduit devant l'homme qui, avec le gouverneur et le chef militaire, contrôlait tout ce qui se passait à Akbar.

« Qu'es-tu venu faire ici ? demanda-t-il. Ne vois-tu pas que tu es un ennemi de notre pays ?

— Pendant des années j'ai négocié avec le Liban, et je respecte ton peuple et tes coutumes. Je suis ici parce que je suis persécuté en Israël.

— J'en connais la raison, dit le prêtre. C'est une femme qui t'a fait fuir ?

— Cette femme est la plus belle créature que j'aie rencontrée, quoique je me sois trouvé quelques minutes seulement devant elle. Mais son cœur est de pierre, et derrière ses yeux verts se cache l'ennemi qui entend détruire mon pays. Je n'ai pas fui : j'attends simplement le moment opportun de retourner là-bas. »

Le prêtre rit.

« Alors, prépare-toi à rester à Akbar le reste de ta vie. Nous ne sommes pas en guerre avec ton pays. Tout ce que nous désirons, c'est que la foi authentique se répande — par des moyens pacifiques — à travers le monde entier. Nous ne voulons pas répéter les atrocités que vous avez commises quand vous vous êtes installés en Canaan.

— Assassiner les prophètes est-il un moyen pacifique ?

— Si l'on coupe la tête du monstre, il cesse d'exister. Quelques-uns peuvent mourir, mais les guerres de religion seront évitées pour toujours. Et, d'après ce que m'ont raconté les commerçants, c'est un prophète nommé Elie qui est à l'origine de tout cela et qui ensuite s'est enfui. »

Le prêtre le regarda fixement, avant de poursuivre :

« Un homme qui te ressemblait.

— C'est moi, répondit Elie.

— Parfait. Sois le bienvenu dans la cité d'Akbar. Lorsque nous aurons besoin d'obtenir quelque chose de Jézabel, nous la paierons avec ta tête — la meilleure monnaie d'échange que nous ayons. En attendant, cherche un emploi et apprends à subvenir à tes besoins, ici il n'y a pas de place pour les prophètes. »

Elie se préparait à partir quand le prêtre reprit :

« On dirait qu'une jeune femme de Sidon est plus puissante que ton Dieu unique. Elle a réussi à ériger un autel à Baal, et les anciens prêtres s'agenouillent maintenant devant lui.

— Tout se passera ainsi que le Seigneur l'a écrit, répliqua le prophète. A certains moments, nos vies connaissent des tribulations et nous ne pouvons les éviter. Mais elles ont un motif.

— Lequel ?

— A cette question nous ne pouvons répondre avant, ou pendant, les difficultés. C'est seulement une fois que nous les avons surmontées que nous comprenons pourquoi elles sont survenues. »

*

Sitôt qu'Elie fut parti, le grand prêtre convoqua la commission de citoyens qui était venue le trouver le matin.

« Ne vous en faites pas, dit-il. La tradition nous commande de donner refuge aux étrangers. En outre, ici, il est sous notre contrôle et nous pourrons surveiller ses allées et venues. La meilleure manière de connaître et de détruire un ennemi, c'est de feindre de devenir son ami. Quand arrivera le bon moment, il sera livré à Jézabel, et notre cité recevra de l'or et des récompenses. D'ici là, nous aurons appris comment anéantir ses idées ; pour le moment, nous savons seulement comment détruire son corps. »

Bien qu'Elie fût un adorateur du Dieu unique et un ennemi potentiel de la princesse, le prêtre exigea que le droit d'asile fût respecté. Tous connaissaient la vieille tradition : si une cité refusait d'accueillir un voyageur, les fils de ses habitants connaîtraient semblable malheur. Comme la progéniture de bon nombre des citoyens d'Akbar était dispersée sur la gigantesque flotte marchande du pays, nul n'osa braver la loi de l'hospitalité.

En outre, cela ne coûtait rien d'attendre le jour où la tête du prophète juif serait échangée contre de grandes quantités d'or.

*

Ce soir-là, Elie dîna en compagnie de la veuve et de son fils. Comme le prophète israélite constituait désormais une précieuse monnaie d'échange susceptible d'être négociée plus tard, certains commerçants avaient envoyé suffisamment de nourriture pour permettre à la famille de s'alimenter pendant une semaine.

« On dirait que le Seigneur d'Israël tient sa parole, remarqua la veuve. Depuis que mon mari est mort, jamais ma table n'a été aussi opulente. »

Elie s'intégra peu à peu à la vie de Sarepta. Comme tous ses habitants, il se mit à l'appeler Akbar. Il fit la connaissance du gouverneur, du commandant de la garnison, du grand prêtre, des maîtres artisans qui travaillaient le verre et que l'on admirait dans toute la région. Quand on lui demandait ce qu'il faisait là, il disait la vérité : Jézabel tuait tous les prophètes en Israël.

« Tu es un traître à ton pays, et un ennemi de la Phénicie, rétorquait-on. Mais nous sommes une nation de commerçants, et nous savons que, plus un homme est dangereux, plus élevé est le prix de sa tête. »

Ainsi passèrent quelques mois.

A l'entrée de la vallée, des patrouilles assyriennes avaient installé leur campement et semblaient bien disposées à y rester. C'était un petit groupe de soldats qui ne représentait aucune menace. Néanmoins, le commandant invita le gouverneur à prendre des mesures.

« Ils ne nous ont rien fait, remarqua le gouverneur. Ils sont sans doute en mission commerciale, cherchant un meilleur itinéraire pour acheminer leurs produits. S'ils décident d'utiliser nos routes, ils paieront des impôts, et nous serons encore plus riches. Pourquoi les provoquer ? »

Pour aggraver la situation, le fils de la veuve tomba malade, sans aucune raison apparente. Les voisins attribuèrent l'événement à la présence de l'étranger, et la femme pria Elie de s'en aller. Mais il n'en fit rien — le Seigneur ne l'avait pas encore appelé. Le bruit commença à se répandre que cet étranger avait apporté avec lui la colère des dieux de la Cinquième Montagne.

On pouvait contrôler l'armée et rassurer la population sur l'arrivée des patrouilles assyriennes. Mais lorsque le fils de la veuve tomba malade, le gouverneur eut de plus en plus de mal à apaiser les gens, que la présence d'Elie inquiétait.

Une commission d'habitants vint le trouver pour lui faire une proposition :

« Nous pouvons construire une maison pour l'Israélite de l'autre côté des murailles. Ainsi, nous ne violons pas la loi de l'hospitalité, mais nous nous protégeons contre la colère divine. Les dieux sont mécontents de la présence de cet homme.

— Laissez-le où il est, répondit le gouverneur. Je préfère ne pas créer de problèmes politiques avec Israël.

— Comment ! s'exclamèrent les habitants. Jézabel

pourchasse tous les prophètes qui adorent le Dieu unique, elle veut leur mort.

— Notre princesse est une femme courageuse, et fidèle aux dieux de la Cinquième Montagne. Mais, malgré tout son pouvoir actuel, elle n'est pas israélite. Elle peut tomber en disgrâce demain, et il nous faudra affronter la colère de nos voisins. Si nous montrons que nous traitons bien un de leurs prophètes, ils seront complaisants à notre égard. »

Les habitants partirent contrariés, car le grand prêtre avait dit qu'Élie serait un jour échangé contre de l'or et des récompenses. D'ici là, même si le gouverneur faisait erreur, ils ne pouvaient rien faire : selon la tradition, on devait respecter la famille gouvernante.

Au loin, à l'entrée de la vallée, les tentes des guerriers assyriens commencèrent à se multiplier.

Le commandant s'en inquiétait, mais il n'avait le soutien ni du prêtre, ni du gouverneur. Il obligeait ses guerriers à s'entraîner en permanence, tout en sachant qu'aucun d'eux — pas plus que leurs aïeux — n'avait l'expérience du combat. Les guerres appartenaient au passé d'Akbar, et toutes les stratégies qu'il avait apprises étaient rendues obsolètes par les techniques et les armes nouvelles qu'utilisaient les pays étrangers.

« Akbar a toujours négocié sa paix, affirmait le gouverneur. Ce n'est pas cette fois que nous serons envahis. Laisse les pays étrangers se battre entre eux : nous, nous avons une arme beaucoup plus puissante, l'argent. Lorsqu'ils auront fini de se détruire mutuellement, nous entrerons dans leurs cités — et nous vendrons nos produits. »

Le gouverneur réussit à tranquilliser la population

au sujet des Assyriens. Mais le bruit courait toujours que l'Israélite avait attiré la malédiction des dieux sur Akbar. Elie représentait un problème qui s'aggravait chaque jour.

*

Un après-midi, l'état du petit garçon empira. Il ne parvenait déjà plus à se tenir debout, ni à reconnaître les gens qui venaient lui rendre visite. Avant que le soleil ne descendît sur l'horizon, Elie et la femme s'agenouillèrent près du lit de l'enfant.

« Seigneur tout-puissant, Toi qui as dévié les flèches du soldat et m'as mené jusqu'ici, fais que cet enfant soit sauf. Il est innocent de mes péchés et des péchés de ses parents. Sauve-le, Seigneur. »

L'enfant ne bougeait presque plus ; ses lèvres étaient blanches, ses yeux perdaient rapidement leur éclat.

« Adresse une prière à ton Dieu unique, demanda la femme. Parce que seule une mère est capable de reconnaître le moment où l'âme de son fils est en train de s'en aller. »

Elie eut envie de lui prendre la main, de lui dire qu'elle n'était pas seule, et que le Dieu tout-puissant devrait exaucer son souhait. Il était prophète, il avait accepté cette mission sur les rives du Kerith, et désormais les anges se tenaient à ses côtés.

« Je n'ai plus de larmes, continua-t-elle. S'Il n'a pas de compassion, s'Il a besoin d'une vie, alors prie-Le de m'emporter et de laisser mon fils se promener dans la vallée et par les rues d'Akbar. »

Elie fit son possible pour se concentrer sur son oraison ; mais la souffrance de cette mère était si intense qu'elle semblait emplir la chambre et pénétrer partout, dans les murs et les portes.

Il toucha le corps du gamin. Sa température n'était plus aussi élevée que les jours précédents, et c'était mauvais signe.

*

Le prêtre était passé à la maison le matin et, comme il l'avait fait durant deux semaines, il avait appliqué des cataplasmes d'herbes sur le visage et la poitrine de l'enfant. Ces jours derniers, les femmes d'Akbar avait apporté des remèdes dont les recettes s'étaient transmises de génération en génération au fil des siècles et dont le pouvoir de guérison avait été démontré en maintes occasions. Tous les après-midi, elles se réunissaient au pied de la Cinquième Montagne et faisaient des sacrifices pour que l'âme du petit ne quittât pas son corps.

Emu par tous ces événements, un marchand égyptien de passage dans la cité remit sans se faire payer une poudre rouge, très onéreuse, qui devait être mélangée à la nourriture de l'enfant. Selon la légende, le secret de fabrication de cette poudre avait été confié aux médecins égyptiens par les dieux eux-mêmes.

Elie avait prié sans arrêt tout ce temps.

Mais rien, absolument rien, aucun progrès.

*

« Je sais pourquoi ils t'ont permis de rester ici », dit la femme, d'une voix de plus en plus éteinte parce qu'elle avait passé plusieurs jours sans dormir. « Je sais que ta tête est mise à prix et qu'un jour tu seras envoyé en Israël, où on t'échangera contre de l'or. Si tu sauves mon fils, je jure par Baal et par les dieux de la Cinquième Montagne que tu ne seras jamais capturé. Je connais des chemins que cette génération a oubliés, et je t'apprendrai comment t'enfuir d'Akbar sans que l'on te voie. »

Elie resta silencieux.

« Adresse une prière à ton Dieu unique, supplia de nouveau la femme. S'Il sauve mon fils, je jure que je renierai Baal et que je croirai en Lui. Explique à ton Seigneur que je t'ai donné refuge quand tu en as eu besoin, que j'ai fait exactement ce qu'Il avait ordonné. »

Elie pria encore, et il implora de toutes ses forces. A ce moment précis, l'enfant bougea.

« Je veux sortir d'ici », dit l'enfant d'une voix faible.

Les yeux de la mère brillaient de contentement, et ses larmes coulaient.

« Viens, mon fils. Allons où tu veux, fais ce que tu désires. »

Elie tenta de prendre l'enfant dans ses bras, mais le petit écarta sa main.

« Je veux sortir seul. »

Il se leva lentement et se dirigea vers la salle. Au bout de quelques pas, il tomba sur le sol, comme foudroyé.

Elie et la veuve s'approchèrent. Le gamin était mort.

Il y eut un instant pendant lequel ni l'un ni l'autre ne parlèrent. Tout à coup, la femme se mit à hurler.

« Maudits soient les dieux, maudits soient ceux qui ont emporté l'âme de mon fils ! Maudit soit l'homme qui a porté le malheur sur ma maison ! Mon fils unique ! criait-elle. J'ai respecté la volonté des cieux, j'ai été généreuse avec un étranger, et finalement mon fils est mort ! »

Les voisins écoutèrent les lamentations de la veuve et virent son fils étendu sur le sol. Elle continuait à crier, donnant des coups de poing au prophète israélite qui se tenait debout à côté d'elle — il semblait avoir perdu toute capacité de réaction et ne faisait rien pour se défendre. Pendant que les femmes essayaient de la calmer, les hommes saisirent Elie par le bras et l'emmenèrent devant le gouverneur.

« Cet homme a rétribué la générosité par la haine. Il a jeté un sortilège sur la maison de la veuve dont le fils est mort. Nous donnons refuge à un individu maudit par les dieux. »

L'Israélite pleurait : « Seigneur, mon Dieu, même à cette veuve qui a été généreuse avec moi Tu veux du mal ? songeait-il. Si Tu as fait mourir son fils, c'est parce que je n'accomplis pas la mission qui m'a été confiée, et je mérite la mort. »

*

Dans la soirée, le conseil de la cité d'Akbar fut réuni, sous la présidence du prêtre et du gouverneur. Elie fut traduit en jugement.

« Tu as décidé de rétribuer l'amour par la haine. Pour cela, je te condamne à mort, décréta le gouverneur.

— Même si ta tête vaut un sac d'or, nous ne pouvons pas réveiller la colère des dieux de la Cinquième Montagne. Sinon, après cela, plus personne en ce monde ne sera capable de rendre la paix à cette cité », ajouta le prêtre.

Elie baissa la tête. Il méritait toute la souffrance qu'il pourrait supporter, parce que le Seigneur l'avait abandonné.

« Tu partiras gravir la Cinquième Montagne, ordonna le prêtre. Tu demanderas pardon aux dieux offensés. Ils feront descendre le feu des cieux pour te tuer. S'ils s'en abstiennent, c'est qu'ils désirent que la justice soit accomplie par nos mains ; nous attendrons ton retour, et demain tu seras exécuté, selon le rituel. »

Elie connaissait bien les exécutions sacrées : on arrachait le cœur de la victime et on lui coupait la tête. Selon la coutume, un homme qui n'avait plus de cœur ne pouvait entrer au Paradis.

« Pourquoi m'as-Tu choisi pour cela, Seigneur ? » s'écria-t-il à voix haute, sachant que les hommes qui l'entouraient ne comprendraient pas le choix que le Seigneur avait fait pour lui. « Ne vois-tu pas que je suis incapable d'accomplir ce que tu exiges ? »

Il n'entendit pas de réponse.

Les hommes et les femmes d'Akbar suivirent en procession le groupe de gardes qui emmenait l'Israélite jusqu'au pied de la Cinquième Montagne. Ils criaient des insultes et lui jetaient des pierres. Les soldats parvinrent à grand-peine à contenir la fureur de la foule. Au bout d'une demi-heure de marche, ils atteignirent la montagne sacrée.

Le groupe s'arrêta devant les autels de pierre sur lesquels le peuple avait coutume de déposer les offrandes, de consommer les sacrifices, de prononcer vœux et prières. Tous connaissaient la légende des géants qui vivaient là et se souvenaient des individus qui, bravant l'interdit, avaient été frappés par le feu du ciel. Les voyageurs qui empruntaient de nuit le chemin de la vallée assuraient avoir entendu les rires des dieux et des déesses. Bien que l'on n'eût aucune certitude de tout cela, personne ne se risquait à défier les dieux.

« Allons-y, dit un soldat, en poussant Elie de la pointe de sa lance. Celui qui a tué un enfant mérite le pire des châtiments. »

*

Elie foula le sol interdit et commença à gravir la pente. Quand il eut marché assez longtemps pour ne plus percevoir les cris des habitants d'Akbar, il s'assit sur un rocher et pleura : depuis cet après-midi, dans la charpenterie, où il avait vu des lumières scintiller dans l'obscurité, il n'avait réussi qu'à porter malheur aux autres. Le Seigneur avait perdu ses porte-parole en Israël et le culte des dieux phéniciens s'était renforcé. La première nuit qu'il avait passée près du ruisseau du Kerith, Elie avait cru que Dieu l'avait choisi pour qu'il devînt un martyr, comme cela s'était produit pour tant d'autres.

Bien au contraire, le Seigneur avait envoyé un corbeau — un oiseau de mauvais augure —, qui l'avait nourri jusqu'à ce que le Kerith fût asséché. Pourquoi un corbeau, et pas une colombe, ou un ange ? Tout cela n'avait-il été que le délire d'un homme désireux de cacher sa peur, ou dont la tête était restée trop longtemps exposée au soleil ? Elie n'était maintenant plus sûr de rien : peut-être le Mal avait-il trouvé son instrument et était-il, lui, cet instrument. Pourquoi, au lieu de s'en retourner et d'en finir avec la princesse qui causait tellement de tort à son peuple, Dieu lui avait-il ordonné de se rendre à Akbar ?

Il s'était senti lâche mais il avait obéi. Il avait lutté pour s'adapter à ce peuple inconnu, gentil, mais dont la culture lui était complètement étrangère. Au moment où il croyait accomplir son destin, le fils de la veuve était mort.

« Pourquoi moi ? » se demandait-il.

*

Il se leva, se remit en marche et pénétra dans le brouillard qui enveloppait le sommet de la montagne. Il pouvait profiter de l'absence de visibilité pour échapper à ses poursuivants, mais à quoi bon ? Il était fatigué de fuir, il savait que jamais il ne réussirait à trouver sa place dans ce monde. Même s'il parvenait à se sauver maintenant, la malédiction l'accompagnerait dans une autre cité, et de nouvelles tragédies se produiraient. Il emporterait avec lui, où qu'il allât, l'ombre de ces morts. Il valait mieux qu'on lui arrache le cœur de la poitrine et qu'on lui coupe la tête.

Il s'assit de nouveau, cette fois au beau milieu du brouillard. Il était décidé à attendre un peu, de façon à laisser croire aux hommes en bas qu'il était monté jusqu'au sommet du mont. Ensuite il retournerait à Akbar et se laisserait capturer.

« Le feu du ciel. » Beaucoup en étaient morts, bien qu'Elie doutât qu'il fût envoyé par le Seigneur. Les nuits sans lune, son éclat traversait le firmament, apparaissant puis disparaissant brusquement. Peut-être brûlait-il. Peut-être tuait-il instantanément, sans souffrance.

*

La nuit tomba et le brouillard se dissipa. Il aperçut la vallée, en bas, les lumières d'Akbar et les feux du campement assyrien. Il écouta l'aboiement des chiens et le chant de guerre des guerriers.

« Je suis prêt, se dit-il. J'ai accepté d'être un prophète, et j'ai fait de mon mieux. Mais j'ai échoué, et maintenant Dieu a besoin de quelqu'un d'autre. »

A ce moment, une lumière descendit jusqu'à lui.

« Le feu du ciel ! »

La lumière, cependant, ne le toucha pas et demeura devant lui. Une voix dit :

« Je suis un ange du Seigneur. »

Elie s'agenouilla, le visage contre terre.

« Je t'ai déjà vu plusieurs fois, et j'ai obéi à l'ange du Seigneur qui me fait semer le malheur partout où je passe », répliqua Elie, toujours prosterné.

Mais l'ange reprit :

« Lorsque tu regagneras la cité, prie trois fois pour que l'enfant revienne à la vie. Le Seigneur t'entendra la troisième fois.

— Pour quoi ferais-je cela ?

— Pour la grandeur de Dieu.

— Quoi qu'il advienne, j'ai douté de moi-même. Je ne suis plus digne de ma tâche, rétorqua Elie.

— Tout homme a le droit de douter de sa tâche et d'y faillir de temps en temps. La seule chose qu'il ne puisse faire, c'est l'oublier. Celui qui ne doute pas de soi est indigne — car il a une confiance aveugle dans sa valeur et pèche par orgueil. Béni soit celui qui traverse des moments d'indécision.

— Il y a un instant, tu as pu voir que je n'étais même plus sûr que tu sois un émissaire de Dieu.

— Va, et fais ce que je dis. »

*

Un long moment s'écoula, puis Elie redescendit de la montagne. Les gardes l'attendaient près des autels de sacrifice, mais la foule s'en était déjà retournée à Akbar.

« Je suis prêt à mourir, déclara-t-il. J'ai imploré le pardon des dieux de la Cinquième Montagne, et ils exigent, avant que mon âme ne quitte mon corps, que je passe chez la veuve qui m'a accueilli et que je lui demande d'avoir pitié de mon âme. »

Les soldats le ramenèrent devant le prêtre. Là, ils transmirent sa requête.

« Je te l'accorde, dit le prêtre au prisonnier. Puisque tu as sollicité le pardon des dieux, tu dois aussi implorer celui de la veuve. Pour que tu ne t'enfuies pas, quatre soldats en armes t'accompagneront. Mais ne crois pas que tu réussiras à la convaincre de réclamer la clémence pour ta vie. Au lever du jour, nous t'exécuterons au centre de la place. »

Le prêtre voulut l'interroger sur ce qu'il avait vu là-haut. Mais, en présence des soldats, la réponse risquait de le mettre dans l'embarras. Il décida donc de ne rien dire. Il songeait toutefois que c'était une bonne idée qu'Elie demandât pardon publiquement ; plus personne ne mettrait en doute le pouvoir des dieux de la Cinquième Montagne.

Elie et les soldats s'engagèrent dans la ruelle misérable où il avait habité pendant quelques mois. La porte et les fenêtres de la maison de la veuve étaient grandes ouvertes, afin que — selon la coutume — l'âme de son fils pût s'en aller rejoindre le séjour des dieux. Le corps était placé au centre de la petite salle, veillé par tous les voisins.

Quand ils virent apparaître l'Israélite, hommes et femmes furent horrifiés.

« Faites-le sortir d'ici ! crièrent-ils aux gardes. Le mal qu'il a déjà causé ne suffit-il pas ? Cet homme est tellement mauvais que les dieux de la Cinquième Montagne n'ont pas voulu souiller leurs mains de son sang !

— Laissez-nous la tâche de le tuer ! cria un autre. Nous allons le faire sur-le-champ, sans attendre l'exécution rituelle ! »

Affrontant les bourrades et les gifles, Elie se libéra des mains qui le retenaient, et il courut jusqu'à la veuve qui pleurait dans un coin.

« Je peux faire revenir ton fils d'entre les morts. Laisse-moi le toucher. Juste un instant. »

La veuve ne releva même pas la tête.

« Je t'en prie, insista-t-il. Même si c'est la dernière chose que tu fais pour moi dans cette vie, donne-moi une chance de te récompenser pour ta générosité. »

Des hommes s'emparèrent de lui, voulant l'éloigner. Mais Elie se débattait et luttait de toutes ses forces, implorant qu'on le laissât toucher l'enfant mort.

Malgré sa vigueur, on parvint à le repousser sur le seuil. « Ange du Seigneur, où es-tu ? » s'écria-t-il à l'adresse des cieux.

Tous s'arrêtèrent. La veuve s'était levée et elle se dirigeait vers lui. Elle le prit par la main, le conduisit jusqu'à la dépouille de son fils et retira le drap qui la recouvrait.

« Voici le sang de mon sang, dit-elle. Qu'il descende sur la tête de tes parents si tu ne réussis pas ce que tu désires. »

Il s'approcha pour le toucher.

« Un instant, dit la veuve. Prie ton Dieu que ma malédiction s'accomplisse. »

Le cœur d'Elie battait la chamade. Mais il croyait aux paroles de l'ange.

« Que le sang de cet enfant descende sur mes parents, sur mes frères et sur les fils et les filles de mes frères si j'échoue. »

Alors, malgré tous ses doutes, sa culpabilité et ses craintes,

« *il le prit des bras de la femme, et le porta dans la chambre haute où il logeait. Puis il invoqua les cieux en disant :*

"Veux-tu du mal, Seigneur, même à cette veuve qui m'a donné l'hospitalité, au point que tu fasses mourir son fils ?"

Il s'étendit trois fois sur l'enfant et invoqua le Seigneur en disant : "Seigneur mon Dieu, que le souffle de cet enfant revienne en lui !" »

Pendant quelques instants, rien ne se passa. Elie se vit de nouveau à Galaad, devant le soldat, la flèche pointée sur son cœur. Il savait que très souvent le destin d'un homme n'a rien à voir avec ce qu'il croit ou redoute. Il se sentait tranquille et confiant comme cet après-midi-là, car il savait que, quelle que fût l'issue, il y avait une raison à tout cela. Au sommet de la Cinquième Montagne, l'ange avait appelé cette raison « la grandeur de Dieu ». Il espérait comprendre un jour pourquoi le Créateur avait besoin de Ses créatures pour montrer cette gloire.

C'est alors que l'enfant ouvrit les yeux.

« Où est ma mère ? demanda-t-il.

— Là en bas, elle t'attend, répondit Elie en souriant.

— J'ai fait un rêve étrange. Je voyageais dans un tunnel noir, à une vitesse bien plus grande que le cheval de course le plus rapide d'Akbar. J'ai vu un homme, dont je sais qu'il était mon père, bien que je ne l'aie jamais connu. Alors je suis arrivé dans un endroit magnifique, où j'aurais beaucoup aimé rester. Mais un autre homme — je ne le connais pas, mais il m'a paru très bon et très brave — m'a demandé doucement de revenir. J'aurais voulu aller plus loin, mais tu m'as réveillé. »

L'enfant semblait triste. Ce lieu dans lequel il était presque entré devait être fort beau.

« Ne me laisse pas seul, car tu m'as fait revenir d'un endroit où je savais que j'étais protégé.

— Descendons, dit Elie. Ta mère veut te voir. »

L'enfant essaya de se lever, mais il était trop faible pour marcher. Elie le prit contre lui, et ils descendirent.

*

En bas, dans la salle, les gens semblaient saisis d'une profonde terreur.

« Pourquoi y a-t-il tant de monde ici ? » demanda l'enfant.

Avant qu'Elie ait pu répondre, la veuve prit son fils dans ses bras et l'embrassa en pleurant.

« Qu'est-ce qu'ils t'ont fait, maman ? Pourquoi es-tu triste ?

— Je ne suis pas triste, mon fils, répondit-elle en séchant ses larmes. Je n'ai jamais été aussi heureuse de ma vie. »

La veuve se jeta à genoux et se mit à crier :

« Je sais maintenant que tu es un homme de Dieu ! La vérité du Seigneur sort de tes paroles ! »

Elie la serra dans ses bras et lui demanda de se relever.

« Libérez cet homme ! dit-elle aux soldats. Il a combattu le mal qui s'était abattu sur ma maison ! »

Les gens réunis là ne pouvaient en croire leurs yeux. Une jeune fille de vingt ans, qui était peintre, s'agenouilla près de la veuve. Peu à peu, tous l'imitèrent — même les soldats qui étaient chargés de conduire Elie en captivité.

« Levez-vous, pria-t-il. Et adorez le Seigneur. Je ne suis qu'un de Ses serviteurs, peut-être le plus mal préparé. »

Mais tous restaient à genoux, tête baissée.

Il entendit quelqu'un qui disait : « Tu as conversé avec les dieux de la Cinquième Montagne. Et maintenant tu peux faire des miracles.

— Il n'y a pas de dieux là-bas, répliqua-t-il. J'ai vu un ange du Seigneur, qui m'a ordonné de faire cela.

— Tu as rencontré Baal et ses frères », renchérit un autre.

Elie se fraya un chemin parmi les gens à genoux et sortit dans la rue. Son cœur cognait toujours dans sa poitrine, comme s'il n'avait pas correctement accompli la tâche que l'ange lui avait assignée. « A quoi bon ressusciter un mort, si personne ne comprend d'où vient tant de pouvoir ? » L'ange lui avait demandé de crier trois fois le nom du Seigneur mais il ne lui avait rien dit sur la façon d'expliquer le miracle à la foule amassée en bas. « Serait-ce que, comme les anciens prophètes, je me suis contenté de faire preuve de vanité ? » se demandait-il.

Il entendit la voix de son ange gardien, avec lequel il conversait depuis son enfance :

« Tu as rencontré aujourd'hui un ange du Seigneur.

— Oui, répondit Elie. Mais les anges du Seigneur ne conversent pas avec les hommes. Ils ne font que transmettre les ordres de Dieu.

— Sers-toi de ton pouvoir », commanda l'ange gardien.

Elie ne comprit pas ce qu'il entendait par là. « Je n'ai pas de pouvoir qui ne vienne du Seigneur.

— Personne n'en a. Tout le monde possède le pouvoir du Seigneur, mais personne ne s'en sert. »

Et l'ange ajouta :

« Désormais, et jusqu'à ce que tu retournes dans le pays que tu as quitté, aucun autre miracle ne te sera accordé.

— Et quand y retournerai-je ?

— Le Seigneur a besoin de toi pour reconstruire Israël. Tu fouleras de nouveau son sol lorsque tu auras appris à reconstruire. »

Et il n'en dit pas plus.

Seconde partie

Le grand prêtre adressa ses prières au soleil qui se levait et demanda au dieu de la tempête, ainsi qu'à la déesse des animaux, d'avoir pitié des fous. On lui avait raconté, ce matin-là, qu'Elie avait ramené le fils de la veuve du royaume des morts.

La cité en était effrayée et excitée tout à la fois. Ils croyaient tous que l'Israélite avait reçu son pouvoir des dieux sur la Cinquième Montagne, si bien que désormais il était beaucoup plus difficile d'en finir avec lui. « Mais l'heure viendra », se dit le prêtre.

Les dieux lui donneraient l'occasion de tuer cet homme. Pourtant, la colère divine avait un autre motif, et la présence des Assyriens à l'entrée de la vallée était un signe. Pourquoi des siècles de paix prendraient-ils fin ainsi ? Il connaissait la réponse à cette question : à cause de l'invention de Byblos. Son pays avait développé une forme d'écriture accessible à tous — même à ceux qui n'étaient pas préparés à l'utiliser. N'importe qui pouvait l'apprendre en peu de temps, et ce serait la fin de la civilisation.

Le prêtre savait que, de toutes les armes de destruction inventées par l'homme, la plus terrible — et la plus puissante — était la parole. Poignards et lances laissaient des traces de sang ; les flèches se voyaient de loin ; on finissait par détecter les poisons et par les éviter. Mais la parole parvenait à détruire sans laisser de traces. Si les rituels sacrés pouvaient être diffusés, bien des gens s'en serviraient pour tenter de transformer l'univers, et les dieux en seraient perturbés. Jusque-là, seule la caste sacerdotale détenait la mémoire des ancêtres — que l'on se transmettait oralement, sous le serment que les informations seraient maintenues secrètes. Ou alors, il fallait des années d'étude pour arriver à déchiffrer les caractères que les Egyptiens avaient répandus de par le monde ; ainsi, seuls ceux qui étaient très préparés, scribes et prêtres, étaient en mesure d'échanger des informations.

D'autres cultures avaient leurs méthodes pour enregistrer l'Histoire, mais elles étaient tellement compliquées que nul ne s'était préoccupé de les apprendre hors des régions où elles étaient en usage. L'invention de Byblos, elle, risquait d'avoir des effets considérables : n'importe quel pays pouvait l'utiliser, quelle que soit sa langue. Même les Grecs, qui en général rejetaient tout ce qui n'était pas originaire de leurs cités, avaient déjà adopté l'écriture de Byblos et la pratiquaient couramment dans leurs transactions commerciales. Comme ils étaient spécialistes dans l'art de s'approprier tout ce qui avait un caractère novateur, ils l'avaient baptisée du nom grec d'*alphabet*.

Les secrets gardés pendant des siècles de civilisation couraient le risque d'être exposés au grand jour. En comparaison, le sacrilège d'Elie — qui avait ramené un être de l'autre rive du fleuve de la Mort, comme les Egyptiens avaient coutume de le faire — était insignifiant.

« Nous sommes punis parce que nous sommes incapables de protéger soigneusement ce qui est sacré, pensa-t-il. Les Assyriens sont à nos portes, ils traverseront la vallée et ils détruiront la civilisation de nos ancêtres. »

Et ils mettraient fin à l'écriture. Le prêtre savait que la présence de l'ennemi n'était pas fortuite. C'était le prix à payer. Les dieux avaient organisé les choses afin que personne ne devinât qu'ils étaient les véritables responsables ; ils avaient placé au pouvoir un gouverneur qui s'inquiétait davantage des affaires que de l'armée, excité la convoitise des Assyriens, fait en sorte que la pluie se raréfiât, et envoyé un infidèle pour diviser la cité. Bientôt, le combat final s'engagerait. Akbar continuerait d'exister, mais la menace que représentaient les caractères de Byblos serait à tout jamais rayée de la surface de la terre.

Le prêtre nettoya avec soin la pierre qui signalait l'endroit où, des générations plus tôt, un pèlerin étranger avait trouvé le lieu indiqué par les cieux et fondé la cité. « Comme elle est belle ! » pensa-t-il. Les pierres étaient une image des dieux — dures, résistantes, survivant à toutes les situations, et n'ayant nul besoin d'expliquer la raison de leur présence. La tradition orale rapportait que le centre du monde était marqué d'une pierre et, dans son enfance, il avait parfois pensé à en chercher l'emplacement. Il avait nourri ce projet jusqu'à cette année. Mais quand il avait constaté la présence des Assyriens au fond de la vallée, il avait compris que jamais il ne réaliserait son rêve.

« Cela n'a pas d'importance. Le sort a voulu que ma génération fût offerte en sacrifice pour avoir offensé les dieux. Il y a des choses inévitables dans l'histoire du monde, il nous faut les accepter. »

Il se promit d'obéir aux dieux : il ne chercherait pas à empêcher la guerre.

« Peut-être sommes-nous arrivés à la fin des temps. Il n'y a pas moyen de contourner les crises qui sont de plus en plus nombreuses. »

Le prêtre prit son bâton et sortit du petit temple ; il avait rendez-vous avec le commandant de la garnison d'Akbar.

Il avait presque atteint le rempart sud quand Elie l'aborda.

« Le Seigneur a fait revenir un enfant d'entre les morts, dit l'Israélite. La cité croit en mon pouvoir.

— L'enfant n'était sans doute pas mort, répliqua le grand prêtre. Cela s'est déjà produit d'autres fois ; le cœur s'arrête, et bientôt se remet à battre. Aujourd'hui, toute la cité en parle. Demain, les gens se souviendront que les dieux sont proches et qu'ils peuvent écouter leurs paroles. Alors, leurs bouches redeviendront muettes. Je dois y aller, parce que les Assyriens se préparent au combat.

— Ecoute ce que j'ai à te dire : après le miracle de la nuit dernière, je suis allé dormir à l'extérieur des murailles, parce que j'avais besoin d'un peu de tranquillité. Alors l'ange que j'avais vu en haut de la Cinquième Montagne m'est apparu de nouveau. Et il m'a dit : "Akbar sera détruite par la guerre."

— Les cités ne peuvent pas être détruites. Elles seront reconstruites soixante-dix-sept fois, parce que les dieux savent où ils les ont placées, et ils ont besoin qu'elles soient là. »

Le gouverneur s'approcha, accompagné d'un groupe de courtisans :

« Qu'est-ce que tu dis ? demanda-t-il.

— Recherchez la paix, reprit Elie.

— Si tu as peur, retourne d'où tu viens, rétorqua sèchement le prêtre.

— Jézabel et son roi attendent les prophètes fugitifs pour les mettre à mort, dit le gouverneur. Mais j'aimerais que tu m'expliques comment tu as pu gravir la Cinquième Montagne sans être détruit par le feu du ciel ? »

Le prêtre devait absolument interrompre cette conversation : le gouverneur avait l'intention de négocier avec les Assyriens et peut-être chercherait-il à se servir d'Elie pour parvenir à ses fins.

« Ne l'écoute pas, dit le prêtre au gouverneur. Hier, quand on l'a amené devant moi pour qu'il soit jugé, je l'ai vu pleurer de peur.

— Je pleurais pour le mal que je pensais avoir causé. Car je n'ai peur que du Seigneur et de moi-même. Je n'ai pas fui Israël et je suis prêt à y retourner dès que le Seigneur le permettra. Je détruirai sa belle princesse et la foi d'Israël survivra à cette nouvelle menace.

— Il faut avoir le cœur très dur pour résister aux charmes de Jézabel, ironisa le gouverneur. Mais en ce cas nous enverrions une autre femme encore plus belle, comme nous l'avons déjà fait avant Jézabel. »

Le prêtre disait vrai. Deux cents ans auparavant, une princesse de Sidon avait séduit le plus sage de tous les gouvernants d'Israël, le roi Salomon. Elle lui avait demandé de construire un autel en hommage à la déesse Astarté, et Salomon avait obéi. A cause de ce sacrilège, le Seigneur avait levé les armées voisines contre son pays et Salomon avait été maudit par Dieu.

« La même chose arrivera à Achab, le mari de Jézabel », songea Elie. Le Seigneur lui ferait accomplir sa tâche quand l'heure serait venue. Mais à quoi bon tenter de convaincre ces hommes ? Ils étaient comme ceux qu'il avait vus la nuit précédente, agenouillés sur le sol dans la maison de la veuve, priant les dieux de la Cinquième Montagne. Jamais la tradition ne leur permettrait de penser autrement.

« Il est regrettable que nous devions respecter la loi de l'hospitalité », remarqua le gouverneur qui, apparemment, avait déjà oublié les commentaires d'Elie sur la paix. « Sinon, nous aiderions Jézabel dans sa tâche de destruction des prophètes.

— Ce n'est pas pour cela que vous épargnez ma vie. Vous savez que je représente une précieuse monnaie d'échange, et vous voulez donner à Jézabel le plaisir de me tuer de ses propres mains. Mais — depuis hier — le peuple m'a attribué des pouvoirs miraculeux. Les gens pensent que j'ai rencontré les dieux au sommet de la Cinquième Montagne ; quant à vous, cela ne vous dérangerait pas d'offenser les dieux, mais vous ne voulez pas irriter les habitants de la cité. »

Le gouverneur et le prêtre laissèrent Elie monologuer et se dirigèrent vers les murailles. A ce moment précis, le prêtre décida qu'il tuerait le prophète israélite à la première occasion ; celui qui jusque-là ne représentait qu'une monnaie d'échange était devenu une menace.

*

En les voyant s'éloigner, Elie se désespéra. Que pouvait-il faire pour aider le Seigneur ? Alors il se mit à crier au milieu de la place :

« Peuple d'Akbar ! Hier soir, j'ai gravi la Cinquième

Montagne et j'ai conversé avec les dieux qui habitent là-haut. A mon retour, j'ai pu ramener un enfant du royaume des morts ! »

Les gens se groupèrent autour de lui. L'histoire était déjà connue dans toute la cité. Le gouverneur et le grand prêtre s'arrêtèrent en chemin et firent demi-tour pour voir ce qui se passait : le prophète israélite racontait qu'il avait vu les dieux de la Cinquième Montagne adorer un Dieu supérieur.

« Je le ferai tuer, déclara le prêtre.

— Et la population se rebellera contre nous », répliqua le gouverneur, qui s'intéressait aux propos de l'étranger. « Mieux vaut attendre qu'il commette une erreur.

— Avant que je ne descende de la montagne, les dieux m'ont chargé de venir en aide au gouverneur contre la menace des Assyriens, poursuivait Elie. Je sais que c'est un homme d'honneur et qu'il veut bien m'entendre. Mais il y a des gens qui ont tout intérêt à ce que la guerre se produise, et ils ne me laissent pas l'approcher.

— L'Israélite est un homme saint, dit un vieillard au gouverneur. Personne ne peut monter sur la Cinquième Montagne sans être foudroyé par le feu du ciel, mais cet homme a réussi, et maintenant il ressuscite les morts.

— Tyr, Sidon et toutes les cités phéniciennes ont une tradition de paix, dit un autre vieillard. Nous avons connu de pires menaces, et nous les avons surmontées. »

Des malades et des estropiés s'approchèrent, se frayant un passage dans la foule, touchant les vêtements d'Elie et lui demandant de guérir leurs maux.

« Avant de conseiller le gouverneur, guéris les malades, ordonna le prêtre. Alors nous croirons que les dieux de la Cinquième Montagne sont avec toi. »

Elie se souvint de ce que lui avait dit l'ange la nuit précédente : seule la force des personnes ordinaires lui serait accordée.

« Les malades appellent à l'aide, insista le prêtre. Nous attendons.

— Nous veillerons d'abord à éviter la guerre. Il y

aura beaucoup d'autres malades et d'autres infirmes si nous n'y parvenons pas. »

Le gouverneur interrompit la discussion :

« Elie viendra avec nous. Il a été touché par l'inspiration divine. »

Bien qu'il ne crût pas qu'il existât des dieux sur la Cinquième Montagne, il avait besoin d'un allié pour convaincre le peuple que la paix avec les Assyriens était la seule issue.

Tandis qu'ils allaient à la rencontre du commandant, le prêtre s'expliqua avec Elie.

« Tu ne crois en rien de ce que tu affirmes.

— Je crois que la paix est la seule issue. Mais je ne crois pas que les hauteurs de cette montagne soient habitées par des dieux. J'y suis allé.

— Et qu'as-tu vu ?

— Un ange du Seigneur. Je l'avais déjà vu auparavant, dans plusieurs lieux où je suis passé. Et il n'existe qu'un seul Dieu. »

Le prêtre rit.

« Tu veux dire que, selon toi, le dieu qui a fait la tempête a fait aussi le blé, même si ce sont des choses complètement différentes ?

— Tu vois la Cinquième Montagne ? demanda Elie. De quelque côté que tu regardes, elle te semble différente, pourtant c'est la même montagne. Il en est ainsi de tout ce qui a été créé : ce sont les nombreuses faces du même Dieu. »

Ils arrivèrent au sommet de la muraille, d'où l'on apercevait au loin le campement de l'ennemi. Dans la vallée désertique, la blancheur des tentes sautait aux yeux.

Quelque temps auparavant, lorsque des sentinelles avaient remarqué la présence des Assyriens à une extrémité de la vallée, les espions avaient affirmé qu'ils étaient là en mission de reconnaissance ; le commandant avait suggéré qu'on les fît prisonniers et qu'on les vendît comme esclaves. Le gouverneur avait opté pour une autre stratégie : ne rien faire. Il misait sur le fait qu'en établissant de bonnes relations avec les Assyriens, il pourrait ouvrir un nouveau marché pour le commerce du verre fabriqué à Akbar. En outre, même s'ils étaient là pour préparer une guerre, les Assyriens savaient bien que les petites cités se rangent toujours du côté des vainqueurs. Les généraux assyriens désiraient simplement traverser ces villes, sans qu'elles opposent de résistance, pour atteindre Tyr et Sidon où l'on conservait le trésor et le savoir de leur peuple.

La patrouille campait à l'entrée de la vallée et, peu à peu, des renforts étaient arrivés. Le prêtre affirmait en connaître la raison : la cité possédait un puits, le seul à plusieurs jours de marche dans le désert. Si les Assyriens voulaient conquérir Tyr ou Sidon, ils avaient besoin de cette eau pour approvisionner leurs armées.

Au bout d'un mois, ils pouvaient encore les chasser. Au bout de deux, ils pouvaient encore les vaincre facilement et négocier une retraite honorable des soldats assyriens.

Ils étaient prêts au combat, mais ils n'attaquaient pas. Au bout de cinq mois, ils pouvaient encore gagner la bataille. « Les Assyriens vont bientôt attaquer, parce qu'ils doivent souffrir de la soif », se disait le gouverneur. Il demanda au commandant d'élaborer des stratégies de défense et d'entraîner constamment ses hommes pour réagir à une attaque surprise.

Mais il ne se concentrait que sur la préparation de la paix.

*

Six mois avaient passé et l'armée assyrienne ne bougeait toujours pas. La tension à Akbar, croissante durant les premières semaines d'occupation, avait totalement disparu ; les gens s'étaient remis à vivre, les agriculteurs retournaient aux champs, les artisans fabriquaient le vin, le verre et le savon, les commerçants continuaient à vendre et à acheter leurs marchandises. Tous croyaient que, comme Akbar n'avait pas attaqué l'ennemi, la crise serait rapidement résolue par des négociations. Tous savaient que le gouverneur était conseillé par les dieux et connaissait toujours la meilleure décision à prendre.

Lorsque Elie était arrivé dans la cité, le gouverneur avait fait répandre des rumeurs sur la malédiction que l'étranger apportait avec lui ; de cette manière, si la menace de guerre devenait insupportable, il pourrait l'accuser d'être la cause principale du désastre. Les habitants d'Akbar seraient convaincus qu'avec la mort de l'Israélite tout rentrerait dans l'ordre. Le gouverneur expliquerait alors qu'il était désormais trop tard pour exiger le départ des Assyriens ; il ferait tuer Elie, et il expliquerait à son peuple que la paix constituait la meilleure solution. A son avis, les marchands — qui désiraient eux aussi la paix — forceraient les autres à admettre cette idée.

Pendant tous ces mois, il avait lutté contre la pression du prêtre et du commandant, exigeant une attaque rapide. Mais les dieux de la Cinquième Montagne ne l'avaient jamais abandonné. Après la miraculeuse résurrection de l'autre nuit, la vie d'Elie était plus importante que son exécution.

*

« Que fait cet étranger avec vous ? demanda le commandant.

— Il est inspiré par les dieux, répondit le gouverneur. Et il va nous aider à trouver la meilleure issue. »

Il changea rapidement de sujet de conversation.

« On dirait que le nombre de tentes a augmenté aujourd'hui.

— Et il augmentera encore demain, dit le commandant. Si nous avions attaqué alors qu'ils n'étaient qu'une patrouille, ils ne seraient probablement pas revenus.

— Tu te trompes. L'un d'eux aurait fini par s'échapper, et ils seraient revenus pour se venger.

— Lorsque l'on tarde pour la cueillette, les fruits pourrissent, insista le commandant. Mais quand on repousse les problèmes, ils ne cessent de croître. »

Le gouverneur expliqua que la paix régnait en Phénicie depuis presque trois siècles et que c'était la grande fierté de son peuple. Que diraient les générations futures s'il interrompait cette ère de prospérité ?

« Envoie un émissaire négocier avec eux, conseilla Elie. Le meilleur guerrier est celui qui parvient à faire de l'ennemi un ami.

— Nous ne savons pas exactement ce qu'ils veulent. Nous ne savons même pas s'ils désirent conquérir notre cité. Comment pouvons-nous négocier ?

— Il y a des signes de menace. Une armée ne perd pas son temps à faire des exercices militaires loin de son pays. »

Chaque jour arrivaient de nouveaux soldats — et le gouverneur imaginait la quantité d'eau qui serait nécessaire à tous ces hommes. En peu de temps, la cité serait sans défense devant l'armée ennemie.

« Pouvons-nous attaquer maintenant ? demanda le prêtre au commandant.

— Oui, nous le pouvons. Nous allons perdre beaucoup d'hommes mais la cité sera sauve. Cependant, il nous faut prendre rapidement une décision.

— Nous ne devons pas faire cela, gouverneur. Les dieux de la Cinquième Montagne m'ont affirmé que nous avions encore le temps de trouver une solution pacifique », dit Elie.

Bien qu'il eût écouté la conversation entre le prêtre et l'Israélite, le gouverneur feignit de l'approuver. Pour lui, peu importait que Sidon et Tyr fussent gouvernées par les Phéniciens, par les Cananéens ou par les Assyriens. L'essentiel était que la cité pût continuer à faire le commerce de ses produits.

« Attaquons, insista le prêtre.

— Encore un jour, pria le gouverneur. La situation va peut-être se résoudre. »

Il lui fallait décider rapidement de la meilleure façon d'affronter la menace des Assyriens. Il descendit de la muraille, se dirigea vers le palais et demanda à l'Israélite de l'accompagner.

En chemin, il observa le peuple autour de lui : les bergers menant les brebis aux pâturages, les agriculteurs allant aux champs, essayant d'arracher à la terre desséchée un peu de nourriture pour eux et leur famille. Les soldats faisaient des exercices avec leurs lances et des marchands arrivés récemment exposaient leurs produits sur la place. Aussi incroyable que cela pût paraître, les Assyriens n'avaient pas fermé la route qui traversait la vallée dans toute sa longueur ; les commerçants continuaient à circuler avec leurs marchandises, payant à la cité l'impôt sur le transport.

« Maintenant qu'ils ont réussi à rassembler une force puissante, pourquoi ne ferment-ils pas la route ? s'enquit Elie.

— L'empire assyrien a besoin des produits qui arrivent aux ports de Sidon et de Tyr, répondit le gouverneur. Si les commerçants étaient menacés, le flux de ravitaillement se tarirait. Et les conséquences seraient plus graves qu'une défaite militaire. Il doit y avoir un moyen d'éviter la guerre.

— Oui, renchérit Elie. S'ils désirent de l'eau, nous pouvons la vendre. »

Le gouverneur resta silencieux. Mais il comprit qu'il pouvait faire de l'Israélite une arme contre ceux qui désiraient la guerre. Il avait gravi la Cinquième Montagne, il avait défié les dieux et, au cas où le prêtre persisterait dans l'idée de faire la guerre aux Assyriens, seul Elie pourrait lui tenir tête. Il lui proposa de sortir faire un tour avec lui, pour discuter un peu.

Le prêtre resta immobile à observer l'ennemi du haut de la muraille.

« Que peuvent faire les dieux pour arrêter les envahisseurs ? demanda le commandant.

— J'ai accompli les sacrifices devant la Cinquième Montagne. J'ai prié pour qu'on nous envoie un chef plus courageux.

— Nous aurions dû agir comme Jézabel et tuer les prophètes. Cet Israélite qui hier était condamné à mort, le gouverneur se sert aujourd'hui de lui pour convaincre la population de choisir la paix. »

Le commandant regarda en direction de la montagne.

« Nous pouvons faire assassiner Elie. Et recourir à mes guerriers pour éloigner le gouverneur de ses fonctions.

— Je donnerai l'ordre de mettre à mort Elie, répliqua le prêtre. Quant au gouverneur, nous ne pouvons rien faire : ses ancêtres sont au pouvoir depuis plusieurs générations. Son grand-père a été notre chef, il a donné le pouvoir des dieux à son père, qui le lui a transmis à son tour.

— Pourquoi la tradition nous empêche-t-elle de placer au gouvernement un personnage plus efficace ?

— La tradition existe pour maintenir le monde en ordre. Si nous nous en mêlons, le monde prend fin. »

Le prêtre regarda autour de lui, le ciel et la terre, les montagnes et la vallée, chaque élément accomplissant ce qui avait été écrit pour lui. Parfois la terre tremblait, d'autres fois — comme à présent — il ne pleuvait pas pendant très longtemps. Mais les étoiles restaient à leur place et le soleil n'était pas tombé sur la tête des hommes. Tout cela parce que, depuis le Déluge, les hommes avaient appris qu'il était impossible de modifier l'ordre de la Création.

Autrefois, il n'y avait que la Cinquième Montagne. Hommes et dieux vivaient ensemble, se promenaient dans les jardins du Paradis, conversaient et riaient. Mais les êtres humains avaient péché et les dieux les en avaient chassés ; comme ils n'avaient nulle part où les envoyer, ils avaient finalement créé la terre autour de la montagne, pour pouvoir les y précipiter, les garder sous surveillance et faire en sorte qu'ils se souviennent toujours de se trouver sur un plan bien inférieur à celui des occupants de la Cinquième Montagne.

Mais ils avaient pris soin de laisser entrouverte une porte de retour. Si l'humanité suivait le bon chemin, elle finirait par revenir au sommet de la montagne. Et, pour que cette idée ne fût pas oubliée, les dieux avaient chargé les prêtres et les gouvernants de la maintenir vivante dans l'imagination du monde.

Tous les peuples partageaient la même croyance : si les familles ointes par les dieux s'éloignaient du pouvoir, les conséquences seraient graves. Nul ne se rappelait pourquoi ces familles avaient été choisies, mais tous savaient qu'elles avaient un lien de parenté avec les familles divines. Akbar existait depuis des centaines d'années, et elle avait toujours été administrée par les ancêtres de l'actuel gouverneur. Envahie plusieurs fois, elle était tombée aux mains d'oppresseurs et de barbares, mais avec le temps les envahisseurs s'en allaient ou ils étaient chassés. Alors, l'ordre ancien se rétablissait et les hommes reprenaient leur vie d'antan.

Les prêtres étaient tenus de préserver cet ordre : le monde avait un destin et il était régi par des lois. Il n'était plus temps de chercher à comprendre les dieux. Il fallait désormais les respecter et faire tout ce qu'ils voulaient. Ils étaient capricieux et s'irritaient facilement.

Sans les rituels de la récolte, la terre ne donnerait pas de fruits. Si certains sacrifices étaient oubliés, la cité serait infestée par des maladies mortelles. Si le dieu du Temps était de nouveau provoqué, il pourrait mettre fin à la croissance du blé et des hommes.

« Regarde la Cinquième Montagne, dit le grand prêtre au commandant. De son sommet, les dieux gouvernent la vallée et nous protègent. Ils ont de toute éternité un plan pour Akbar. L'étranger sera mis à mort, ou bien il retournera dans son pays, le gouverneur disparaîtra un jour, et son fils sera plus sage que lui. Ce que nous vivons maintenant est passager.

— Il nous faut un nouveau chef, déclara le commandant. Si nous restons aux mains de ce gouverneur, nous serons détruits. »

Le prêtre savait que c'était ce que voulaient les dieux, pour mettre fin à la menace de l'écriture de Byblos. Mais il ne dit rien. Il se réjouit de constater une fois de plus que les gouvernants accomplissent toujours — qu'ils le veuillent ou non — le destin de l'univers.

Elie se promena dans la cité, expliqua ses plans de paix au gouverneur et fut nommé son auxiliaire. Quand ils arrivèrent au milieu de la place, de nouveaux malades s'approchèrent — mais il déclara que les dieux de la Cinquième Montagne lui avaient interdit d'accomplir des guérisons. A la fin de l'après-midi, il retourna chez la veuve. L'enfant jouait au milieu de la rue et il le remercia d'avoir été l'instrument d'un miracle du Seigneur.

La femme l'attendait pour dîner. A sa surprise, il y avait une carafe de vin sur la table.

« Les gens ont apporté des présents pour te remercier, dit-elle. Et je veux te demander pardon pour mon injustice.

— Quelle injustice ? s'étonna Elie. Ne vois-tu pas que tout fait partie des desseins de Dieu ? »

La veuve sourit, ses yeux brillèrent, et il put constater à quel point elle était belle. Elle avait au moins dix ans de plus que lui, mais il éprouvait pour elle une profonde tendresse. Ce n'était pas son habitude et il eut peur ; il se rappela les yeux de Jézabel, et la prière qu'il avait faite en sortant du palais d'Achab — il aurait aimé se marier avec une femme du Liban.

74

« Même si ma vie a été inutile, au moins j'ai eu mon fils. Et l'on se souviendra de son histoire parce qu'il est revenu du royaume des morts, dit-elle.

— Ta vie n'est pas inutile. Je suis venu à Akbar sur ordre du Seigneur et tu m'as accueilli. Si l'on se souvient un jour de l'histoire de ton fils, sois certaine que l'on n'oubliera pas la tienne. »

La femme remplit les deux coupes. Ils burent tous deux au soleil qui se cachait et aux étoiles dans le ciel.

« Tu es venu d'un pays lointain en suivant les signes d'un Dieu que je ne connaissais pas, mais qui est désormais mon Seigneur. Mon fils aussi est revenu d'une contrée lointaine et il aura une belle histoire à raconter à ses petits-enfants. Les prêtres recueilleront ses paroles et les transmettront aux générations à venir. »

C'était grâce à la mémoire des prêtres que les cités avaient connaissance de leur passé, de leurs conquêtes, de leurs dieux anciens, des guerriers qui avaient défendu la terre de leur sang. Même s'il existait désormais de nouvelles méthodes pour enregistrer le passé, les habitants d'Akbar n'avaient confiance qu'en la mémoire des prêtres. Tout le monde peut écrire ce qu'il veut ; mais personne ne parvient à se souvenir de choses qui n'ont jamais existé.

« Et moi, qu'ai-je à raconter ? » continua la femme en remplissant la coupe qu'Elie avait vidée rapidement. « Je n'ai pas la force ni la beauté de Jézabel. Ma vie ressemble à toutes les autres : le mariage arrangé par les parents lorsque j'étais encore enfant, les tâches domestiques quand je suis devenue adulte, le culte, les jours sacrés, le mari toujours occupé à autre chose. De son vivant, nous n'avons jamais eu de conversation sur un sujet important. Lui était tout le temps préoccupé par ses affaires, moi, je prenais soin de la maison, et nous avons passé ainsi les meilleures années de notre vie.

« Après sa mort, il ne m'est resté que la misère et l'éducation de mon fils. Quand il sera grand, il ira traverser les mers, et je ne compterai plus pour personne. Je n'ai pas de haine, ni de ressentiment, seulement la conscience de mon inutilité. »

Elie remplit encore un verre. Son cœur commençait à donner des signaux d'alarme. Il aimait la compagnie de cette femme. L'amour pouvait être une expérience plus redoutable que lorsqu'il s'était trouvé devant un soldat d'Achab, une flèche pointée vers son cœur ; si la flèche l'avait atteint, il serait mort — et Dieu se serait chargé du reste. Mais si l'amour l'atteignait, il devrait lui-même en assumer les conséquences.

« J'ai tant désiré l'amour dans ma vie », pensa-t-il. Et pourtant, maintenant qu'il l'avait devant lui — aucun doute, il était là, il suffisait de ne pas le fuir —, il n'avait qu'une idée, l'oublier le plus vite possible.

Sa pensée revint au jour où il était arrivé à Akbar, après son exil dans la région du Kerith. Il était tellement fatigué et assoiffé qu'il ne se souvenait de rien, sauf du moment où il s'était remis de son évanouissement et où il avait vu la femme lui verser un peu d'eau entre les lèvres. Son visage était proche du sien, plus proche que ne l'avait jamais été celui d'une autre femme. Il avait remarqué qu'elle avait les yeux du même vert que ceux de Jézabel, mais d'un éclat différent, comme s'ils pouvaient refléter les cèdres, l'océan dont il avait tant rêvé sans le connaître, et même — comment était-ce possible ? — son âme.

« J'aimerais tant le lui dire, pensa-t-il. Mais je ne sais comment m'y prendre. Il est plus facile de parler de l'amour de Dieu. »

*

Elie but encore un peu. Elle devina qu'elle avait dit quelque chose qui lui avait déplu, et elle décida de changer de sujet.

« Tu as gravi la Cinquième Montagne ? » demanda-t-elle.

Il acquiesça.

Elle aurait aimé lui demander ce qu'il avait vu

là-haut, et comment il avait réussi à échapper au feu des cieux. Mais il semblait mal à l'aise.

« C'est un prophète. Il lit dans mon cœur », pensat-elle.

Depuis que l'Israélite était entré dans sa vie, tout avait changé. Même la pauvreté était plus facile à supporter — parce que cet étranger avait éveillé un sentiment qu'elle n'avait jamais connu : l'amour. Lorsque son fils était tombé malade, elle avait lutté contre tous les voisins pour qu'il restât chez elle.

Elle savait que, pour lui, le Seigneur comptait plus que tout ce qui advenait sous les cieux. Elle avait conscience que c'était un rêve impossible, car cet homme pouvait s'en aller à tout moment, faire couler le sang de Jézabel et ne jamais revenir pour lui raconter ce qui s'était passé.

Pourtant, elle continuerait de l'aimer car, pour la première fois de sa vie, elle avait conscience de ce qu'était la liberté. Elle pouvait l'aimer — quand bien même il ne le saurait jamais. Elle n'avait pas besoin de sa permission pour sentir qu'il lui manquait, penser à lui à longueur de journée, l'attendre pour dîner, et s'inquiéter de ce que les gens pouvaient comploter contre un étranger. C'était cela la liberté : sentir ce que son cœur désirait, indépendamment de l'opinion des autres. Elle s'était opposée à ses amis et à ses voisins au sujet de la présence de l'étranger dans sa maison. Elle n'avait pas besoin de lutter contre elle-même.

Elie but un peu de vin, prit congé et gagna sa chambre. Elle sortit, se réjouit de voir son fils jouer devant la maison et décida d'aller faire une courte promenade.

Elle était libre, car l'amour libère.

*

Elie demeura très longtemps à regarder le mur de sa chambre. Finalement, il décida d'invoquer son ange.

« Mon âme est en danger », dit-il.

L'ange resta silencieux. Elie hésita à poursuivre,

mais il était maintenant trop tard : il ne pouvait pas l'invoquer sans motif.

« Quand je suis devant cette femme, je ne me sens pas bien.

— Au contraire, répliqua l'ange. Et cela te dérange. Parce que tu es peut-être sur le point de l'aimer. »

Elie eut honte, parce que l'ange connaissait son âme.

« L'amour est dangereux, dit-il.

— Très, renchérit l'ange. Et alors ? »

Puis il disparut.

*

Son ange n'éprouvait pas les doutes qui le tourmentaient. Oui, il connaissait l'amour ; il avait vu le roi d'Israël abandonner le Seigneur parce que Jézabel, une princesse de Sidon, avait conquis son cœur. La tradition racontait que le roi Salomon avait perdu son trône à cause d'une étrangère. Le roi David avait envoyé l'un de ses meilleurs amis à la mort parce qu'il était tombé amoureux de son épouse. A cause de Dalila, Samson avait été fait prisonnier et les Philistins lui avaient crevé les yeux.

Comment, il ne connaissait pas l'amour ? L'Histoire abondait en exemples tragiques. Et même s'il n'avait pas connu les Ecritures saintes, il avait l'exemple d'amis — et d'amis de ses amis — perdus dans de longues nuits d'attente et de souffrance. S'il avait eu une femme en Israël, il aurait difficilement pu quitter sa cité quand le Seigneur l'avait ordonné, et maintenant il serait mort.

« Je mène un combat inutile, pensa-t-il. L'amour va gagner cette bataille, et je l'aimerai pour le reste de mes jours. Seigneur, renvoie-moi en Israël pour que jamais il ne me faille dire à cette femme ce que je ressens. Elle ne m'aime pas, et elle va me rétorquer que son cœur a été enterré avec le corps de son mari, ce héros. »

Le lendemain, Elie retourna voir le commandant. Il apprit que de nouvelles tentes avaient été installées.

« Quelle est actuellement la proportion des guerriers ? demanda-t-il.

— Je ne donne pas d'informations à un ennemi de Jézabel.

— Je suis conseiller du gouverneur. Il m'a nommé son auxiliaire hier soir, tu en as été informé et tu me dois une réponse. »

Le commandant eut envie de mettre fin à la vie de l'étranger.

« Les Assyriens ont deux soldats pour un des nôtres », répondit-il enfin.

Elie savait que l'ennemi avait besoin d'une force très supérieure.

« Nous approchons du moment idéal pour entreprendre les négociations de paix, dit-il. Ils comprendront que nous sommes généreux et nous obtiendrons de meilleures conditions. N'importe quel général sait que, pour conquérir une cité, il faut cinq envahisseurs pour un défenseur.

— Ils atteindront ce nombre si nous n'attaquons pas maintenant.

— Malgré toutes les mesures d'approvisionnement, ils n'auront pas assez d'eau pour ravitailler tous ces hommes. Et ce sera le moment d'envoyer nos ambassadeurs.

— Quand cela ?

— Laissons le nombre de guerriers assyriens augmenter encore un peu. Lorsque la situation sera insupportable, ils seront forcés d'attaquer mais, dans la proportion de trois ou quatre pour un des nôtres, ils savent qu'ils seront mis en déroute. C'est alors que nos émissaires leur proposeront la paix, la liberté de passage et la vente d'eau. Telle est l'idée du gouverneur. »

Le commandant resta silencieux et laissa partir l'étranger. Même si Elie mourait, le gouverneur pouvait s'accrocher à cette idée. Il se jura que si la situation en arrivait à ce point, il tuerait le gouverneur ; puis il se suiciderait pour ne pas assister à la fureur des dieux. Cependant, en aucune manière il ne permettrait que son peuple fût trahi par l'argent.

*

« Renvoie-moi en terre d'Israël, Seigneur ! criait Elie tous les soirs en marchant dans la vallée. Ne laisse pas mon cœur devenir prisonnier à Akbar ! »

Selon une coutume des prophètes qu'il avait connue enfant, il se donnait des coups de fouet chaque fois qu'il pensait à la veuve. Son dos était à vif et, pendant deux jours, il délira de fièvre. A son réveil, la première chose qu'il vit fut le visage de la femme ; elle soignait ses blessures à l'aide d'onguent et d'huile d'olive. Comme il était trop faible pour descendre jusqu'à la salle, elle montait ses aliments à la chambre.

*

Dès qu'il se sentit bien, il reprit ses marches dans la vallée.

« Renvoie-moi en terre d'Israël, Seigneur ! disait-il. Mon cœur est prisonnier à Akbar, mais mon corps peut encore poursuivre le voyage. »

L'ange apparut. Ce n'était pas l'ange du Seigneur qu'il avait vu au sommet de la montagne, mais celui qui le protégeait et dont la voix lui était familière.

« Le Seigneur écoute les prières de ceux qui prient pour oublier la haine. Mais il est sourd à ceux qui veulent échapper à l'amour. »

*

Tous les trois, ils dînaient ensemble chaque soir. Ainsi que le Seigneur l'avait promis, jamais la farine n'avait manqué dans la cruche, ni l'huile dans la jarre.

Ils conversaient rarement pendant les repas. Mais un soir, l'enfant demanda :

« Qu'est-ce qu'un prophète ?

— C'est un homme qui écoute encore les voix qu'il entendait lorsqu'il était enfant et qui croit toujours en elles. Ainsi, il peut savoir ce que pensent les anges.

— Oui, je sais de quoi tu parles, dit le gamin. J'ai des amis que personne d'autre ne voit.

— Ne les oublie jamais, même si les adultes te disent que c'est une sottise. Ainsi, tu sauras toujours ce que Dieu veut.

— Je connaîtrai l'avenir, comme les devins de Babylone, affirma le gamin.

— Les prophètes ne connaissent pas l'avenir. Ils ne font que transmettre les paroles que le Seigneur leur inspire dans le présent. C'est pourquoi je suis ici, sans savoir quand je retournerai vers mon pays. Il ne me le dira pas avant que cela ne soit nécessaire. »

Les yeux de la femme s'emplirent de tristesse. Oui, un jour il partirait.

*

Elie n'implorait plus le Seigneur. Il avait décidé que, lorsque ce serait le moment de quitter Akbar, il emmènerait la veuve et son fils. Il n'en dirait rien jusqu'à ce que l'heure fût venue.

Peut-être ne désirait-elle pas s'en aller. Peut-être n'avait-elle pas deviné ce qu'il ressentait pour elle — car il avait lui-même tardé à le comprendre. Dans ce cas, et cela vaudrait mieux, il pourrait se consacrer entièrement à l'expulsion de Jézabel et à la reconstruction d'Israël. Son esprit serait trop occupé pour penser à l'amour.

« *Le Seigneur est mon berger*, dit-il, se rappelant une vieille prière du roi David. *Apaise mon âme, et mène-moi auprès des eaux reposantes*. Et tu ne me laisseras pas perdre le sens de ma vie », conclut-il avec ses mots à lui.

*

Un après-midi, il revint à la maison plus tôt que d'habitude et il trouva la veuve assise sur le seuil.

« Que fais-tu ?

— Je n'ai rien à faire.

— Alors apprends quelque chose. En ce moment, beaucoup de gens ont renoncé à vivre. Ils ne s'ennuient pas, ils ne pleurent pas, ils se contentent d'attendre que le temps passe. Ils n'ont pas accepté les défis de la vie et elle ne les défie plus. Tu cours ce risque. Réagis, affronte la vie, mais ne renonce pas.

— Ma vie a retrouvé un sens, dit-elle en baissant les yeux. Depuis que tu es arrivé. »

Pendant une fraction de seconde, il sentit qu'il pouvait lui ouvrir son cœur. Mais il n'osa pas — elle faisait certainement allusion à autre chose.

« Trouve une occupation, dit-il pour changer de sujet. Ainsi, le temps sera un allié, non un ennemi.

— Que puis-je apprendre ? »

Elie réfléchit.

« L'écriture de Byblos. Elle te sera utile si tu dois voyager un jour. »

La femme décida de se consacrer corps et âme à cet apprentissage. Jamais elle n'avait songé à quitter Akbar mais, à la manière dont il en parlait, peut-être pensait-il l'emmener avec lui.

De nouveau elle se sentit libre. De nouveau elle se réveilla tôt le matin et marcha en souriant dans les rues de la cité.

« Elie est toujours en vie, dit le commandant au prêtre, deux mois plus tard. Tu n'as pas réussi à le faire assassiner.

— Il n'y a pas, dans tout Akbar, un seul homme qui veuille accomplir cette mission. L'Israélite a consolé les malades, rendu visite aux prisonniers, nourri les affamés. Quand quelqu'un a une querelle à résoudre avec son voisin, il a recours à lui, et tous acceptent ses jugements — parce qu'ils sont justes. Le gouverneur se sert de lui pour accroître sa popularité, mais personne ne s'en rend compte.

— Les marchands ne désirent pas la guerre. Si le gouverneur est populaire au point de convaincre la population que la paix est préférable, nous ne parviendrons jamais à chasser les Assyriens d'ici. Il faut qu'Elie soit mis à mort sans tarder. »

Le prêtre indiqua la Cinquième Montagne, son sommet toujours dissimulé par les nuages.

« Les dieux ne permettront pas que leur pays soit humilié par une puissance étrangère. Ils vont trouver une astuce : un incident se produira, et nous saurons profiter de l'occasion.

— Laquelle ?

— Je l'ignore. Mais je serai attentif aux signes. Abstiens-toi de fournir les chiffres exacts concernant les forces assyriennes. Si l'on t'interroge, dis que la proportion des guerriers envahisseurs est encore de quatre pour un. Et continue à entraîner tes troupes.

— Pourquoi dois-je faire cela ? S'ils atteignent la proportion de cinq pour un, nous sommes perdus.

— Non : nous serons en situation d'égalité. Lorsque le combat aura lieu, tu ne lutteras pas contre un ennemi inférieur, et on ne pourra pas te considérer comme un lâche qui abuse des faibles. L'armée d'Akbar affrontera un adversaire aussi puissant qu'elle et elle gagnera la bataille — parce que son commandant a mis au point la meilleure stratégie. »

Piqué par la vanité, le commandant accepta cette proposition. Et dès lors il commença à dissimuler des informations au gouverneur et à Elie.

Deux mois encore avaient passé et, ce matin-là, l'armée assyrienne avait atteint la proportion de cinq soldats pour un défenseur d'Akbar. A tout moment elle pouvait attaquer.

Depuis quelque temps, Elie soupçonnait le commandant de mentir à propos des forces ennemies, mais cela finirait par se retourner à son avantage : quand la proportion atteindrait le point critique, il serait facile de convaincre la population que la paix était la seule issue.

Il songeait à cela en se dirigeant vers la place où, tous les sept jours, il aidait les habitants à résoudre leurs différends. En général il s'agissait de problèmes sans importance : des querelles de voisinage, des vieux qui ne voulaient plus payer d'impôts, des commerçants qui se jugeaient victimes de préjudices dans leurs affaires.

Le gouverneur était là ; il faisait une apparition de temps en temps, pour le voir en action. L'antipathie qu'Elie ressentait pour lui avait complètement disparu ; il découvrait en lui un homme sage, désireux de régler les difficultés avant qu'elles ne surviennent — même s'il ne croyait pas dans le monde spirituel et avait très peur de mourir. A plusieurs reprises il avait usé de son autorité pour donner à une décision d'Elie valeur de loi. D'autres fois, il s'était opposé à une sentence et, avec le temps, Elie avait compris qu'il avait raison.

Akbar devenait un modèle de cité phénicienne. Le gouverneur avait créé un système d'impôts plus juste, il avait rénové les rues, et il savait administrer avec intelligence les profits provenant des taxes sur les marchandises. A une certaine époque Elie avait réclamé l'interdiction de la consommation de vin et de bière, parce que la majorité des affaires qu'il avait à résoudre concernait des agressions commises par des individus ivres. Mais le gouverneur avait fait valoir que c'était ce genre de choses qui faisait une grande cité. Selon la tradition, les dieux se réjouissaient quand les hommes se divertissaient à la fin d'une journée de travail, et ils protégeaient les ivrognes. De plus, la région avait la réputation de produire un des meilleurs vins du monde, et les étrangers se méfieraient si ses propres habitants ne le consommaient plus. Elie respecta la décision du gouverneur et, finalement, il dut admettre que, joyeux, les gens produisaient mieux.

« Tu n'as pas besoin de faire tant d'efforts », dit le gouverneur, avant qu'Elie entreprît le travail de la journée. « Un auxiliaire aide le gouvernement simplement en lui faisant part de ses opinions.

— J'ai la nostalgie de mon pays et je veux y retourner. Occupé à ces activités, j'arrive à me sentir utile et j'oublie que je suis un étranger », répondit-il.

« Et je réussis mieux à contrôler mon amour pour elle », pensa-t-il en lui-même.

*

Le tribunal populaire était désormais suivi par une assistance toujours très attentive. Petit à petit, les gens arrivèrent : les uns étaient des vieillards qui n'avaient plus la force de travailler aux champs et venaient applaudir, ou huer, les décisions d'Elie ; d'autres avaient un intérêt direct dans les affaires qui seraient traitées — soit parce qu'ils avaient été victimes, soit parce qu'ils pourraient tirer profit du jugement. Il y avait aussi des femmes et des enfants qui, faute de travail, devaient occuper leur temps libre.

Elie présenta les affaires de la matinée. Le premier cas était celui d'un berger qui avait rêvé d'un trésor caché en Egypte près des pyramides et qui avait besoin d'argent pour s'y rendre. Elie n'était jamais allé en Egypte mais il savait que c'était loin. Il expliqua au berger qu'il lui serait difficile de trouver les moyens nécessaires auprès d'autrui, mais que, s'il se décidait à vendre ses brebis et à payer le prix de son rêve, il trouverait assurément ce qu'il cherchait.

Ensuite vint une femme qui désirait apprendre l'art de la magie d'Israël. Elie rappela qu'il n'était pas un maître, seulement un prophète.

Alors qu'il se préparait à trouver une solution à l'amiable dans l'affaire d'un agriculteur qui avait maudit la femme d'un autre, un soldat ruisselant de sueur s'avança, écartant la foule, et s'adressa au gouverneur :

« Une patrouille a réussi à capturer un espion. On le conduit ici ! »

Un frisson parcourut l'assemblée ; c'était la première fois qu'on allait assister à un jugement de ce genre.

« A mort ! cria quelqu'un. Mort aux ennemis ! »

Tous les participants semblaient d'accord, à en croire leurs mugissements. En un clin d'œil, la nouvelle se répandit dans toute la cité et la place se remplit encore. Les autres affaires furent jugées à grand-peine. A tout instant on interrompait Elie, en demandant que l'étranger fût présenté sur-le-champ.

« Je ne peux pas juger ce genre d'affaire, expliquait-il. Cela relève des autorités d'Akbar.

— Qu'est-ce que les Assyriens sont venus faire ici ? s'exclamait l'un. Ils ne voient pas que nous sommes en paix depuis des générations ?

— Pourquoi veulent-ils notre eau ? criait un autre. Pourquoi menacent-ils notre cité ? »

Depuis des mois personne n'osait évoquer en public la présence de l'ennemi. Tout le monde voyait un nombre croissant de tentes se dresser à l'horizon, les marchands affirmaient qu'il fallait entreprendre aussitôt les négociations de paix, pourtant le peuple d'Akbar se refusait à croire qu'il vivait sous la menace d'une invasion. Excepté l'incursion ponctuelle d'une tribu insignifiante, dont on venait à bout rapidement, les guerres n'existaient que dans la mémoire des prêtres. Ceux-ci évoquaient un pays nommé Egypte, ses chevaux, ses chars de guerre et ses dieux aux formes d'animaux. Mais cela s'était passé voilà fort longtemps, l'Egypte n'était plus une nation puissante, et les guerriers à la peau sombre qui parlaient une langue inconnue avaient regagné leurs terres. Maintenant les habitants de Tyr et de Sidon dominaient les mers, étendant un nouvel empire sur le monde, et, bien qu'ils fussent des guerriers expérimentés, ils avaient découvert une nouvelle façon de lutter : le commerce.

« Pourquoi sont-ils nerveux ? demanda le gouverneur à Elie.

— Parce qu'ils sentent que quelque chose a changé. Tu sais comme moi que désormais les Assyriens peuvent attaquer à tout moment. Et que le commandant ment sur le nombre des troupes ennemies.

— Mais il ne peut pas être assez fou pour dire la vérité ! Il sèmerait la panique.

— Les gens devinent lorsqu'ils sont en danger ; ils ont des réactions étranges, des pressentiments, ils sentent quelque chose dans l'air. Ils essaient de se cacher la réalité, se croyant incapables de faire face à la situation. Jusqu'à maintenant, eux se sont raconté des histoires ; mais le moment approche où il leur faudra affronter la vérité. »

Le prêtre arriva.

« Allons au palais réunir le Conseil d'Akbar. Le commandant est en route.

— Ne fais pas cela, dit Elie à voix basse au gouverneur. Ils te forceront à faire ce que tu ne veux pas faire.

— Allons-y, insista le prêtre. Un espion a été arrêté et il faut prendre des mesures d'urgence.

— Rends le jugement au milieu du peuple, chuchota Elie. Le peuple t'aidera, parce qu'il désire la paix — même s'il réclame la guerre.

— Qu'on amène cet homme ici ! » ordonna le gouverneur.

La foule poussa des cris de joie. Pour la première fois, elle allait assister à une réunion du Conseil.

« Nous ne pouvons pas faire cela ! s'exclama le prêtre. C'est une affaire délicate, qui doit être résolue dans le calme ! »

Quelques huées. De nombreuses protestations.

« Qu'on l'amène ici, répéta le gouverneur. Il sera jugé sur cette place, au milieu du peuple. Nous travaillons ensemble à transformer Akbar en une cité prospère, et ensemble nous jugerons tout ce qui la menace. »

La décision fut accueillie par une salve d'applaudissements. Un groupe de soldats apparut, traînant un homme à demi nu, couvert de sang. Il avait sans doute été frappé abondamment avant d'arriver jusque-là.

Les bruits cessèrent. Un silence pesant s'abattit sur l'assistance, et l'on entendait le grognement des porcs et le bruit des enfants qui jouaient dans le coin opposé de la place.

« Pourquoi avez-vous fait cela au prisonnier ? s'écria le gouverneur.

— Il s'est débattu, répondit un garde. Il a déclaré qu'il n'était pas un espion. Qu'il était venu jusqu'ici pour vous parler. »

Le gouverneur envoya chercher trois sièges. Ses domestiques apportèrent également le manteau de la justice, qu'il portait chaque fois que devait se réunir le Conseil d'Akbar.

Le gouverneur et le grand prêtre prirent place. Le troisième siège était réservé au commandant, qui n'était pas encore arrivé.

« Je déclare solennellement ouvert le tribunal de la cité d'Akbar. Que les anciens s'approchent. »

Un groupe de vieillards se présenta et se plaça en demi-cercle derrière les sièges. Ils formaient le Conseil des anciens ; autrefois, leurs opinions étaient respectées et suivies d'effet, mais aujourd'hui ce groupe n'avait plus qu'un rôle décoratif : ils étaient là pour entériner toutes les décisions du gouvernement.

Une fois accomplies certaines formalités — une prière aux dieux de la Cinquième Montagne et la déclamation des noms de quelques héros du passé —, le gouverneur s'adressa au prisonnier :

« Que veux-tu ? »

L'homme ne répondit pas. Il le dévisageait d'une manière étrange, comme s'il était son égal.

« Que veux-tu ? » insista le gouverneur.

Le prêtre lui toucha le bras.

« Nous avons besoin d'un interprète. Il ne parle pas notre langue. »

L'ordre fut donné et un garde partit à la recherche

d'un commerçant qui pût servir d'interprète. Toujours très occupés par leurs affaires et leurs profits, les marchands n'allaient jamais assister aux séances qu'organisait Elie.

Tandis qu'ils attendaient, le prêtre murmura :
« Ils ont frappé le prisonnier parce qu'ils ont peur. Laisse-moi conduire ce procès et ne dis rien : la panique les rend tous agressifs et, si nous ne faisons pas preuve d'autorité, nous risquons de perdre le contrôle de la situation. »

Le gouverneur ne répondit pas. Lui aussi avait peur. Il chercha Elie des yeux mais, de l'endroit où il était assis, il ne le voyait pas.

*

Un commerçant arriva, amené de force par le garde. Il protesta contre le tribunal parce qu'il perdait son temps et qu'il avait beaucoup d'affaires à régler. Mais le prêtre, d'un regard sévère, lui intima l'ordre de se tenir tranquille et de traduire la conversation.

« Que viens-tu faire ici ? interrogea le gouverneur.
— Je ne suis pas un espion, répondit l'homme. Je suis un général de l'armée. Je suis venu discuter avec vous. »

L'assistance, qui était totalement silencieuse, se mit à crier à peine la phrase traduite. Le public affirmait que c'était un mensonge et exigeait la peine de mort immédiate.

Le prêtre réclama le silence et se tourna de nouveau vers le prisonnier :

« De quoi veux-tu discuter ?
— Le gouverneur a la réputation d'être un homme sage, répondit l'Assyrien. Nous ne voulons pas détruire cette cité : ce qui nous intéresse, c'est Tyr et Sidon. Mais Akbar se trouve au milieu du chemin et contrôle cette vallée. Si nous sommes obligés de combattre, nous perdrons du temps et des hommes. Je viens proposer un règlement. »

« Cet homme dit la vérité », songea Elie. Il avait remarqué qu'il était entouré par un groupe de soldats qui l'empêchaient de voir l'endroit où le gouverneur était assis. « Il pense comme nous. Le Seigneur a réalisé un miracle, et il va mettre un point final à cette situation périlleuse. »

Le prêtre se leva et cria au peuple :

« Vous voyez ? Ils veulent nous détruire sans combat !

— Continue ! » reprit le gouverneur.

Mais le prêtre s'interposa une fois de plus :

« Notre gouverneur est un homme bon, qui refuse de faire couler le sang. Mais nous sommes dans une situation de guerre et le prévenu qui se tient devant vous est un ennemi !

— Il a raison ! » s'écria quelqu'un dans l'assistance.

Elie comprit son erreur. Le prêtre jouait avec l'auditoire tandis que le gouverneur ne cherchait qu'à faire justice. Il tenta de s'approcher mais on le bouscula. Un soldat le saisit par le bras.

« Attends ici. En fin de compte, l'idée était de toi. »

Elie se retourna : c'était le commandant, et il souriait.

« Nous ne pouvons écouter aucune proposition, poursuivit le prêtre, laissant l'émotion émaner de ses gestes et de ses propos. Si nous montrons que nous voulons négocier, ce sera la preuve que nous avons peur. Et le peuple d'Akbar est courageux. Il est en mesure de résister à n'importe quelle invasion.

— Cet homme recherche la paix », dit le gouverneur, en s'adressant à la foule.

Une voix s'éleva :

« Les marchands recherchent la paix. Les prêtres désirent la paix. Les gouverneurs administrent la paix. Mais une armée ne souhaite qu'une chose : la guerre !

— Ne voyez-vous pas que nous parvenons à faire face à la menace religieuse d'Israël sans mener aucune guerre ? hurla le gouverneur. Nous n'avons pas envoyé d'armées, ni de navires, mais Jézabel. Maintenant ils adorent Baal sans que nous ayons eu besoin de sacrifier un seul homme au front.

— Eux, ils n'ont pas envoyé une belle femme, mais leurs guerriers ! » cria le prêtre encore plus fort.

Le peuple exigeait la mort de l'Assyrien. Le gouverneur retint le prêtre par le bras.

« Assieds-toi, ordonna-t-il. Tu vas trop loin.

— C'est toi qui as eu l'idée d'un procès public. Ou, mieux, c'est le traître israélite, qui semble dicter les actes du gouverneur d'Akbar.

— Je m'expliquerai plus tard avec lui. Maintenant nous devons apprendre ce que veut l'Assyrien. Pendant des générations, les hommes ont cherché à imposer leur volonté par la force ; ils disaient ce qu'ils voulaient, mais ils ne tenaient aucun compte de ce que pensait le peuple, et tous ces empires ont finalement été détruits. Notre peuple est devenu grand parce qu'il a appris à écouter. Ainsi, nous avons développé le commerce, en écoutant ce que l'autre désire et en faisant notre possible pour l'obtenir. Le résultat est le profit. »

Le prêtre hocha la tête.

« Tes propos semblent sages, et c'est le pire de tous les dangers. Si tu disais des sottises, il serait facile de prouver que tu te trompes. Mais ce que tu viens d'affirmer nous conduit tout droit à un piège. »

Les gens qui se trouvaient au premier rang intervenaient dans la discussion. Jusque-là, le gouverneur s'était toujours efforcé de tenir compte de l'opinion du Conseil, et Akbar avait une excellente réputation ; Tyr et Sidon avaient envoyé des émissaires pour observer comment elle était administrée ; le nom du gouverneur était parvenu aux oreilles de l'empereur et, avec un peu de chance, il pourrait terminer ses jours comme ministre de la Cour. Mais aujourd'hui, on avait bravé publiquement son autorité. S'il ne prenait pas rapidement des mesures, il perdrait le respect du peuple — et il ne pourrait plus prendre de décisions capitales parce que personne ne lui obéirait.

« Continue », lança-t-il au prisonnier, ignorant le regard furieux du prêtre et exigeant que l'interprète traduisît sa question.

« Je suis venu proposer un arrangement, dit l'Assyrien. Vous nous laissez passer, et nous marcherons contre Tyr et Sidon. Une fois que ces cités seront vaincues — elles le seront certainement, car une grande partie de leurs guerriers sont sur les navires pour surveiller le commerce —, nous serons généreux avec Akbar. Et nous te garderons comme gouverneur.

— Vous voyez ? s'exclama le prêtre en se relevant. Ils pensent que notre gouverneur est capable d'échanger l'honneur d'Akbar contre un poste élevé ! »

La foule en colère se mit à gronder. Ce prisonnier blessé, à moitié nu, voulait imposer ses conditions ! Un homme vaincu qui proposait la reddition de la cité ! Certains se levèrent et s'apprêtèrent à l'agresser. Les gardes eurent bien du mal à maîtriser la situation.

« Attendez ! reprit le gouverneur, qui tentait de parler plus fort que tous. Nous avons devant nous un homme sans défense, il ne peut donc pas nous faire peur. Nous savons que notre armée est la mieux préparée et que nos guerriers sont les plus vaillants. Nous n'avons rien à prouver à personne. Si nous décidons de combattre, nous vaincrons, mais les pertes seront énormes. »

Elie ferma les yeux et pria pour que le gouverneur parvînt à convaincre le peuple.

« Nos ancêtres nous parlaient de l'empire égyptien, mais ce temps est révolu, continua-t-il. Maintenant nous revenons à l'âge d'or, nos pères et nos grands-pères ont vécu en paix. Pourquoi devrions-nous rompre cette tradition ? Les guerres modernes se font dans le commerce, non sur les champs de bataille. »

Peu à peu, la foule redevint silencieuse. Le gouverneur était sur le point de réussir.

Quand le bruit cessa, il s'adressa à l'Assyrien.

« Ce que tu proposes ne suffit pas. Vous devrez payer les taxes dont les marchands s'acquittent pour traverser nos territoires.

— Crois-moi, gouverneur, vous n'avez pas le choix, répliqua le prisonnier. Nous avons suffisamment d'hommes pour raser cette cité et tuer tous ses habitants. Vous êtes en paix depuis très longtemps et vous ne savez plus lutter, alors que, nous, nous sommes en train de conquérir le monde. »

Les murmures reprirent dans l'assistance. Elie pensait : « Il ne peut pas flancher maintenant. » Mais il devenait difficile d'affronter le prisonnier assyrien qui, même dominé, imposait ses conditions. A chaque minute, la foule augmentait — Elie remarqua que les commerçants avaient abandonné leur travail et s'étaient mêlés aux spectateurs, inquiets du déroulement des événements. Le jugement revêtait une importance considérable ; il n'y avait plus moyen de reculer, la décision fût-elle la négociation ou la mort.

*

Les spectateurs commencèrent à se diviser ; les uns défendaient la paix, les autres exigeaient la résistance d'Akbar. Le gouverneur dit tout bas au prêtre :

« Cet homme m'a défié publiquement. Mais toi aussi. »

Le prêtre se tourna vers lui. Et, parlant de manière que personne ne pût l'entendre, il lui ordonna de condamner immédiatement l'Assyrien à mort.

« Je ne demande pas, j'exige. C'est moi qui te maintiens au pouvoir et je peux mettre fin quand je veux à cette situation, tu comprends ? Je connais des sacrifices qui peuvent apaiser la colère des dieux lorsque nous sommes contraints de remplacer la famille gouvernante. Ce ne sera pas la première fois : même en Egypte, un empire qui a duré des milliers d'années, de nombreuses dynasties ont été remplacées. Et pourtant l'univers est resté en ordre et le ciel ne nous est pas tombé sur la tête. »

Le gouverneur pâlit.

« Le commandant se trouve dans l'assistance, avec une partie de ses soldats. Si tu persistes à négocier avec cet homme, je dirai à tout le monde que les dieux t'ont abandonné. Et tu seras déposé. Nous allons poursuivre le procès. Et tu vas faire exactement ce que je t'ordonnerai. »

Si Elie avait été en vue, le gouverneur aurait encore eu une solution : il aurait demandé au prophète israélite d'affirmer qu'il avait vu un ange au sommet de la Cinquième Montagne, ainsi qu'il le lui avait raconté. Il aurait rappelé l'histoire de la résurrection du fils de la veuve. Et cela aurait été la parole d'Elie, un homme qui s'était déjà montré capable de faire des miracles, contre la parole d'un homme qui jamais n'avait fait la preuve d'aucune sorte de pouvoir surnaturel.

Mais Elie l'avait abandonné, et il n'avait plus le choix. En outre, ce n'était qu'un prisonnier — et aucune armée au monde n'entreprend une guerre parce qu'elle a perdu un soldat.

« Tu gagnes cette partie », dit-il au prêtre. Un jour, il négocierait une contrepartie.

Le prêtre hocha la tête. Le verdict fut rendu peu après.

« Personne ne défie Akbar, proclama le gouverneur. Et personne n'entre dans notre cité sans la permission de son peuple. Tu as tenté de le faire et tu es condamné à mort. »

Là où il se trouvait, Elie baissa les yeux. Le commandant souriait.

On conduisit le prisonnier, accompagné d'une foule de plus en plus nombreuse, jusqu'à un terrain non loin des remparts. Là, on lui arracha ce qui lui restait de vêtements et on le laissa nu. Un soldat le poussa au fond d'une fosse. Les gens, agglutinés tout autour, se bousculaient à celui qui le verrait le mieux.

« Un soldat porte avec fierté son uniforme de guerre et se rend visible à l'ennemi parce qu'il a du courage. Un espion s'habille en femme, car il est lâche ! cria le gouverneur, pour être entendu de tous. C'est pourquoi je te condamne à quitter cette vie sans la dignité des braves. »

Le peuple hua le prisonnier et applaudit le gouverneur.

Le prisonnier parlait, mais l'interprète n'était plus là et personne ne le comprenait. Elie parvint à se frayer un chemin pour rejoindre le gouverneur, mais il était trop tard. Quand il toucha son manteau, il fut violemment repoussé.

« C'est ta faute. Tu as voulu un procès public.

— C'est *ta* faute, rétorqua Elie. Même si le Conseil d'Akbar s'était réuni en secret, le commandant et le prêtre auraient obtenu ce qu'ils désiraient. J'étais entouré de gardes pendant tout le procès. Ils avaient tout arrangé. »

La coutume voulait qu'il revînt au prêtre de déterminer la durée du supplice. Celui-ci se baissa, ramassa une pierre et la tendit au gouverneur : elle n'était pas assez grosse pour entraîner une mort rapide, ni assez petite pour prolonger la souffrance très longtemps.

« A toi l'honneur.

— J'y suis obligé, murmura le gouverneur afin que seul le prêtre l'entendît. Mais tu sais que ce n'est pas la bonne voie.

— Pendant toutes ces années, tu m'as forcé à adopter les positions les plus dures, tandis que tu tirais profit des décisions qui faisaient plaisir au peuple, répliqua le prêtre, lui aussi à voix basse. J'ai dû affronter le doute et la culpabilité, et j'ai passé des nuits d'insomnie, poursuivi par le fantôme des erreurs que j'aurais pu commettre. Mais comme je ne suis pas un lâche, Akbar est aujourd'hui une cité enviée du monde entier. »

Les gens étaient allés chercher des pierres de la taille requise. Pendant quelque temps, on n'entendit plus que le bruit des cailloux qui s'entrechoquaient. Le prêtre poursuivit :

« Je peux me tromper en condamnant à mort cet homme. Mais je suis sûr de l'honneur de notre cité ; nous ne sommes pas des traîtres. »

*

Le gouverneur leva la main et jeta la première pierre ; le prisonnier l'esquiva. Mais aussitôt, la foule, au milieu des cris et des huées, se mit à le lapider.

L'homme tentait de protéger son visage de ses bras, et les pierres atteignaient sa poitrine, son dos, son ventre. Le gouverneur voulut s'en aller ; il avait tant de fois vu ce spectacle, il savait que la mort était lente et douloureuse, que le visage deviendrait une bouillie d'os, de cheveux et de sang, que les gens continueraient à jeter des pierres bien après que la vie aurait abandonné ce corps. Dans quelques minutes, le prisonnier cesserait de se défendre et baisserait les bras. S'il avait été un homme bon dans cette vie, les dieux guideraient l'une des pierres, qui atteindrait le devant du crâne, provoquant l'évanouissement. En revanche, s'il avait commis des cruautés, il resterait conscient jusqu'à la dernière minute.

La foule criait, lançait des pierres avec une férocité croissante, et le condamné cherchait à se défendre de son mieux. Soudain, l'homme écarta les bras et parla dans une langue que tous pouvaient comprendre. Surprise, la foule s'interrompit.

« Vive l'Assyrie ! s'exclama-t-il. En ce moment, je contemple l'image de mon peuple et je meurs heureux, car je meurs comme un général qui a tenté de sauver la vie de ses guerriers. Je vais rejoindre la compagnie des dieux et je suis content car je sais que nous conquerrons cette terre !

— Tu as entendu ? dit le prêtre. Il a écouté et compris toute notre conversation au cours du procès ! »

Le gouverneur l'admit. L'homme parlait leur langue, et maintenant il savait que le Conseil d'Akbar était divisé.

« Je ne suis pas en enfer, parce que la vision de mon pays me donne dignité et force. La vision de mon pays me donne la joie ! Vive l'Assyrie ! » cria l'homme de nouveau.

Revenue de sa stupeur, la foule se remit à le lapider. L'homme gardait les bras écartés sans chercher à se protéger — c'était un guerrier vaillant. Quelques secondes plus tard, la miséricorde des dieux se manifesta : une pierre le frappa au front et il s'évanouit.

« Nous pouvons nous en aller maintenant, déclara le prêtre. Le peuple d'Akbar se chargera d'achever la tâche. »

*

Elie ne retourna pas chez la veuve. Il se promena sans but dans le désert.

« Le Seigneur n'a rien fait, disait-il aux plantes et aux rochers. Et Il aurait pu intervenir. »

Il regrettait sa décision, il se jugeait encore une fois coupable de la mort d'un homme. S'il avait accepté l'idée d'une réunion secrète du Conseil d'Akbar, le gouverneur aurait pu l'emmener avec lui ; ils auraient été deux face au prêtre et au commandant. Leurs chances auraient été minces mais tout de même plus sérieuses que dans un procès public.

Pire encore : il avait été impressionné par la manière dont le prêtre s'était adressé à la foule ; même s'il n'était pas d'accord avec tous ses propos, il était bien obligé de reconnaître que cet homme avait une profonde connaissance du commandement. Il tâcherait de se rappeler chaque détail de cette scène pour le jour où — en Israël — il devrait affronter le roi et la princesse de Tyr.

Il marcha sans but, regardant les montagnes, la cité et le campement assyrien au loin. Il n'était qu'un point dans cette vallée et un monde immense l'entourait — un monde si vaste que, même s'il voyageait sa vie entière, il n'en atteindrait pas le bout. Ses amis, et ses ennemis, avaient peut-être mieux compris que lui la terre où ils vivaient : ils pouvaient voyager vers des pays lointains, naviguer sur des mers inconnues, aimer une femme sans se sentir coupables. Aucun d'eux n'écoutait plus les anges de l'enfance, ni ne se proposait de lutter au nom du Seigneur. Ils vivaient dans le présent et ils étaient heureux. Elie était une personne comme les autres, et, à ce moment, alors qu'il se promenait dans la vallée, il désirait n'avoir jamais entendu la voix du Seigneur et de Ses anges.

Mais la vie n'est pas faite de désirs, elle est faite des actes de chacun. Il se souvint qu'il avait déjà tenté à plusieurs reprises de renoncer à sa mission, et pourtant il était là, au milieu de cette vallée, parce que le Seigneur l'avait exigé ainsi.

« J'aurais pu n'être qu'un charpentier, mon Dieu, et j'aurais été encore utile à Ton entreprise. »

Mais Elie accomplissait ce qu'on avait exigé de lui, portant le poids de la guerre à venir, le massacre des prophètes par Jézabel, la lapidation du général assyrien, la peur de son amour pour une femme d'Akbar. Le Seigneur lui avait fait un cadeau, et il ne savait qu'en faire.

Au milieu de la vallée surgit la lumière. Ce n'était pas son ange gardien — celui qu'il écoutait toujours, mais voyait rarement. C'était un ange du Seigneur, qui venait le consoler.

« Je ne peux rien faire de plus ici, dit Elie. Quand retournerai-je en Israël ?

— Quand tu auras appris à reconstruire, répondit l'ange. Rappelle-toi ce que Dieu a enseigné à Moïse avant un combat. Profite de chaque moment, si tu ne veux pas plus tard avoir des regrets, et te dire que tu as perdu ta jeunesse. A chaque âge, le Seigneur donne à l'homme ses inquiétudes particulières. »

« *Le Seigneur dit à Moïse :*
"N'aie pas peur, ne laisse pas ton cœur faiblir avant le combat, ne sois pas terrifié devant tes ennemis. L'homme qui a planté une vigne et n'en a pas encore profité, qu'il le fasse vite, afin que, s'il meurt dans la lutte, ce ne soit pas un autre qui en profite. L'homme

qui aime une femme, et ne l'a pas encore reçue, qu'il retourne chez elle, afin que, s'il meurt dans la lutte, ce ne soit pas un autre homme qui la reçoive." »

Elie marcha encore quelque temps, cherchant à comprendre ce qu'il venait d'entendre. Alors qu'il se préparait à retourner à Akbar, il aperçut la femme qu'il aimait assise sur un rocher au pied de la Cinquième Montagne — à quelques minutes de l'endroit où il se trouvait.

« Que fait-elle ici ? Serait-elle au courant du procès, de la condamnation à mort, et des risques que nous courons désormais ? »

Il devait l'avertir immédiatement. Il décida de la rejoindre.

Elle remarqua sa présence et lui fit signe. Elie semblait avoir oublié les paroles de l'ange, car d'un seul coup son inquiétude revint. Il feignit d'être préoccupé par les problèmes de la cité, afin qu'elle ne devinât pas la confusion qui régnait dans son cœur et dans son esprit.

« Que fais-tu ici ? demanda-t-il en arrivant près d'elle.

— Je suis venue chercher un peu d'inspiration. L'écriture que j'apprends me fait penser à la Main qui a dessiné les vallées, les monts, la cité d'Akbar. Des commerçants m'ont donné des encres de toutes les couleurs car ils désirent que j'écrive pour eux. J'ai songé à les utiliser pour décrire le monde qui m'entoure mais je sais que c'est difficile : même si je dispose des couleurs, seul le Seigneur parvient à les mélanger avec une telle harmonie. »

Elle gardait les yeux fixés sur la Cinquième Montagne. Elle était devenue complètement différente de la personne qu'il avait rencontrée quelques mois auparavant, ramassant du bois à la porte de la cité.

Sa présence solitaire, au milieu du désert, lui inspirait confiance et respect.

« Pourquoi toutes les montagnes ont-elles un nom, sauf la Cinquième Montagne, que l'on désigne par un nombre ? demanda Elie.

— Pour ne pas susciter de querelle entre les dieux, répondit-elle. La tradition raconte que si l'homme avait donné à cette montagne le nom d'un dieu particulier, les autres, furieux, auraient détruit la terre. C'est pour cela qu'elle s'appelle le Mont Cinq. Parce que c'est le cinquième mont que nous apercevons au-delà des murailles. Ainsi, nous n'offensons personne, et l'Univers reste en ordre. »

Ils se turent quelque temps. Puis la femme rompit le silence :

« Je réfléchis sur les couleurs, mais je pense aussi au danger que représente l'écriture de Byblos. Elle peut offenser les dieux phéniciens et le Seigneur notre Dieu.

— Seul existe le Seigneur, l'interrompit Elie. Et tous les pays civilisés ont leur écriture.

— Mais celle-ci est différente. Quand j'étais enfant, j'allais souvent sur la place assister au travail que le peintre de mots réalisait pour les marchands. Ses dessins, fondés sur l'écriture égyptienne, exigeaient adresse et savoir. Maintenant, l'antique et puissante Egypte est décadente, elle n'a plus d'argent pour acheter quoi que ce soit, et personne n'utilise plus son langage. Les navigateurs de Tyr et de Sidon répandent l'écriture de Byblos dans le monde entier. On peut inscrire les mots et les cérémonies sacrées sur les tablettes d'argile et les transmettre d'un peuple à l'autre. Qu'adviendra-t-il du monde si des gens sans scrupules se mettent à utiliser les rituels pour intervenir dans l'univers ? »

Elie comprenait ce que la femme voulait dire. L'écriture de Byblos était fondée sur un système très simple : il suffisait de transformer les dessins égyptiens en sons, puis de désigner une lettre pour chaque son. Selon l'ordre dans lequel on plaçait ces lettres, on pouvait créer tous les sons possibles et décrire tout ce qui existait dans l'univers. Certains sons étant malaisés à prononcer, les Grecs avaient résolu la difficulté en ajoutant cinq lettres — appelées *voyelles* — aux vingt et quelques caractères de Byblos. Ils avaient baptisé cette innovation *alphabet*, nom qui maintenant servait à désigner la nouvelle forme d'écriture.

Les relations commerciales entre les différentes cultures en avaient été grandement facilitées. Avec l'écriture égyptienne, il fallait beaucoup d'espace et d'habileté pour parvenir à exprimer ses idées, et une profonde connaissance pour les interpréter ; elle avait été imposée aux peuples conquis, mais n'avait pas survécu à la décadence de l'empire. Le système de Byblos, pendant ce temps, se répandait rapidement à travers le monde, et son adoption ne dépendait plus de la puissance économique de la Phénicie.

La méthode de Byblos, avec son adaptation grecque, avait plu aux marchands de diverses nations ; depuis les temps anciens, c'étaient eux qui décidaient de ce qui devait demeurer dans l'Histoire, et de ce qui disparaîtrait à la mort de tel roi ou de tel haut personnage. Tout indiquait que l'invention phénicienne était destinée à devenir le langage courant des affaires, survivant à ses navigateurs, ses rois, ses princesses séductrices, ses producteurs de vin, ses maîtres verriers.

« Dieu disparaîtra des mots ? s'enquit la femme.

— Il sera toujours en eux, répondit Elie. Mais chacun sera responsable devant Lui de tout ce qu'il écrira. »

Elle retira de la manche de son vêtement une tablette d'argile portant une inscription.

« Qu'est-ce que cela signifie ? demanda Elie.

— C'est le mot *amour*. »

Elie prit la tablette, mais il n'eut pas le courage de demander pourquoi elle la lui avait tendue. Sur ce morceau d'argile, quelques traits griffonnés résumaient pourquoi les étoiles restaient suspendues dans les cieux et pourquoi les hommes marchaient sur la terre.

Il voulut la lui rendre mais elle refusa.

« J'ai écrit cela pour toi. Je connais ta responsabilité, je sais qu'un jour il te faudra partir, et que tu te transformeras en ennemi de mon pays car tu désires anéantir Jézabel. Ce jour-là, je serai peut-être à ton côté, t'apportant mon soutien pour que tu accomplisses ta tâche. Ou peut-être lutterai-je contre toi, parce que le sang de Jézabel est celui de mon pays ; ce mot, que tu tiens dans tes mains, est empli de mystères. Personne ne peut savoir ce qu'il éveille dans le cœur d'une femme — pas même les prophètes qui conversent avec Dieu.

— Je connais ce mot, dit Elie en rangeant la tablette dans son manteau. J'ai lutté jour et nuit contre lui, car si j'ignore ce qu'il éveille dans le cœur d'une femme, je sais ce qu'il peut faire d'un homme. J'ai suffisamment de courage pour affronter le roi d'Israël, la princesse de Sidon, le Conseil d'Akbar, mais ce seul mot, *amour*, me cause une terreur profonde. Avant que tu ne le dessines sur la tablette, tes yeux l'avaient déjà écrit dans mon cœur. »

Ils restèrent tous deux silencieux. Il y avait la mort de l'Assyrien, le climat de tension dans la cité, l'appel du Seigneur qui pouvait survenir à tout moment ; mais le mot qu'elle avait inscrit était plus puissant que tout cela.

Elie tendit la main, et elle la prit. Ils restèrent ainsi jusqu'à ce que le soleil se cache derrière la Cinquième Montagne.

« Merci, dit-elle sur le chemin du retour. Il y a longtemps que je désirais passer une fin d'après-midi avec toi. »

Quand ils arrivèrent à la maison, un émissaire du gouverneur attendait : il demandait à Elie d'aller le retrouver immédiatement.

« Je t'ai soutenu, et pour me remercier tu t'es montré lâche, dit le gouverneur. Que dois-je faire de ta vie ?

— Je ne vivrai pas une seconde de plus que le Seigneur ne le désire, répondit Elie. C'est Lui qui décide, pas toi. »

Le gouverneur s'étonna du courage d'Elie.

« Je peux te faire décapiter sur-le-champ. Ou te traîner par les rues de la cité, en disant que tu as porté malheur à notre peuple, répliqua-t-il. Et ce ne sera pas une décision de ton Dieu unique.

— Quel que soit mon destin, il se réalisera. Mais je veux que tu saches que je n'ai pas fui ; les soldats du commandant m'ont empêché d'arriver jusqu'à toi. Il voulait la guerre, et il a tout fait pour y parvenir. »

Le gouverneur décida de mettre un terme à cette discussion stérile. Il lui fallait expliquer son plan au prophète israélite.

« Ce n'est pas le commandant qui désire la guerre ; en bon militaire, il a conscience que son armée est inférieure, qu'elle manque d'expérience et sera décimée par l'ennemi. En homme d'honneur, il sait que cela risque d'être un motif de honte pour ses descendants. Mais l'orgueil et la vanité ont endurci son cœur.

— Il pense que l'ennemi a peur. Il ne sait pas que les guerriers assyriens sont bien entraînés : dès qu'ils entrent dans l'armée, ils plantent un arbre, et chaque jour ils sautent par-dessus l'endroit où la graine est enfouie. La graine se transforme en pousse et ils sautent toujours par-dessus. La pousse devient plante et ils continuent de sauter. Ils ne s'ennuient pas, ils ne trouvent pas que ce soit une perte de temps. Peu à peu, l'arbre grandit — et les guerriers sautent de plus en plus haut. Ils se préparent ainsi aux obstacles avec patience et dévouement.

— Ils sont habitués à reconnaître un défi. Ils nous observent depuis des mois. »

Elie interrompit le gouverneur :

« Qui a intérêt à cette guerre ?

— Le prêtre. Je l'ai compris pendant le procès du prisonnier assyrien.

— Pour quelle raison ?

— Je l'ignore. Mais il a été suffisamment habile pour persuader le commandant et le peuple. Maintenant, la cité entière est de son côté, et je ne vois qu'une issue à la difficile situation dans laquelle nous nous trouvons. »

Il fit une longue pause et fixa l'Israélite dans les yeux :

« Toi. »

Le gouverneur se mit à marcher de long en large, parlant vite et laissant paraître sa nervosité.

« Les commerçants aussi désirent la paix, mais ils ne peuvent rien faire. En outre, ils sont assez riches pour s'installer dans une autre cité ou attendre que les conquérants commencent à acheter leurs produits. Le reste de la population a perdu la raison et exige que nous attaquions un ennemi infiniment supérieur. La seule chose qui puisse les convaincre de changer d'avis, c'est un miracle. »

Elie était tendu.

« Un miracle ?

— Tu as ressuscité un enfant que la mort avait déjà emporté. Tu as aidé le peuple à trouver son chemin et, bien qu'étant étranger, tu es aimé de presque tout le monde.

— La situation était celle-là jusqu'à ce matin, dit Elie. Mais maintenant elle est différente : dans le contexte que tu viens de décrire, quiconque défendra la paix sera considéré comme un traître.

— Il ne s'agit pas de défendre quoi que ce soit. Je veux que tu fasses un miracle aussi grand que la résurrection de l'enfant. Alors, tu diras au peuple que la paix est la seule issue et il t'écoutera. Le prêtre perdra complètement son pouvoir. »

Il y eut un moment de silence. Le gouverneur reprit :

« Je suis prêt à passer un accord : si tu fais ce que je te demande, la religion du Dieu unique sera obligatoire à Akbar. Tu plairas à Celui que tu sers, et moi je parviendrai à négocier les conditions de paix. »

Elie monta à l'étage de la maison, où se trouvait sa chambre. Il avait, à ce moment-là, une opportunité qu'aucun prophète n'avait eue auparavant : convertir une cité phénicienne. Ce serait la manière la plus cuisante de montrer à Jézabel qu'il y avait un prix à payer pour ce qu'elle avait fait dans son pays.

Il était excité par la proposition du gouverneur. Il pensa même réveiller la femme, qui dormait en bas, mais il changea d'avis ; elle devait rêver du bel après-midi qu'ils avaient passé ensemble.

Il invoqua son ange. Et celui-ci apparut.

« Tu as entendu la proposition du gouverneur, dit Elie. C'est une chance unique.

— Aucune chance n'est unique, répondit l'ange. Le Seigneur offre aux hommes de nombreuses occasions. En outre, rappelle-toi ce qui a été annoncé : aucun autre miracle ne te sera permis jusqu'à ce que tu sois retourné au sein de ta patrie. »

Elie baissa la tête. A ce moment, l'ange du Seigneur surgit et fit taire son ange gardien. Et il déclara :

« Voici ton prochain miracle :

« Tu iras réunir tout le peuple devant la montagne. D'un côté, tu ordonneras que soit élevé un autel à Baal, et un bouvillon lui sera présenté. De l'autre côté, tu élèveras un autel au Seigneur ton Dieu, et sur lui aussi tu placeras un bouvillon.

« Et tu diras aux adorateurs de Baal : "Invoquez le nom de votre dieu, tandis que j'invoquerai le nom du Seigneur." Laisse-les faire d'abord ; qu'ils passent toute la matinée à prier et à crier, demandant à Baal de descendre pour recevoir ce qui lui est offert.

« Ils crieront à haute voix et ils se tailladeront avec leurs poignards et ils prieront que le bouvillon soit reçu par le dieu, mais il ne se passera rien.

« Quand ils seront fatigués, tu empliras quatre jarres d'eau et tu les verseras sur ton bouvillon. Tu le feras une seconde fois. Et tu le feras encore une troisième fois. Alors tu imploreras le Dieu d'Abraham, d'Isaac et d'Israël de montrer à tous Son pouvoir.

« A ce moment, le Seigneur enverra le feu du ciel et il dévorera ton sacrifice. »

Elie s'agenouilla et rendit grâces.

« Cependant, poursuivit l'ange, ce miracle ne peut avoir lieu qu'une seule fois dans ta vie. Choisis si tu désires le réaliser ici, pour empêcher une bataille, ou si tu préfères le réaliser dans ton pays, pour délivrer les tiens de la menace de Jézabel. »

Et l'ange du Seigneur s'en fut.

La femme se réveilla tôt et vit Elie assis sur le seuil. Il avait les yeux cernés de quelqu'un qui n'a pas dormi.

Elle aurait aimé lui demander ce qui s'était passé la nuit précédente, mais elle redoutait sa réponse. Son insomnie pouvait avoir été causée par sa conversation avec le gouverneur, et par la menace de guerre ; mais il y avait peut-être un autre motif, la tablette d'argile qu'elle lui avait offerte. Alors, si elle soulevait la question, elle risquait d'entendre que l'amour d'une femme ne convenait pas aux desseins de Dieu.

« Viens manger quelque chose », fut son seul commentaire.

Son fils se réveilla à son tour. Ils se mirent tous les trois à table et mangèrent.

« J'aurais aimé rester avec toi hier, dit Elie. Mais le gouverneur avait besoin de moi.

— Ne t'en fais pas pour lui, dit-elle, sentant que son

cœur se calmait. Sa famille gouverne Akbar depuis des générations, et il saura quoi faire devant la menace.

— J'ai aussi conversé avec un ange. Et il a exigé de moi une décision très difficile.

— Tu ne dois pas non plus t'inquiéter à cause des anges. Peut-être vaut-il mieux croire que les dieux changent avec le temps. Mes ancêtres adoraient les dieux égyptiens qui avaient forme d'animaux. Ces dieux sont partis et, jusqu'à ton arrivée, on m'a appris à faire des sacrifices à Astarté, à El, à Baal et à tous les habitants de la Cinquième Montagne. Maintenant j'ai connaissance du Seigneur mais il se peut que lui aussi nous quitte un jour, et que les prochains dieux soient moins exigeants. »

L'enfant réclama un peu d'eau. Il n'y en avait pas.

« Je vais en chercher, dit Elie.

— Je viens avec toi », proposa l'enfant.

*

Ils prirent ensemble la direction du puits. En chemin, ils passèrent là où, tôt le matin, le commandant entraînait ses soldats.

« Allons jeter un coup d'œil, dit le gamin. Je serai soldat quand je serai grand. »

Elie acquiesça.

« Lequel d'entre nous est le meilleur au maniement de l'épée ? demandait un guerrier.

— Va jusqu'à l'endroit où l'espion a été lapidé hier, dit le commandant. Ramasse une grosse pierre et insulte-la.

— Pourquoi cela ? La pierre ne me répondra pas.

— Alors attaque-la avec ton épée.

— Mon épée se brisera, dit le soldat. Et ce n'était pas ma question ; je veux savoir qui est le meilleur au maniement de l'épée.

— Le meilleur est celui qui ressemble à une pierre, répondit le commandant. Sans sortir la lame du fourreau, il réussit à prouver que personne ne pourra le vaincre. »

« Le gouverneur a raison : le commandant est un

sage, pensa Elie. Mais même la plus grande sagesse peut être occultée par l'éclat de la vanité. »

*

Ils poursuivirent leur chemin. L'enfant lui demanda pourquoi les soldats s'entraînaient autant.

« Pas seulement les soldats, mais ta mère aussi, et moi, et ceux qui suivent leur cœur. Tout, dans la vie, exige de l'entraînement.

— Même pour être prophète ?

— Même pour comprendre les anges. Nous voulons tellement leur parler que nous n'écoutons pas ce qu'ils disent. Il n'est pas facile d'écouter : dans nos prières, nous cherchons toujours à expliquer en quoi nous nous sommes trompés et ce que nous aimerions qu'il nous arrive. Mais le Seigneur sait déjà tout cela, et parfois Il nous demande seulement d'entendre ce que nous dit l'univers. Et d'avoir de la patience. »

Le gamin le regardait, surpris. Il ne devait rien comprendre, et pourtant Elie éprouvait le besoin de poursuivre la conversation. Peut-être — quand il serait grand — ces propos l'aideraient-ils dans une situation difficile.

« Toutes les batailles de la vie nous enseignent quelque chose, même celles que nous perdons. Lorsque tu seras grand, tu découvriras que tu as soutenu des mensonges, que tu t'es menti à toi-même, ou que tu as souffert pour des bêtises. Si tu es un bon guerrier, tu ne te sentiras pas coupable, mais tu ne laisseras pas non plus tes erreurs se répéter. »

Il décida de se taire ; un enfant de cet âge ne pouvait pas comprendre ce qu'il disait. Ils marchaient lentement, et Elie regardait les rues de la cité qui un jour l'avait accueilli et qui, maintenant, était près de disparaître. Tout dépendait de la décision qu'il prendrait.

Akbar était plus silencieuse que de coutume. Sur la place centrale, les gens discutaient à voix basse — comme s'ils redoutaient que le vent ne transportât leurs propos jusqu'au campement assyrien. Les plus vieux affirmaient qu'il n'arriverait rien, les jeunes étaient excités par l'éventualité de la lutte, les marchands et les artisans projetaient d'aller à Tyr et à Sidon en attendant que les choses se calment.

« Pour eux il est facile de partir, pensa-t-il. Les marchands peuvent transporter leurs biens dans n'importe quelle partie du monde. Les artisans peuvent travailler même là où l'on parle une langue étrangère. Mais moi, il me faut la permission du Seigneur. »

*

Ils arrivèrent au puits et remplirent deux jarres d'eau. En général, cet endroit était plein de monde ; les femmes se réunissaient pour laver, teindre les étoffes et épiloguaient sur tout ce qui se passait dans la cité. Aucun secret n'existait plus quand il parvenait près du puits ; les nouvelles concernant le commerce, les trahisons familiales, les problèmes de voisinage, la vie intime des gouvernants, tous les sujets — sérieux ou superficiels — y étaient débattus, commentés, critiqués ou applaudis. Même durant les mois où la force ennemie n'avait cessé de croître, Jézabel — la princesse qui avait conquis le roi d'Israël — restait le sujet préféré. Les femmes faisaient l'éloge de son audace, de sa bravoure, certaines que, si un malheur arrivait à la cité, elle reviendrait dans son pays pour les venger.

Mais, ce matin-là, il n'y avait presque personne. Les rares femmes présentes disaient qu'il fallait aller chercher à la campagne le plus de céréales possible parce que les Assyriens allaient bientôt fermer les portes de la cité. Deux d'entre elles projetaient de se rendre jusqu'à la Cinquième Montagne pour offrir un sacrifice aux dieux — elles ne voulaient pas que leurs fils meurent au combat.

« Le prêtre a dit que nous pouvions résister plusieurs mois, expliqua l'une d'elles à Elie. Il suffit que nous ayons le courage nécessaire pour défendre l'honneur d'Akbar, et les dieux nous aideront. »

L'enfant était effrayé.

« L'ennemi va attaquer ? » demanda-t-il.

Elie ne répondit pas ; cela dépendait du choix que l'ange lui avait proposé la nuit précédente.

« J'ai peur, insista le gamin.

— Cela prouve que tu aimes la vie. C'est normal d'avoir peur, aux bons moments. »

*

Elie et l'enfant revinrent à la maison avant la fin de la matinée. La femme avait disposé autour d'elle de petits récipients, contenant des encres de différentes couleurs.

« Je dois travailler, dit-elle en regardant les lettres et les phrases inachevées. A cause de la sécheresse, la cité est envahie par la poussière. Les pinceaux sont toujours sales, et l'encre impure, et tout est plus difficile. »

Elie demeura silencieux : il ne voulait pas lui faire partager ses préoccupations. Il s'assit dans un coin de la salle et resta absorbé dans ses pensées. L'enfant sortit jouer avec ses amis.

« Il a besoin de silence », songea la femme, et elle s'efforça de se concentrer sur son travail.

Elle passa le reste de la matinée à achever quelques mots qui auraient pu être écrits en deux fois moins de temps, et elle se sentit coupable de ne pas faire ce que l'on attendait d'elle ; en fin de compte, pour la première fois de sa vie, elle avait la chance de subvenir aux besoins de sa famille.

Elle se remit au travail ; elle utilisait du papyrus, un matériau qu'un marchand venu d'Egypte lui avait récemment apporté — lui demandant de noter quelques messages commerciaux qu'il devait expédier à Damas. La feuille n'était pas de la meilleure qualité et l'encre débordait sans cesse. « Malgré toutes ces difficultés, c'est mieux que de dessiner sur l'argile. »

Les pays voisins avaient coutume d'envoyer leurs messages sur des plaques d'argile ou sur du parchemin. L'Egypte était peut-être un pays décadent, et son écriture dépassée, mais au moins y avait-on découvert un moyen pratique et léger d'enregistrer le commerce et l'Histoire : on découpait en plusieurs épaisseurs la tige d'une plante qui poussait sur les rives du Nil, et, selon un processus simple, on collait ces couches l'une à côté de l'autre pour former une feuille jaunâtre. Akbar devait importer le papyrus car il était impossible de le cultiver dans la vallée. Même s'il coûtait cher, les marchands le préféraient car ils pouvaient transporter les feuilles écrites dans leur sac — ce qui se révélait impossible avec les tablettes d'argile et les parchemins.

« Tout devient plus simple », pensa-t-elle. Dommage qu'il fallût l'autorisation du gouvernement pour employer l'alphabet de Byblos sur le papyrus. Une loi dépassée soumettait encore les textes écrits au contrôle du Conseil d'Akbar.

Son travail terminé, elle le montra à Elie, qui avait passé tout ce temps à la regarder faire, sans le moindre commentaire.

« Que penses-tu du résultat ? » demanda-t-elle.

Il parut sortir d'une transe.

« Oui, c'est joli », répondit-il sans prêter attention à ce qu'elle disait.

Il devait converser avec le Seigneur. Et elle ne voulait pas l'interrompre. Elle sortit et alla chercher le prêtre.

*

A son retour, Elie était toujours assis au même endroit. Les deux hommes se dévisagèrent. Tous deux restèrent silencieux pendant un long moment. Ce fut le prêtre qui rompit le silence. « Tu es un prophète, et tu parles avec les anges. Je ne fais qu'interpréter les lois anciennes, exécuter des rituels, et tenter de protéger mon peuple des erreurs qu'il commet. C'est pourquoi je sais que ce combat n'oppose pas des hommes. C'est une bataille des dieux, et je ne dois pas l'empêcher.

— J'admire ta foi, même si tu adores des dieux qui n'existent pas, répondit Elie. Si la situation présente est, comme tu l'affirmes, digne d'une bataille céleste, le Seigneur fera de moi Son instrument pour détruire Baal et ses compagnons de la Cinquième Montagne. Il aurait mieux valu que tu ordonnes mon assassinat.

« — J'y ai songé. Mais ce n'était pas nécessaire ; au moment opportun, les dieux m'ont été favorables. »

Elie ne répliqua pas. Le prêtre se retourna et prit le papyrus sur lequel la femme venait d'écrire un texte.

« C'est du bon travail », commenta-t-il. Après l'avoir lu soigneusement, il retira sa bague de son doigt, la trempa dans l'encre et appliqua son sceau dans le coin gauche. Quiconque se faisait prendre avec un papyrus dépourvu du sceau du prêtre pouvait être condamné à mort.

« Pourquoi devez-vous toujours faire cela ? demanda-t-elle.

— Parce que ces papyrus colportent des idées, répondit-il. Et les idées ont un pouvoir.

— Ce ne sont que des transactions commerciales.

— Mais ce pourrait être des plans de bataille. Ou un rapport sur nos richesses. Ou nos prières secrètes. De nos jours, au moyen des lettres et des papyrus, on peut sans peine voler l'inspiration d'un peuple. Il est plus difficile de cacher des tablettes d'argile ou des parchemins ; mais la combinaison du papyrus et de l'alphabet de Byblos peut mettre fin à la culture de chaque pays et détruire le monde. »

Une femme entra.

« Prêtre ! Prêtre ! Viens voir ce qui se passe ! »

Elie et la veuve le suivirent. Des gens affluaient de toutes les directions au même endroit ; la poussière qu'ils soulevaient rendait l'air pratiquement irrespirable. Les enfants couraient en tête, riant et faisant du vacarme. Les adultes avançaient lentement, en silence.

Quand ils atteignirent la porte Sud de la cité, une petite foule s'y trouvait déjà réunie. Le prêtre se fraya un chemin et s'enquit du motif de toute cette confusion.

Une sentinelle d'Akbar se tenait à genoux, les bras écartés, les mains clouées sur un morceau de bois placé en travers de ses épaules. Ses vêtements étaient déchirés et un morceau de bois lui avait crevé l'œil gauche.

Sur sa poitrine, quelques caractères assyriens

avaient été tracés avec la lame d'un poignard. Le prêtre comprenait l'égyptien mais la langue assyrienne n'était pas encore assez répandue pour être enseignée et sue par cœur ; il dut faire appel à un commerçant qui assistait à la scène.

« *Nous déclarons la guerre*, voilà ce qui est écrit », traduisit l'homme.

Les gens tout autour n'avaient dit mot. Elie pouvait lire la panique sur leurs visages.

« Donne-moi ton épée », dit le prêtre à un soldat.

Le soldat obéit. Le prêtre demanda qu'on avertît le gouverneur et le commandant de ce qui était arrivé. Puis, d'un geste rapide, il enfila la lame dans le cœur de la sentinelle agenouillée.

L'homme poussa un gémissement et tomba à terre, mort, libéré de la douleur et de la honte de s'être laissé capturer.

« Demain je me rendrai sur la Cinquième Montagne pour offrir des sacrifices, dit-il au peuple effrayé. Et les dieux de nouveau se souviendront de nous. »

Avant de partir, il se tourna vers Elie :

« Tu le vois de tes propres yeux : les cieux continuent de nous venir en aide.

— Une seule question, dit Elie. Pourquoi veux-tu voir sacrifier ton peuple ?

— Parce qu'il faut en passer par là pour tuer une idée. »

Lorsqu'il l'avait entendu converser avec la femme ce matin-là, Elie avait déjà compris de quelle idée il s'agissait : l'alphabet.

« Il est trop tard. Il est déjà répandu de par le monde, et les Assyriens ne peuvent pas conquérir la terre entière.

— Qui t'a dit cela ? En fin de compte, les dieux de la Cinquième Montagne sont du côté de leurs armées. »

*

Pendant des heures, il marcha dans la vallée, comme il l'avait fait l'après-midi précédent. Il savait qu'il y aurait encore au moins une soirée et une nuit de paix : on ne fait pas la guerre dans l'obscurité, car les guerriers ne peuvent y distinguer l'ennemi. Cette nuit-là, le Seigneur lui laissait une chance de changer le destin de la cité qui l'avait accueilli.

« Salomon saurait quoi faire maintenant, expliqua-t-il à son ange. Et David, et Moïse, et Isaac. Ils étaient des hommes de confiance du Seigneur, mais moi, je ne suis qu'un serviteur indécis. Le Seigneur me donne un choix qui aurait dû être le Sien.

— L'histoire de nos ancêtres abonde apparemment en hommes qui étaient la bonne personne au bon endroit, répliqua l'ange. Ne crois pas cela : le Seigneur n'exige de chacun que ce qui est du domaine de ses possibilités.

— Alors, Il s'est trompé avec moi.

— Tous les malheurs ont une fin. Ainsi en est-il aussi des gloires et des tragédies du monde.

— Je ne l'oublierai pas, dit Elie. Mais, quand elles se retirent, les tragédies laissent des marques éternelles, et les gloires laissent de vains souvenirs. »

L'ange ne répondit pas.

« Pourquoi, pendant tout le temps que j'ai passé à Akbar, ai-je été incapable de trouver des alliés pour lutter en faveur de la paix ? Quelle importance a un prophète solitaire ?

— Quelle importance a le soleil qui poursuit sa course dans le ciel ? Quelle importance a une montagne qui surgit au milieu d'une vallée ? Quelle importance a un puits isolé ? Ce sont pourtant eux qui indiquent le chemin que doit suivre la caravane.

— Mon cœur suffoque de tristesse, dit Elie en s'agenouillant et en tendant les bras vers le ciel. Si seulement je pouvais mourir ici et ne jamais avoir les mains tachées du sang de mon peuple, ou d'un peuple étranger. Regarde là-derrière : que vois-tu ?

— Tu sais bien que je suis aveugle, dit l'ange. Mes yeux gardent encore la lumière de la gloire du Seigneur, et je ne peux rien voir d'autre. Tout ce que je perçois, c'est ce que ton cœur me raconte. Tout ce que je peux entrevoir, ce sont les vibrations des dangers qui te menacent. Je ne peux pas savoir ce qui se trouve derrière toi.

— Eh bien, je vais te le dire : il y a Akbar. A cette heure, le soleil de l'après-midi illuminant son profil, elle est belle. Je me suis habitué à ses rues et à ses murailles, à son peuple généreux et accueillant. Même si les habitants de la cité sont encore prisonniers du commerce et des superstitions, ils ont le cœur aussi pur que celui de n'importe quelle autre nation du monde. J'ai appris grâce à eux beaucoup de choses que j'ignorais ; en échange, j'ai écouté leurs plaintes et, inspiré par Dieu, j'ai réussi à résoudre leurs conflits internes. Souvent j'ai été en danger, et toujours quelqu'un m'a aidé. Pourquoi dois-je choisir entre sauver cette cité ou racheter mon peuple ?

— Parce qu'un homme doit choisir, répondit l'ange. En cela réside sa force : le pouvoir de ses décisions.

— C'est un choix difficile : il exige d'accepter la mort d'un peuple pour en sauver un autre.

— Il est encore plus difficile de définir sa propre voie. Celui qui ne fait pas de choix meurt aux yeux du Seigneur, même s'il continue à respirer et à marcher dans les rues. En outre, personne ne meurt. L'Eternité accueille toutes les âmes et chacune poursuivra sa tâche. Il y a une raison pour tout ce qui se trouve sous le soleil. »

Elie leva de nouveau les bras vers les cieux :

« Mon peuple s'est éloigné du Seigneur à cause de la beauté d'une femme. La Phénicie peut être détruite parce qu'un prêtre pense que l'écriture constitue une menace pour les dieux. Pourquoi Celui qui a créé le monde préfère-t-Il se servir de la tragédie pour écrire le livre du destin ? »

Les cris d'Elie résonnèrent dans la vallée et l'écho revint à ses oreilles.

« Tu ne sais pas ce que tu dis, rétorqua l'ange. Il n'y a pas de tragédie, il y a seulement l'inévitable. Tout a sa raison d'être : c'est à toi de savoir distinguer ce qui est passager de ce qui est définitif.

— Qu'est-ce qui est passager ? demanda Elie.

— L'inévitable.
— Et qu'est-ce qui est définitif ?
— Les leçons de l'inévitable. »
Sur ces mots, l'ange s'éloigna.

Cette nuit-là, au cours du dîner, Elie dit à la femme et à l'enfant :
« Préparez vos affaires. Nous pouvons partir à tout moment.
— Voilà deux jours que tu ne dors pas, remarqua la femme. Un émissaire du gouverneur est venu cet après-midi ; il demandait que tu te rendes au palais. J'ai dit que tu étais parti dans la vallée et que tu y dormirais.
— Tu as bien fait », répliqua-t-il. Puis il gagna directement sa chambre et sombra dans un profond sommeil.

Il fut réveillé le lendemain matin par le son d'instruments de musique. Quand il descendit voir ce qui se passait, l'enfant était déjà sur le seuil.
« Regarde ! disait-il, les yeux brillants d'excitation. C'est la guerre ! »
Un bataillon de soldats, imposants avec leurs uniformes de guerre et leur armement, se dirigeait vers la porte Sud d'Akbar. Un groupe de musiciens les suivait, marquant le pas au rythme des tambours.
« Hier tu avais peur, dit Elie au gamin.
— Je ne savais pas que nous avions tant de soldats. Nos guerriers sont les meilleurs ! »
Elie quitta l'enfant et sortit dans la rue ; il lui fallait à tout prix rencontrer le gouverneur. Les habitants de la cité, réveillés au son des hymnes de guerre, étaient hypnotisés ; pour la première fois de leur vie, ils assistaient au défilé d'un bataillon organisé, en uniforme militaire, lances et boucliers reflé-

116

tant les premiers rayons du soleil. Le commandant avait réussi un tour de force ; il avait préparé son armée à l'insu de tous, et maintenant — Elie le redoutait — il pouvait laisser croire que la victoire sur les Assyriens était possible.

Il se fraya un chemin parmi les soldats et parvint jusqu'au devant de la colonne. Là, montés sur leurs chevaux, le commandant et le gouverneur ouvraient la marche.

« Nous avons passé un accord, lança Elie tout en courant à côté du gouverneur. Je peux faire un miracle ! »

Le gouverneur ne lui répondit pas. La garnison franchit les remparts de la cité et sortit en direction de la vallée.

« Tu sais que cette armée est une chimère, insista-t-il. Les Assyriens sont cinq fois plus nombreux, et ils ont l'expérience de la guerre ! Ne laisse pas détruire Akbar !

— Qu'attends-tu de moi ? demanda le gouverneur, sans arrêter sa monture. Hier soir, j'ai envoyé un émissaire te chercher pour que nous discutions, et on m'a fait dire que tu étais absent de la cité. Que pouvais-je faire de plus ?

— Affronter les Assyriens en terrain ouvert est un suicide ! Vous le savez bien ! »

Le commandant écoutait la conversation sans faire le moindre commentaire. Il avait déjà discuté de sa stratégie avec le gouverneur ; le prophète israélite serait surpris.

Elie courait à côté des chevaux, sans savoir exactement ce qu'il devait faire. La colonne de soldats s'éloignait de la cité et se dirigeait vers le centre de la vallée.

« Aide-moi, Seigneur, pensait-il. De même que tu as caché le soleil pour aider Josué au combat, arrête le temps et fais que je réussisse à persuader le gouverneur de son erreur. »

A peine avait-il eu cette pensée que le commandant cria : « Halte ! »

« C'est peut-être un signal, se dit Elie. Je dois en profiter. »

Les soldats formèrent deux lignes, semblables à des murs d'hommes, les boucliers prenant solidement appui sur le sol et les armes pointées en avant.

« Tu crois voir les guerriers d'Akbar, dit le gouverneur à Elie.

— Je vois des jeunes gens qui rient devant la mort.

— Mais sache qu'ici il n'y a qu'un seul bataillon. La plupart de nos hommes sont restés dans la cité, en haut des murailles. Nous avons disposé des chaudrons d'huile bouillante prêts à être versés sur la tête de quiconque tenterait de les escalader. Nous avons réparti des réserves dans différentes maisons pour éviter que des flèches incendiaires ne détruisent nos provisions. Selon les calculs du commandant, nous pouvons résister presque deux mois au siège de la cité. Pendant que les Assyriens se préparaient, nous faisions la même chose.

— On ne m'a jamais raconté cela, dit Elie.

— Rappelle-toi : même si tu as aidé le peuple d'Akbar, tu restes un étranger, et certains militaires pouvaient te prendre pour un espion.

— Mais toi, tu désires la paix !

— La paix reste possible, même après le commencement d'un combat. Seulement, nous négocierons en position d'égalité. »

Le gouverneur raconta que des messagers avaient été envoyés à Tyr et à Sidon pour rendre compte de la gravité de la situation. Il lui en coûtait de réclamer du secours : on pouvait le croire incapable de maîtriser la situation. Mais il était parvenu à la conclusion que c'était la seule solution.

Le commandant avait mis au point un plan ingénieux ; dès que le combat s'engagerait, il retournerait dans la cité pour organiser la résistance. De son côté, la troupe qui se trouvait maintenant sur le terrain devait tuer le plus d'ennemis possible, puis se retirer dans les montagnes. Les soldats connaissaient cette vallée mieux que personne et ils pouvaient attaquer les Assyriens par de petites escarmouches, diminuant ainsi la pression du siège.

Les secours arriveraient rapidement, et l'armée assyrienne serait écrasée.

« Nous pouvons résister soixante jours, mais ce ne sera pas nécessaire, dit le gouverneur à Elie.

— Mais il y aura beaucoup de morts.

— Nous sommes tous en présence de la mort. Et personne n'a peur, pas même moi. »

Le gouverneur était étonné de son propre courage. Il ne s'était jamais trouvé à la veille d'une bataille et, à mesure que le combat approchait, il avait dressé des plans pour fuir la cité. Ce matin-là, il avait combiné avec les plus fidèles de ses hommes la meilleure manière de battre en retraite. Il ne pourrait pas aller à Tyr ou à Sidon, parce qu'il serait considéré comme un traître, mais Jézabel l'accueillerait puisqu'elle avait besoin d'hommes de confiance à ses côtés.

Cependant, en foulant le champ de bataille, il percevait dans les yeux des soldats une joie immense — comme s'ils s'étaient entraînés leur vie entière pour un objectif et qu'enfin ce grand moment était arrivé.

« La peur existe jusqu'au moment où survient l'inévitable, dit-il à Elie. Après, nous ne devons plus perdre notre énergie à cause d'elle. »

Elie était troublé. Il ressentait la même chose, bien qu'il eût honte de le reconnaître ; il se souvint de l'excitation de l'enfant au passage de la troupe.

« Va-t'en, ordonna le gouverneur. Tu es un étranger, désarmé, et tu n'as pas besoin de combattre pour une idée à laquelle tu ne crois pas. »

Elie demeura immobile.

« Ils vont venir, insista le commandant. Tu n'en reviens pas, mais nous sommes prêts. »

Mais Elie resta là.

Ils regardèrent l'horizon ; pas la moindre poussière, l'armée assyrienne ne bougeait pas.

Les soldats du premier rang tenaient fermement leurs lances pointées en avant ; les archers avaient déjà tendu la corde de leurs arcs pour décocher leurs flèches dès que le commandant en donnerait l'ordre. Des hommes qui s'entraînaient fendaient l'air de leurs épées, pour garder leurs muscles échauffés.

« Tout est prêt, répéta le commandant. Ils vont attaquer. »

Elie nota l'euphorie dans sa voix. Il était sans doute impatient que la bataille commençât ; il voulait lutter et montrer sa bravoure. Assurément, il imaginait les guerriers assyriens, les coups d'épée, les cris et la confusion, il se figurait que les prêtres phéniciens le citeraient en exemple pour son efficacité et son courage.

Le gouverneur interrompit ses pensées :

« Ils ne bougent pas. »

Elie se rappela ce qu'il avait demandé au Seigneur : que le soleil s'arrêtât dans les cieux, comme il l'avait fait pour Josué. Il tenta de converser avec son ange, mais il n'entendit pas sa voix.

Peu à peu, les lanciers baissèrent leurs armes, les archers relâchèrent la tension de leurs arcs, les hommes remirent leurs épées au fourreau. Ce fut le soleil brûlant de midi, et des guerriers s'évanouirent sous l'effet de la chaleur ; pourtant, le détachement se tint prêt jusqu'à la fin de l'après-midi.

Quand le soleil se cacha, les guerriers retournèrent à Akbar. Ils semblaient désappointés d'avoir survécu un jour de plus.

Seul Elie resta au cœur de la vallée. Il marcha sans but quelque temps ; soudain il vit la lumière. L'ange du Seigneur apparut devant lui.

« Dieu a entendu tes prières. Et Il a vu le tourment de ton âme. »

Elie se tourna vers les cieux et remercia des bénédictions.

« Le Seigneur est la source de la gloire et du pouvoir. Il a retenu l'armée assyrienne.

— Non, répliqua l'ange. Tu as dit que le choix devait être le Sien. Et Il a fait le choix pour toi. »

« Partons, dit-il à la femme et à son fils.

— Je ne veux pas m'en aller, répliqua l'enfant. Je suis fier des soldats d'Akbar. »

Sa mère l'obligea à rassembler ses affaires : « Emporte seulement ce que tu peux porter.

— Tu oublies, ma mère, que nous sommes pauvres et que je n'ai pas grand-chose. »

Elie monta à sa chambre. Il en fit le tour du regard, comme si c'était la première et la dernière fois qu'il la voyait ; puis il redescendit et observa la veuve qui rangeait ses encres.

« Merci de m'emmener avec toi, dit-elle. Quand je me suis mariée, j'avais à peine quinze ans, et je ne savais rien de la vie. Nos familles avaient tout arrangé, j'avais été élevée dès l'enfance pour ce moment et soigneusement préparée à assister mon mari en toute circonstance.

— Tu l'aimais ?

— J'ai éduqué mon cœur pour cela. Puisque je n'avais pas le choix, je me suis convaincue que c'était la meilleure voie. Quand j'ai perdu mon mari, je me suis habituée aux jours et aux nuits identiques, et j'ai demandé aux dieux de la Cinquième Montagne — à cette époque je croyais encore en eux — de m'emporter lorsque mon fils serait en âge de vivre seul.

« C'est alors que tu es venu. Je te l'ai déjà dit, et je le répète : à partir de ce jour-là, j'ai découvert la beauté de la vallée, la sombre silhouette des montagnes se projetant sur le ciel, la lune qui change de forme pour que le blé puisse pousser. Souvent, la nuit, pendant que tu dormais, je me promenais dans Akbar, j'écoutais les pleurs des nouveau-nés, les chansons des hommes qui avaient bu après le travail, les pas fermes des sentinelles en haut de la muraille. Combien de fois avais-je vu ce paysage sans remarquer comme il était beau ? Combien de fois avais-je regardé le ciel sans voir sa profondeur ? Combien de fois avais-je entendu les bruits d'Akbar autour de moi sans comprendre qu'ils faisaient partie de ma vie ? J'ai retrouvé une immense envie de vivre. Tu m'as conseillé d'étudier les caractères de Byblos, et je l'ai fait. Je pensais seulement te faire plaisir mais je me suis enthousiasmée pour ce que je faisais et j'ai découvert ceci : *le sens de ma vie était celui que je voulais lui donner.* »

Elie lui caressa les cheveux. C'était la première fois.

« Pourquoi n'as-tu pas toujours été ainsi ? demanda-t-elle.

— Parce que j'avais peur. Mais aujourd'hui, en attendant la bataille, j'ai entendu les paroles du gouverneur et j'ai pensé à toi. La peur va jusqu'où commence l'inévitable ; dès lors, elle n'a plus de sens. Et il ne nous reste que l'espoir de prendre la bonne décision.

— Je suis prête, dit-elle.

— Nous retournerons en Israël. Le Seigneur m'a indiqué ce que je dois faire, et je le ferai. Jézabel sera écartée du pouvoir. »

Elle resta silencieuse. Comme toutes les femmes de Phénicie, elle était fière de sa princesse. Quand ils arriveraient à destination, elle tenterait de le convaincre de changer d'avis.

« Ce sera un long voyage et nous n'aurons pas de repos jusqu'à ce que j'aie fait ce qu'Il m'a demandé, dit Elie, comme s'il devinait sa pensée. Cependant, ton amour sera mon soutien, et aux moments où je serai fatigué des batailles en Son nom, je pourrai me reposer entre tes bras. »

L'enfant s'approcha, un petit sac sur l'épaule. Elie le prit et dit à la femme :

« L'heure est venue. Quand tu traverseras les rues d'Akbar, grave en toi le souvenir de chaque maison, de chaque bruit. Parce que tu ne la reverras jamais.

— Je suis née à Akbar, dit-elle. Et la cité restera toujours dans mon cœur. »

L'enfant entendit, et il se promit que jamais il n'oublierait les paroles de sa mère. Si un jour il pouvait revenir, il verrait la cité comme s'il voyait son visage.

Il faisait nuit lorsque le prêtre arriva au pied de la Cinquième Montagne. Il tenait dans la main droite un bâton et portait un sac dans la gauche.

Il sortit du sac l'huile sacrée et s'en frotta le front et les poignets. Puis, avec le bâton, il dessina sur le sable le taureau et la panthère, symboles du dieu de la Tempête et de la Grande Déesse. Il récita les prières rituelles ; enfin il leva ses bras écartés vers le ciel pour recevoir la révélation divine.

Les dieux se taisaient. Ils avaient dit tout ce qu'ils avaient à dire et maintenant ils n'exigeaient plus que l'accomplissement des rituels. Les prophètes avaient disparu partout dans le monde — sauf en Israël, un pays arriéré, superstitieux, où l'on croyait encore que les hommes peuvent communiquer avec les créateurs de l'Univers.

Il se rappela que, deux générations auparavant, Tyr et Sidon avaient fait du négoce avec un roi de Jérusalem appelé Salomon. Il faisait construire un grand temple et voulait l'orner de ce que le monde offrait de meilleur ; aussi avait-il fait acheter des cèdres de la Phénicie, qu'on appelait Liban. Le roi de Tyr avait fourni le matériau nécessaire et reçu en échange vingt cités de Galilée, mais celles-ci ne lui avaient pas plu. Salomon, alors, l'avait aidé à construire ses premiers navires, et désormais la Phénicie possédait la plus grande flotte commerciale du monde.

A cette époque, Israël était encore une grande nation — bien qu'elle rendît un culte à un dieu unique, dont on ne connaissait même pas le nom et qu'on appelait seulement le « Seigneur ». Une princesse de Sidon avait réussi à faire revenir Salomon à la foi authentique, et il avait édifié un autel aux dieux de la Cinquième Montagne. Les Israélites persistaient à affirmer que le « Seigneur » avait puni le plus sage de leurs rois en faisant en sorte que les guerres l'éloignent du pouvoir.

Mais Jéroboam, qui régna après lui, poursuivit le culte que Salomon avait initié. Il fit faire deux veaux d'or que le peuple d'Israël adorait. C'est alors que les prophètes entrèrent en scène et entreprirent une lutte sans trêve contre le souverain.

Jézabel avait raison : la seule manière de maintenir vivante la foi authentique était de tuer les prophètes. Cette femme douce, élevée dans la tolérance et l'horreur de la guerre, savait qu'il y a un moment où la violence est la seule issue. Le sang qui lui salissait maintenant les mains serait pardonné par les dieux qu'elle servait.

« Bientôt, moi aussi j'aurai du sang sur les mains, dit le prêtre à la montagne silencieuse devant lui. De même que les prophètes sont la malédiction d'Israël, l'écriture est la malédiction de la Phénicie. Elle peut comme eux causer un mal irrémédiable et il faut les arrêter tant que c'est encore possible. Le dieu du Temps ne peut pas nous abandonner maintenant. »

Il était inquiet de ce qui s'était produit le matin ; l'armée ennemie n'avait pas attaqué. Par le passé, le dieu du Temps s'était déjà détourné de la Phénicie, irrité contre ses habitants. En conséquence, le feu des lampes s'était éteint, les brebis et les vaches avaient délaissé leurs petits, le blé et l'orge étaient restés verts. Le dieu Soleil avait envoyé à sa recherche des personnages importants — l'aigle et le dieu de la Tempête — mais en vain. Finalement, la Grande Déesse dépêcha une abeille, qui le découvrit endormi dans un bois et le piqua. Il se réveilla, furieux, et se mit à tout détruire autour de lui. Il fallut s'en emparer et extraire de son âme la haine qui s'y trouvait, puis tout redevint normal.

S'il décidait de se retirer de nouveau, la bataille n'aurait pas lieu. Les Assyriens resteraient à tout jamais à l'entrée de la vallée, et Akbar continuerait d'exister.

« Le courage est la peur qui fait ses prières, dit-il. C'est pour cela que je suis ici ; parce que je ne peux pas fléchir au moment du combat. Je dois montrer aux guerriers d'Akbar qu'il y a une raison de défendre la cité. Ce n'est pas le puits, ce n'est pas le marché, ce n'est pas le palais du gouverneur. Nous allons affronter l'armée assyrienne parce que nous devons donner l'exemple. »

La victoire des Assyriens mettrait fin à tout jamais à la menace de l'alphabet. Les conquérants imposeraient leur langue et leurs coutumes, tout en continuant d'adorer les mêmes dieux sur la Cinquième Montagne ; voilà ce qui importait.

« Plus tard, nos navigateurs emporteront dans d'autres pays les exploits de nos guerriers. Les prêtres se rappelleront leurs noms et le jour où Akbar tenta de résister à l'invasion assyrienne. Les peintres dessineront des caractères égyptiens sur les papyrus, les écrits de Byblos seront morts. Les textes sacrés resteront au seul pouvoir de ceux qui sont nés pour les apprendre. Alors, les générations futures tenteront d'imiter ce que nous avons fait et nous construirons un monde meilleur.

« Mais aujourd'hui, poursuivit-il, nous devons perdre cette bataille. Nous lutterons avec bravoure, mais nous sommes en situation d'infériorité ; et nous mourrons glorieusement. »

A ce moment le prêtre écouta la nuit et comprit qu'il avait raison. Ce silence précédait l'instant d'un combat décisif, mais les habitants d'Akbar l'interprétaient de manière erronée ; ils avaient abaissé leurs lances et se divertissaient au lieu de monter la garde. Ils ne prêtaient pas attention à l'exemple de la nature : les animaux sont silencieux à l'approche du danger.

« Que s'accomplissent les desseins des dieux. Que les cieux ne tombent pas sur la terre, car nous avons fait tout ce qu'il fallait et nous avons obéi à la tradition », ajouta-t-il.

Elie, la femme et l'enfant marchaient sur le chemin qui menait vers Israël ; il n'était pas nécessaire de passer par le campement assyrien, situé au sud.

La pleine lune facilitait leur progression mais, en même temps, elle projetait des ombres étranges et des formes sinistres sur les rochers et les chemins pierreux de la vallée.

Du fond de l'obscurité surgit l'ange du Seigneur. Il tenait une épée de feu dans la main droite.

« Où vas-tu ? demanda-t-il.

— En Israël, répondit Elie.

— Le Seigneur t'a appelé ?

— Je connais déjà le miracle que Dieu attend de moi. Et maintenant je sais où je dois le réaliser.

— Le Seigneur t'a appelé ? » répéta l'ange.

Elie resta silencieux.

« Le Seigneur t'a appelé ? reprit l'ange pour la troisième fois.

— Non.

— Alors retourne d'où tu viens, car tu n'as pas encore accompli ton destin. Le Seigneur ne t'a pas encore appelé.

— Laisse-les au moins partir, ils n'ont rien à faire ici », implora Elie.

Mais l'ange n'était déjà plus là. Elie jeta par terre le sac qu'il portait. Il s'assit au milieu de la route et pleura amèrement.

« Que s'est-il passé ? demandèrent la femme et l'enfant, qui n'avaient rien vu.

— Nous allons retourner, dit-il. Ainsi le veut le Seigneur. »

*

Il ne réussit pas à dormir. Il se réveilla en pleine nuit et sentit une tension dans l'air autour de lui ; un vent méchant soufflait dans les rues, semant la peur et la méfiance.

« Dans l'amour d'une femme j'ai découvert l'amour pour toutes les créatures, priait-il en silence. J'ai besoin d'elle. Je sais que le Seigneur n'oubliera pas que je suis un de Ses instruments, peut-être le plus faible qu'Il ait choisi. Aide-moi, Seigneur, car je dois me reposer tranquille au milieu des batailles. »

Il se rappela le commentaire du gouverneur sur

l'inutilité de la peur. Malgré cela, il ne pouvait trouver le sommeil. « J'ai besoin d'énergie et de calme ; donne-moi le repos tant que c'est possible. »

Il songea à appeler son ange, pour converser un peu avec lui ; mais il risquait d'entendre des choses qu'il ne désirait pas et il changea d'avis. Pour se détendre, il descendit dans la salle ; les sacs que la femme avait préparés pour leur fuite n'étaient même pas défaits.

Il pensa aller jusqu'à la chambre de celle-ci. Il se rappela que le Seigneur avait dit à Moïse avant une bataille : « *L'homme qui aime une femme et ne l'a pas encore reçue, qu'il retourne chez elle, afin que, s'il meurt dans la lutte, ce ne soit pas un autre homme qui la reçoive.* »

Ils n'avaient pas encore cohabité. Mais la nuit avait été épuisante et ce n'était pas le moment.

Il décida de vider les sacs et de ranger chaque chose à sa place. Il découvrit qu'elle avait emporté avec elle, outre les quelques vêtements qu'elle possédait, les instruments dont elle se servait pour dessiner les caractères de Byblos.

Il prit un stylet, mouilla une tablette d'argile et commença à griffonner quelques lettres ; il avait appris à écrire en regardant la femme travailler.

« Que c'est simple et ingénieux ! » pensa-t-il, en essayant de distraire son esprit. Souvent, quand il allait au puits chercher de l'eau, il écoutait les commentaires des femmes : « Les Grecs ont volé notre plus importante invention. » Elie savait que ce n'était pas exact : l'adaptation qu'ils en avaient faite, en introduisant les voyelles, avait transformé l'alphabet en un instrument que les peuples de toutes les nations pourraient utiliser. De surcroît, ils avaient donné à leurs collections de parchemins le nom de *biblia*, en hommage à la cité où était née cette invention.

Les livres grecs étaient rédigés sur des peaux d'animaux. C'était un support bien fragile pour conserver les mots, pensait Elie ; le cuir était moins résistant que les tablettes d'argile, et facile à voler. Quant aux papyrus, ils s'abîmaient au bout d'un certain temps de manipulation, et pouvaient être détruits par l'eau. « Les parchemins et les papyrus sont périssables ; seules les tablettes d'argile sont destinées à durer toujours », songea-t-il.

Si Akbar survivait, il recommanderait au gouverneur de faire consigner l'histoire de son pays et de conserver les tablettes d'argile dans une salle spéciale, afin que les générations futures puissent les consulter. Si jamais les prêtres phéniciens — qui gardaient en mémoire l'histoire de leur peuple — venaient à disparaître un jour, les faits des guerriers et des poètes ne tomberaient pas dans l'oubli.

Il joua ainsi un moment, dessinant les mêmes lettres dans un ordre différent et formant des mots distincts. Il fut émerveillé du résultat. Cette occupation le détendit et il retourna se coucher.

*

Un grand fracas le réveilla peu après ; la porte de sa chambre fut projetée par terre.

« Ce n'est pas un rêve. Ce ne sont pas les armées du Seigneur au combat. »

Des ombres surgissaient de toute part, poussant des cris de déments dans une langue qu'il ne comprenait pas.

« Les Assyriens. »

D'autres portes tombaient, des murs étaient abattus sous de puissants coups de masse, les hurlements des envahisseurs se mêlaient aux appels au secours qui montaient de la place. Il tenta de se lever, mais une ombre le renversa à terre. Un bruit sourd secoua l'étage au-dessous.

« Le feu, pensa Elie. Ils ont mis le feu à la maison. »

« C'est toi ! s'exclama quelqu'un en phénicien. Tu es le chef ! Caché comme un lâche dans la maison d'une femme. »

Elie regarda le visage de celui qui venait de parler ; les flammes illuminaient la pièce, et il put voir un homme avec une longue barbe, en uniforme militaire. Oui, les Assyriens étaient arrivés.

« Vous avez attaqué de nuit ? » demanda-t-il, désorienté.

Mais l'homme ne répondit pas. Elie vit l'éclat des épées sorties de leur fourreau et un guerrier le blessa au bras droit.

Il ferma les yeux ; toute sa vie défila devant lui en une fraction de seconde. Il retourna jouer dans les rues de la cité où il était né, il se rendit pour la première fois à Jérusalem, il sentit l'odeur du bois coupé dans la charpenterie, il fut de nouveau ébloui par l'étendue de la mer et les vêtements que l'on portait dans les cités prospères de la côte. Il se revit parcourant les vallées et les montagnes de la Terre promise, il se rappela qu'il avait connu Jézabel, elle semblait encore une petite fille et elle enchantait tous ceux qui l'approchaient. Il assista de nouveau au massacre des prophètes et entendit la voix du Seigneur qui lui ordonnait de se rendre au désert. Il revit les yeux de la femme qui l'attendait à l'entrée de Sarepta — que ses habitants appelaient Akbar — et comprit qu'il l'avait aimée dès le premier instant. Il gravit encore la Cinquième Montagne, ressuscita un enfant et fut accueilli par le peuple comme un sage et un juste. Il regarda le ciel où les constellations se mouvaient rapidement, s'émerveilla de la lune qui montrait ses quatre phases en même temps, sentit le froid, le chaud, l'automne et le printemps, éprouva encore une fois la pluie et l'éclair de la foudre. Les nuages prirent mille formes différentes et les eaux des rivières coulèrent pour la seconde fois dans le même lit. Il revécut le jour où il avait vu s'installer la première tente assyrienne, puis la deuxième, et d'autres encore, de plus en plus nombreuses, les anges qui allaient et venaient, l'épée de feu sur le chemin d'Israël, les nuits d'insomnie, les dessins sur les tablettes, et...

Il était revenu au présent. Il pensa à ce qui se passait à l'étage au-dessous, il fallait à tout prix sauver la veuve et son fils.

« Au feu ! dit-il aux soldats ennemis. La maison prend feu ! »

Il n'avait pas peur ; son seul souci était pour la

veuve et son fils. Quelqu'un lui poussa la tête contre le sol, et il sentit le goût de la terre dans sa bouche. Il l'embrassa, lui dit combien il l'aimait et expliqua qu'il avait fait son possible pour empêcher cela. Il voulut se libérer de ses assaillants, mais quelqu'un lui maintenait un pied sur la poitrine.

« Elle a dû s'enfuir, pensa-t-il. Ils ne feraient pas de mal à une femme sans défense. »

Un calme profond envahit son cœur. Peut-être le Seigneur s'était-Il rendu compte qu'il n'était pas l'homme de la situation et avait-Il découvert un autre prophète pour sauver Israël du péché. La mort était enfin venue, comme il l'espérait, par le martyre. Il accepta son destin et attendit le coup fatal.

Quelques secondes passèrent ; les guerriers continuaient à vociférer, le sang jaillissait de sa blessure, mais le coup mortel ne venait pas.

« Je vous en prie, tuez-moi vite ! » cria-t-il, convaincu qu'au moins l'un d'eux parlait sa langue.

Personne ne prêta attention à ses paroles. Ils discutaient vivement, comme si une erreur avait été commise. Des soldats se mirent à le frapper et, pour la première fois, Elie constata que l'instinct de survie revenait. Il en fut paniqué.

« Je ne peux pas désirer la vie plus longtemps, pensa-t-il, désespéré. Parce que je ne sortirai pas vivant de cette pièce. »

Mais rien ne se passait. Le monde paraissait s'éterniser dans cette confusion de cris, de bruits et de poussière. Le Seigneur avait peut-être agi comme Il l'avait fait avec Josué, arrêtant le temps en plein milieu du combat.

C'est alors qu'il entendit les cris de la femme en dessous. Dans un effort surhumain, il parvint à repousser un garde et à se lever, mais il fut aussitôt rejeté à terre. Un soldat lui frappa la tête et il s'évanouit.

*

Quelques minutes plus tard, il recouvra ses esprits. Les Assyriens l'avaient traîné dans la rue.

Encore étourdi, il leva la tête : toutes les maisons du quartier étaient en flammes.

« Une femme innocente et sans défense est prisonnière là-dedans ! Sauvez-la ! »

Cris, course, confusion de toutes parts. Il tenta de se redresser mais on le renversa de nouveau.

« Seigneur, Tu peux faire ce que Tu veux de moi, parce que j'ai consacré ma vie et ma mort à Ta cause, pria Elie. Mais sauve celle qui m'a accueilli ! »

Quelqu'un le tira par le bras.

« Viens voir, dit l'officier assyrien qui connaissait sa langue. Tu l'as bien mérité. »

Deux gardes le saisirent et le poussèrent vers la porte. La maison était dévorée par les flammes et le feu illuminait tout alentour. Des cris montaient de tous côtés : un enfant en pleurs, des vieux implorant pardon, des femmes désespérées qui cherchaient leurs enfants. Mais il n'entendait que les appels au secours de celle qui l'avait accueilli.

« Que se passe-t-il ? Il y a une femme et un enfant là-dedans ! Pourquoi leur faites-vous cela ?

— Elle a tenté de cacher le gouverneur d'Akbar.

— Je ne suis pas le gouverneur d'Akbar ! Vous commettez une terrible erreur ! »

L'officier assyrien le poussa sur le seuil. Le toit s'était effondré dans l'incendie, et la femme était à demi ensevelie sous les ruines. Elie n'apercevait que son bras qui s'agitait désespérément. Elle appelait au secours, suppliant qu'on ne la laissât pas brûler vive.

« Pourquoi m'épargner et lui faire cela ? implora-t-il.

— Nous ne t'épargnons pas, nous voulons que tu souffres le plus possible. Notre général est mort lapidé et sans honneur, devant les murailles de la cité. Il venait chercher la vie et il a été condamné à mort. Tu vas connaître le même destin. »

Elie luttait désespérément pour se libérer. Les gardes l'emmenèrent. Ils parcoururent les rues d'Akbar dans une chaleur infernale — les soldats ruisselaient de sueur, et certains semblaient choqués par la scène qu'ils venaient de voir. Elie se débattait et implorait les cieux à grands cris, mais les Assyriens, comme le Seigneur, étaient muets.

Ils allèrent jusqu'au centre de la place. La plupart des édifices de la cité étaient en feu, et le grondement de l'incendie se mêlait aux cris des habitants d'Akbar.

« Heureusement, il y a la mort. »

Combien de fois avait-il pensé cela, depuis ce jour dans l'étable !

Des cadavres — des guerriers d'Akbar, pour la plupart sans uniforme — jonchaient le sol. Des gens couraient dans toutes les directions, ne sachant où ils allaient, ne sachant ce qu'ils cherchaient, poussés par la nécessité de faire semblant d'agir, et de lutter contre la mort et la destruction.

« Où courent-ils ainsi ? pensait-il. Ne voient-ils pas que la cité est aux mains de l'ennemi et qu'ils n'ont nulle part où fuir ? » Tout s'était passé très vite. Les Assyriens avaient profité de leur énorme avantage numérique, et ils avaient réussi à épargner le combat à leurs guerriers. Les soldats d'Akbar avaient été exterminés presque sans lutter.

Au centre de la place, on fit mettre Elie à genoux et on lui attacha les mains. Il n'entendait plus les cris de la femme ; peut-être était-elle morte rapidement, sans connaître la lente torture d'être brûlée vive. Elle était dans les bras du Seigneur. Et elle tenait son fils contre elle.

Un autre groupe de soldats assyriens amenait un prisonnier dont le visage était défiguré par les coups. Elie reconnut pourtant le commandant.

« Vive Akbar ! criait-il. Longue vie à la Phénicie et à ses guerriers qui se battent contre l'ennemi durant le jour ! Mort aux lâches qui attaquent dans l'obscurité ! »

Le commandant eut à peine le temps de terminer sa phrase, l'épée d'un général assyrien s'abattit et sa tête roula à terre.

« Cette fois c'est mon tour, se dit Elie. Je la retrouverai au Paradis, et nous nous promènerons main dans la main. »

C'est alors qu'un homme s'approcha et se mit à discuter avec les officiers. C'était un habitant d'Akbar, un habitué des réunions sur la place. Elie se souvenait qu'il l'avait aidé à résoudre un grave problème avec un voisin.

Les Assyriens discutaient de plus en plus fort, et le montraient du doigt. L'homme s'agenouilla, baisa les pieds de l'un d'entre eux, tendit les mains en direction de la Cinquième Montagne et pleura comme un enfant. La fureur des Assyriens sembla diminuer.

La conversation paraissait interminable. L'homme implorait et ne cessait de pleurer, désignant Elie et la maison où vivait le gouverneur. Les soldats ne semblaient pas satisfaits.

Finalement, l'officier qui parlait sa langue s'approcha :

« Notre espion, dit-il en montrant l'homme, affirme que nous nous trompons. C'est lui qui nous a donné les plans de la cité, et nous pouvons lui faire confiance. Tu n'es pas celui que nous voulions tuer. »

Il poussa Elie du pied et ce dernier tomba à terre.

« Il prétend que tu vas partir en Israël pour renverser la princesse qui a usurpé le trône. C'est vrai ? »

Elie ne répondit pas.

« Dis-moi si c'est vrai, insista l'officier. Et tu pourras t'en aller et retourner chez toi, à temps pour sauver cette femme et son fils.

— Oui, c'est la vérité. »

Peut-être le Seigneur l'avait-Il entendu et l'aiderait-Il à les sauver.

« Nous pourrions t'emmener en captivité à Tyr et à Sidon, poursuivit l'officier. Mais nous avons encore beaucoup de batailles à mener, et tu serais un fardeau. Nous pourrions exiger une rançon, mais à qui ? Tu es un étranger, même dans ton pays. »

De son pied, l'officier lui écrasa le visage.

« Tu n'es d'aucune utilité. Tu ne sers ni aux ennemis, ni aux amis. Tu es comme ta cité ; ce n'est pas la peine de laisser une partie de notre armée ici, pour la maintenir sous notre domination. Quand nous aurons conquis la côte, Akbar sera à nous, de toute façon.

— J'ai une question, dit Elie. Une seule question. »
L'officier le regarda, méfiant.

« Pourquoi avez-vous attaqué de nuit ? Ne savez-vous pas que les guerres se font durant le jour ?

— Nous n'avons pas transgressé la loi. Aucune tradition ne l'interdit, répliqua l'officier. Et nous avons largement eu le temps de reconnaître le terrain. Vous vous souciez tellement de respecter les coutumes que vous avez oublié que les temps changent. »

Sans plus un mot, le groupe le laissa. L'espion s'approcha et lui détacha les mains.

« Je me suis promis qu'un jour je te rendrais ta générosité ; j'ai tenu parole. Quand les Assyriens sont entrés dans le palais, un serviteur les a informés que celui qu'ils cherchaient s'était réfugié dans la maison de la veuve. Le temps qu'ils aillent jusque-là, le véritable gouverneur avait réussi à s'enfuir. »

Elie ne l'écoutait pas. Le feu crépitait de toute part, et les cris s'élevaient toujours.

Au milieu de la confusion, on pouvait remarquer qu'un groupe maintenait la discipline ; obéissant à un ordre invisible, les Assyriens se retiraient en silence.

La bataille d'Akbar était terminée.

*

« Elle est morte, se dit-il. Je ne veux pas y retourner, elle est déjà morte. Ou bien un miracle l'a sauvée, et elle viendra me retrouver. »

Son cœur, cependant, lui commandait de se lever et d'aller jusqu'à la maison où ils habitaient. Elie luttait contre lui-même ; ce n'était pas seulement l'amour d'une femme qui était en jeu à ce moment-là, mais toute sa vie, sa foi dans les desseins du Seigneur, le départ de sa cité natale, l'idée qu'il avait une mission et qu'il était capable de l'accomplir.

Il regarda autour de lui, cherchant une épée pour mettre fin à ses jours, mais les Assyriens avaient emporté toutes les armes d'Akbar. Il pensa se jeter dans les flammes, mais il eut peur de la douleur.

Il resta quelques instants complètement figé. Peu à peu, il retrouva son discernement et put réfléchir à la situation dans laquelle il se trouvait. La femme et son fils avaient sans doute déjà quitté cette terre, mais il devait les enterrer selon la coutume. Œuvrer pour le Seigneur — qu'Il existât ou non — était son seul réconfort en ce moment. Une fois son devoir religieux accompli, il se laisserait aller à la souffrance et au doute.

En outre, il restait une possibilité qu'ils fussent encore en vie. Il ne pouvait pas rester là sans rien faire.

« Je ne veux pas les voir le visage brûlé, la peau détachée de la chair. Leurs âmes se promènent librement dans les cieux. »

Pourtant, il se dirigea vers la maison en suffoquant, aveuglé par la fumée qui l'empêchait de distinguer le chemin. Il put constater peu à peu la situation dans la cité. Bien que les ennemis se fussent déjà retirés, la panique augmentait d'une manière effrayante. Les gens continuaient à errer sans but, pleurant, réclamant aux dieux leurs morts.

Alors qu'il cherchait quelqu'un pour lui demander de l'aide, il ne vit qu'un homme à l'air égaré, en état de choc.

« Mieux vaut y aller directement et ne plus demander d'aide. » Il connaissait Akbar aussi bien que sa ville natale et il réussit à s'orienter, même s'il ne reconnaissait pas la plupart des lieux où il passait d'habitude. Les cris qu'il entendait étaient maintenant plus cohérents. Le peuple commençait à comprendre qu'une tragédie avait eu lieu et qu'il fallait réagir.

« Il y a un blessé ici !

— Nous avons encore besoin d'eau ! Nous n'allons pas pouvoir maîtriser le feu !

— Aidez-moi ! Mon mari est enfermé à l'intérieur ! »

Il atteignit l'endroit où, des mois plus tôt, il avait été reçu et hébergé comme un ami. Une vieille était assise au milieu de la rue, non loin de la maison, complètement nue. Elie voulut lui venir en aide, mais elle le repoussa :

« Elle est en train de mourir, s'écria la vieille. Fais quelque chose ! Ote ce mur qui l'écrase ! » Et elle se mit à pousser des cris hystériques. Elie l'attrapa par les bras et la repoussa, car ses hurlements l'empêchaient d'entendre les gémissements de la femme. Autour de lui tout n'était que désolation — toit et murs s'étant effondrés, il lui était difficile de savoir où exactement il l'avait aperçue pour la dernière fois. Les flammes avaient diminué mais la chaleur était encore insupportable ; il franchit les décombres qui couvraient le sol et gagna l'endroit où auparavant se trouvait la chambre de la femme.

Malgré la confusion au-dehors, il put distinguer un gémissement. C'était sa voix.

Instinctivement, il secoua la poussière de ses vêtements, comme pour arranger son apparence. Il resta silencieux, cherchant à se concentrer. Il entendait le crépitement du feu, les appels au secours de gens enterrés dans les maisons voisines — et il avait envie de leur dire de se taire, car il avait besoin de savoir où se trouvaient la femme et son fils. Très longtemps après, il entendit de nouveau du bruit ; quelqu'un grattait le bois qui se trouvait sous ses pieds.

Il s'agenouilla et commença à creuser comme un fou. Il retourna la terre, les pierres et le bois. Finalement, sa main toucha quelque chose de chaud : c'était du sang.

« Ne meurs pas, je t'en prie, supplia-t-il.

— Laisse les débris sur moi, dit la voix. Je ne veux pas que tu voies mon visage. Va secourir mon fils. »

Il continua à creuser, et la voix répéta :

« Va chercher le corps de mon fils. S'il te plaît, fais ce que je te demande. »

Elie laissa sa tête retomber sur sa poitrine et se mit à pleurer tout bas.

« J'ignore où il est enseveli. Je t'en prie, ne t'en va pas ; je voudrais tant que tu restes avec moi. J'ai besoin que tu m'apprennes à aimer, mon cœur est prêt.

« Avant ton arrivée, j'ai désiré la mort pendant des années. Elle a dû m'entendre et elle est venue me chercher. »

Elle poussa un gémissement. Elie se mordit les lèvres en silence. Quelqu'un lui toucha l'épaule.

Effrayé, il se retourna et vit le gamin. Il était couvert de poussière et de suie, mais il ne semblait pas blessé.

« Où est ma mère ? demanda-t-il.

— Je suis là, mon fils, répondit la voix de sous les ruines. Tu es blessé ? »

L'enfant se mit à pleurer. Elie le prit dans ses bras.

« Tu pleures, mon fils, reprit la voix, plus faiblement. Cesse de pleurer. Ta mère a mis si longtemps à comprendre que la vie a un sens ; j'espère avoir réussi à t'enseigner cela. Dans quel état est la cité où tu es né ? »

Elie et l'enfant étaient calmes, serrés l'un contre l'autre.

« Elle va bien, mentit Elie. Des guerriers sont morts, mais les Assyriens se sont retirés. Ils cherchaient le gouverneur pour venger la mort d'un de leurs généraux. »

De nouveau le silence. Et de nouveau la voix, de plus en plus faible.

« Dis-moi que ma cité est sauve. »

Elie devina qu'elle allait passer d'un instant à l'autre.

« La cité est intacte. Et ton fils va bien.

— Et toi ?

— J'ai survécu. »

Il savait que, par ses mots, il libérait son âme et lui permettait de mourir en paix.

« Dis à mon fils de se mettre à genoux, reprit la femme au bout d'un certain temps. Et je veux que tu me fasses un serment, au nom du Seigneur ton Dieu.

— Ce que tu voudras. Tout ce que tu voudras.

— Un jour, tu m'as dit que le Seigneur était partout, et je l'ai cru. Tu as dit que les âmes n'allaient pas en haut de la Cinquième Montagne, et je l'ai cru aussi. Mais tu ne m'as pas expliqué où elles allaient.

« Voici le serment que je te demande : vous n'allez

pas me pleurer, et vous veillerez l'un sur l'autre — jusqu'à ce que le Seigneur permette à chacun de suivre sa route. A partir de maintenant, mon âme se mêle à tout ce que j'ai connu sur cette terre : je suis la vallée, les montagnes tout autour, la cité, les gens qui marchent dans ses rues. Je suis ses blessés et ses mendiants, ses soldats, ses prêtres, ses commerçants, ses nobles. Je suis le sol que tu foules, et le puits qui étanche la soif de tous. Ne pleurez pas pour moi, car vous n'avez pas de raison d'être tristes. Désormais, je suis Akbar, et la cité est belle. »

Vint le silence de la mort, et le vent cessa de souffler. Elie n'entendait pas les cris au-dehors, ni les flammes qui craquaient dans les maisons voisines ; il n'entendait que le silence, presque palpable tant il était intense.

Alors Elie éloigna l'enfant, déchira ses vêtements et, se tournant vers les cieux, il hurla à pleins poumons :

« Seigneur mon Dieu ! Pour Toi j'ai quitté Israël, et je n'ai pu T'offrir mon sang comme l'ont fait les prophètes restés là-bas. Mes amis m'ont traité de lâche, et mes ennemis, de traître.

« Pour Toi, je n'ai mangé que ce que les corbeaux m'apportaient, et j'ai traversé le désert jusqu'à Sarepta, que ses habitants appellent Akbar. Guidé par Tes mains, j'ai rencontré une femme ; guidé par Toi, mon cœur a appris à l'aimer. Mais à aucun moment je n'ai oublié ma vraie mission ; tous les jours que j'ai passés ici, j'ai toujours été prêt à partir.

« La belle Akbar n'est plus que ruines, et la femme que Tu m'as confiée gît au-dessous. En quoi ai-je péché, Seigneur ? A quel moment me suis-je éloigné de ce que Tu désirais de moi ? Si Tu n'étais pas content de moi, pourquoi ne m'as-Tu pas enlevé à ce monde ? Au contraire, Tu as causé encore une fois le malheur de ceux qui m'avaient aidé et aimé.

« Je ne comprends pas Tes desseins. Je ne vois pas de justice dans Tes actes. Je ne suis pas capable de supporter la souffrance que Tu m'as imposée.

Eloigne-Toi de ma vie, car moi aussi je suis ruines, feu et poussière. »

Au milieu du feu et de la désolation, Elie vit la lumière. Et l'ange du Seigneur apparut.

« Que viens-tu faire ici ? demanda Elie. Ne vois-tu pas qu'il est trop tard ?

— Je suis venu te dire qu'une fois encore le Seigneur a entendu ta prière, et ce que tu demandes te sera accordé. Tu n'écouteras plus ton ange et je ne reviendrai pas te voir tant que tes jours d'épreuves ne seront pas accomplis. »

*

Elie prit l'enfant par la main et ils se mirent à marcher sans but. La fumée, jusque-là dispersée par le vent, se concentrait maintenant dans les rues, rendant l'air irrespirable. « C'est peut-être un rêve, pensa-t-il. C'est peut-être un cauchemar. »

« Tu as menti à ma mère, dit l'enfant. La cité est détruite.

— Quelle importance ? Si elle ne voyait pas ce qui se passait autour d'elle, pourquoi ne pas la laisser mourir heureuse ?

— Parce qu'elle a eu confiance en toi, et elle a dit qu'elle était Akbar. »

Il se blessa le pied dans les débris de verre et de céramique répandus sur le sol ; la douleur lui prouva qu'il n'était pas dans un rêve, que tout, autour de lui, était terriblement réel. Ils parvinrent à gagner la place où — voilà combien de temps ? — le peuple se réunissait et où il aidait les gens à résoudre leurs querelles ; le ciel était doré de la lumière des incendies.

« Je ne veux pas que ma mère soit ce que je vois, insista l'enfant. Tu lui as menti. »

Le gamin parvenait à tenir son serment ; pas une larme ne coulait sur son visage.

« Que puis-je faire ? » se demanda Elie. Son pied saignait, et il décida de se concentrer sur la douleur ; elle l'éloignerait du désespoir.

Il regarda la coupure que l'épée de l'Assyrien avait

faite sur son corps ; elle n'était pas aussi profonde qu'il avait imaginé. Il s'assit avec l'enfant à l'endroit même où il avait été attaché par les ennemis et sauvé par un traître. Les gens ne couraient plus ; ils marchaient lentement au milieu de la fumée, de la poussière et des ruines, tels des morts vivants. On aurait dit des âmes oubliées par les cieux, désormais condamnées à errer éternellement sur la terre. Rien n'avait de sens.

Quelques-uns réagissaient ; on continuait d'entendre les voix de femmes et les ordres contradictoires de soldats qui avaient survécu au massacre. Mais ils étaient peu nombreux et n'obtenaient aucun résultat.

Le grand prêtre avait dit une fois que le monde était le rêve collectif des dieux. Et si, au fond, il avait raison ? Pourrait-il maintenant aider les dieux à se réveiller de ce cauchemar et les endormir de nouveau avec un rêve plus doux ? Quand il avait des visions nocturnes, il se réveillait toujours et se rendormait ; pourquoi la même chose n'arriverait-elle pas aux créateurs de l'univers ?

Il butait sur les morts. Aucun d'eux n'avait plus à se soucier des impôts à payer, des Assyriens qui campaient dans la vallée, des rituels religieux ou de l'existence d'un prophète errant qui, un jour peut-être, leur avait adressé la parole.

« Je ne peux pas rester ici. L'héritage qu'elle m'a laissé est cet enfant, et j'en serai digne, même si c'est la dernière chose que je ferai sur cette terre. »

Péniblement, il se leva, reprit le garçon par la main, et ils se remirent en marche. Des gens pillaient les magasins et les boutiques qui avaient été saccagés. Pour la première fois, Elie tenta de réagir aux événements et leur demanda de ne pas agir ainsi.

Mais ils le bousculaient en disant : « Nous mangeons les restes de ce que le gouverneur a dévoré tout seul. Laisse-nous donc. »

Elie n'avait pas la force de discuter ; il emmena l'enfant hors de la cité et ils avancèrent dans la vallée. Les anges ne reviendraient pas avec leurs épées de feu.

« La pleine lune. »

Loin de la fumée et de la poussière, le clair de lune illuminait la nuit. Quelques heures plus tôt, lorsque Elie avait tenté de quitter la cité en direction de Jérusalem, il avait trouvé son chemin sans difficulté ; la même chose était arrivée aux Assyriens.

L'enfant trébucha sur un corps et poussa un cri. C'était celui du grand prêtre ; il avait les bras et les jambes mutilés mais il était encore vivant et gardait les yeux fixés sur le sommet de la Cinquième Montagne.

« Tu vois, les dieux phéniciens ont remporté la bataille céleste », dit-il avec difficulté mais d'une voix calme. Le sang coulait de sa bouche.

« Laisse-moi mettre fin à ta souffrance, répondit Elie.

— La douleur ne signifie rien auprès de la joie d'avoir accompli mon devoir.

— Ton devoir était-il de détruire une cité d'hommes justes ?

— Une cité ne meurt pas ; seuls meurent ses habitants et les idées qu'ils portaient avec eux. Un jour, d'autres viendront à Akbar, ils boiront son eau, et la pierre de son fondateur sera polie et gardée par de nouveaux prêtres. Va-t'en, ma douleur prendra fin bientôt, tandis que ton désespoir durera le reste de ta vie. »

Le corps mutilé respirait avec difficulté, et Elie le laissa. A cet instant, un groupe de gens — hommes, femmes et enfants — accourut vers lui et l'entoura.

« C'est toi ! criaient-ils. Tu as déshonoré ton pays, et tu as apporté la malédiction sur notre cité !

— Que les dieux en soient témoins ! Qu'ils sachent qui est le coupable ! »

Les hommes le bousculaient et le secouaient par les épaules. L'enfant se protégea de ses mains et disparut. Les gens frappaient Elie au visage, sur la poitrine, dans le dos, mais lui ne pensait qu'à l'enfant ; il n'avait même pas réussi à le garder près de lui.

La correction ne dura pas très longtemps ; peut-être étaient-ils tous fatigués de tant de violence. Elie tomba à terre.

« Va-t'en d'ici ! lança quelqu'un. Tu as rétribué notre amour de ta haine ! »

Le groupe s'éloigna. Il n'avait pas la force de se relever. Quand il parvint à se remettre de la honte éprouvée, il n'était plus le même homme. Il ne voulait ni mourir, ni continuer à vivre. Il ne voulait rien : il n'avait ni amour, ni haine, ni foi.

*

Il fut réveillé par le contact d'une main sur son visage. Il faisait encore nuit mais la lune n'était plus dans le ciel.

« J'ai promis à ma mère que je veillerais sur toi, dit le gamin. Mais je ne sais pas quoi faire.

— Retourne dans la cité. Les gens sont bons et quelqu'un t'accueillera.

— Tu es blessé. Je dois soigner ton bras. Peut-être qu'un ange apparaîtra et me dira quoi faire.

— Tu es ignorant, tu ne sais rien de ce qui se passe ! s'écria Elie. Les anges ne reviendront plus, parce que nous sommes des gens ordinaires, et tout le monde est faible devant la souffrance. Quand surviennent les tragédies, les gens ordinaires doivent se débrouiller par leurs propres moyens ! »

Il respira profondément et tenta de se calmer ; cela n'avançait à rien de discuter.

« Comment es-tu arrivé jusqu'ici ?

— Je ne suis pas parti.

— Alors tu as vu ma honte. Tu as vu que je n'avais plus rien à faire à Akbar.

— Tu m'as dit que toutes les batailles servaient à quelque chose, même celles que nous perdons. »

Il se souvenait de la promenade au puits, le matin précédent. Mais il lui semblait que des années s'étaient écoulées depuis, et il avait envie de rétorquer que les belles paroles ne signifient rien lorsqu'on est confronté à la souffrance ; pourtant il préféra ne pas effrayer le gamin par ces paroles.

« Comment as-tu échappé à l'incendie ? »

L'enfant baissa la tête.

« Je ne dormais pas. J'avais décidé de passer la

nuit éveillé pour savoir si tu irais retrouver ma mère dans sa chambre. J'ai vu quand les premiers soldats sont entrés. »

Elie se leva et se mit en marche. Il cherchait le rocher, devant la Cinquième Montagne, où, un après-midi, il avait assisté au coucher du soleil avec la femme.

« Je ne dois pas y aller, pensa-t-il. Je serai encore plus désespéré. »

Mais une force l'attirait dans cette direction. Une fois arrivé, il pleura amèrement ; comme la cité d'Akbar, l'endroit était marqué par une pierre — mais il était le seul, dans toute cette vallée, à en comprendre la signification ; elle ne serait pas honorée par de nouveaux habitants, ni polie par des couples découvrant le sens de leur amour.

Il prit l'enfant dans ses bras et s'endormit.

« J'ai soif et j'ai faim, dit l'enfant à Elie, à peine éveillé.

— Nous pouvons aller chez des bergers qui vivent près d'ici. Rien n'a dû leur arriver parce qu'ils n'habitaient pas à Akbar.

— Nous devons restaurer la cité. Ma mère a dit qu'elle était Akbar. »

Quelle cité ? Il n'y avait plus de palais, ni de marché, ni de murailles. Les gens de bien s'étaient transformés en brigands, et les jeunes soldats avaient été massacrés. Les anges ne reviendraient plus — mais c'était le cadet de ses soucis.

« Tu trouves que la destruction, la douleur, les morts de la nuit dernière ont un sens ? Tu penses qu'il faut anéantir des milliers de vies pour enseigner à quelqu'un ta façon de voir les choses ? »

Le gamin le regarda d'un air épouvanté.

« Oublie ce que je viens de dire, dit Elie. Allons trouver le berger.

— Et allons restaurer la cité », insista l'enfant.

lie ne répondit pas. Il savait qu'il ne parviendrait plus à imposer son autorité au peuple qui l'accusait d'avoir apporté le malheur. Le gouverneur s'était enfui, le commandant était mort, Tyr et Sidon tomberaient probablement bientôt sous la domination étrangère. La femme avait peut-être raison ; les dieux changeaient toujours — et cette fois c'était le Seigneur qui était parti.

« Quand retournerons-nous là-bas ? » interrogea de nouveau l'enfant.

Elie le prit par les épaules et se mit à le secouer violemment.

« Regarde derrière toi ! Tu n'es pas un ange aveugle, mais un gamin désireux de surveiller ce que faisait sa mère. Qu'est-ce que tu vois ? Tu as remarqué les colonnes de fumée qui montent dans le ciel ? Tu sais ce que cela signifie ?

— Tu me fais mal ! Je veux partir d'ici, je veux m'en aller ! »

Elie s'arrêta, effrayé par sa propre attitude : jamais il n'avait agi de la sorte. L'enfant s'écarta et se mit à courir en direction de la cité. Il parvint à le rattraper et s'agenouilla devant lui.

« Pardonne-moi. Je ne sais pas ce que je fais. »

Le gamin sanglotait, mais pas une larme ne coulait sur son visage. Il s'assit près de lui, en attendant qu'il se calme.

« Ne pars pas, demanda-t-il. Avant que ta mère ne s'en aille, je lui ai promis de rester avec toi jusqu'à ce que tu puisses suivre ton propre chemin.

— Tu as promis aussi que la cité était intacte. Et elle a dit...

— Inutile de le répéter. Je suis honteux, perdu dans ma propre faute. Laisse-moi me retrouver. Excuse-moi, je ne voulais pas te blesser. »

Le gamin le serra dans ses bras. Mais pas une larme ne roula de ses yeux.

*

Ils atteignirent la maison au cœur de la vallée ; une femme se tenait près de la porte et deux petits enfants jouaient devant. Le troupeau était dans l'enclos — ce qui signifiait que le berger n'était pas parti dans les montagnes ce matin-là.

La femme regarda d'un air effrayé l'homme et l'enfant qui marchaient à sa rencontre. Elle eut instinctivement envie de les chasser, mais la tradition — et les dieux — exigeaient qu'elle obéît à la loi universelle de l'hospitalité. Si elle ne les accueillait pas maintenant, un malheur semblable pourrait arriver plus tard à ses enfants.

« Je n'ai pas d'argent, dit-elle. Mais je peux vous donner un peu d'eau et de nourriture. »

Ils s'assirent sur la petite terrasse ombragée par un toit de paille, et elle apporta des fruits secs accompagnés d'un broc d'eau. Ils mangèrent en silence, retrouvant un peu, pour la première fois depuis la nuit précédente, leurs gestes quotidiens. Les enfants, épouvantés par l'aspect des nouveaux venus, s'étaient réfugiés à l'intérieur de la maison.

Son repas terminé, Elie s'enquit du berger.

« Il ne va pas tarder, répondit-elle. Nous avons entendu un grand vacarme, et ce matin quelqu'un est venu nous dire qu'Akbar avait été détruite. Il est parti voir ce qui s'était passé. »

Les enfants l'appelèrent et elle rentra.

« Inutile de chercher à convaincre le gamin, pensa Elie. Tant que je n'aurai pas fait ce qu'il demande, il ne me laissera pas en paix. C'est à moi de lui montrer que c'est impossible. »

La nourriture et l'eau faisaient des miracles ; il se sentait de nouveau faire partie du monde. Ses pensées coulaient avec une incroyable rapidité, cherchant des solutions plutôt que des réponses.

*

Quelque temps après, le berger arriva. Inquiet pour la sécurité de sa famille, il considéra avec crainte l'homme et l'enfant. Mais il comprit bien vite la situation.

« Vous êtes sans doute des réfugiés d'Akbar, dit-il. J'en reviens.

— Que se passe-t-il ? demanda le gamin.

— La cité a été détruite et le gouverneur est en fuite. Les dieux ont désorganisé le monde.

— Nous avons tout perdu, expliqua Elie. Nous aimerions que vous nous accueilliez.

— Ma femme vous a déjà accueillis et nourris. Maintenant, vous devez partir et affronter l'inévitable.

— Je ne sais pas quoi faire de l'enfant. J'ai besoin d'aide.

— Mais si, tu sais. Il est jeune, il a l'air intelligent et il est plein d'énergie. Et toi, tu as l'expérience d'un homme qui a connu beaucoup de victoires et de défaites dans cette vie. C'est une combinaison parfaite car elle peut t'aider à trouver la sagesse. »

Regardant la blessure au bras d'Elie, le berger affirma qu'elle n'était pas grave ; il alla chercher dans la maison des herbes et un morceau de tissu. Le gamin l'aida à maintenir en place le cataplasme. Quand le berger lui fit remarquer qu'il pouvait y arriver tout seul, l'enfant rétorqua qu'il avait promis à sa mère de veiller sur cet homme.

Le berger rit.

« Ton fils est un homme de parole.

— Je ne suis pas son fils. Et lui aussi est un homme de parole. Il va reconstruire la cité parce qu'il doit faire revenir ma mère, tout comme il l'a fait avec moi. »

Elie comprit soudain ce qui préoccupait l'enfant, mais avant qu'il ait pu dire un mot, le berger cria à sa femme qui, à ce moment précis, sortait de la maison, qu'il allait repartir. « Mieux vaut reconstruire la vie sans attendre, déclara-t-il. Cela prendra longtemps pour que tout redevienne comme avant.

— Rien ne sera jamais comme avant.

— Tu sembles être un jeune homme sage, et tu peux comprendre bien des choses que je ne comprends pas. Mais la nature m'a enseigné une leçon que je n'oublierai jamais : un homme qui dépend du temps et des saisons, comme seul en dépend un berger, peut survivre aux événements inévitables. Il soigne son troupeau, traite chaque animal comme s'il était unique, cherche à aider les mères et les petits, ne s'éloigne jamais trop d'un endroit où les bêtes peuvent boire. Cependant, une fois de temps en temps, une brebis à laquelle il a consacré tant d'efforts finit par mourir dans un accident, causé par un serpent, un animal sauvage, ou même une chute dans un précipice. L'inévitable se produit toujours. »

Elie regarda en direction d'Akbar et se rappela la conversation avec l'ange. L'inévitable survient toujours.

« Il faut de la discipline et de la patience pour le surmonter, ajouta le berger.

— Et de l'espoir. Quand l'espoir n'existe plus, il ne faut pas gâcher son énergie à lutter contre l'impossible.

— Ce n'est pas une question d'espoir dans l'avenir. Il s'agit de recréer le passé lui-même. »

Le berger n'était plus pressé, son cœur s'était empli de pitié pour ces réfugiés. Puisque lui et sa famille avaient été épargnés par la tragédie, ça ne lui coûtait rien de leur venir en aide — et de plaire ainsi aux dieux. En outre, il avait entendu parler du prophète israélite qui avait gravi la Cinquième Montagne sans être atteint par le feu du ciel ; tout indiquait que c'était cet homme qui se tenait devant lui.

« Vous pouvez rester un jour de plus, si vous voulez.

— Je n'ai pas compris ce que tu viens de dire, remarqua Elie. A propos de recréer le passé lui-même.

— J'ai toujours vu les gens qui passaient par ici pour aller à Tyr et à Sidon. Certains se plaignaient de n'avoir rien réussi à Akbar, et ils étaient à la recherche d'une nouvelle destinée. Un jour, ces gens revenaient. Ils n'avaient pas trouvé ce qu'ils cherchaient, parce qu'ils avaient emporté avec eux, outre leurs bagages, le poids de leur échec passé. L'un ou l'autre rentrait avec un emploi au gouvernement, ou la joie d'avoir donné une meilleure éducation à ses enfants — mais rien de plus, parce que le passé à

Akbar les avait rendus craintifs, et ils n'avaient pas suffisamment confiance en eux pour prendre des risques.

« Et puis, sont passés aussi devant ma porte des gens pleins d'enthousiasme. Ils avaient profité de chaque minute de leur existence à Akbar et gagné — avec beaucoup d'efforts — l'argent nécessaire au voyage qu'ils voulaient entreprendre. Pour eux, la vie était une victoire permanente, et elle continuerait de l'être. Eux aussi revenaient, mais avec des histoires merveilleuses. Ils avaient conquis tout ce qu'ils désiraient parce qu'ils n'étaient pas limités par les frustrations du passé. »

*

Les propos du berger touchaient le cœur d'Elie.

« Il n'est pas difficile de reconstruire une vie, de même qu'il n'est pas impossible de relever Akbar de ses ruines, poursuivit le berger. Il suffit pour cela d'avoir conscience que nous avons la même force qu'auparavant, et de nous en servir à notre avantage. »

L'homme le regarda dans les yeux.

« Si tu as un passé dont tu n'es pas satisfait, oublie-le maintenant. Imagine une nouvelle histoire pour ta vie et crois en elle. Concentre-toi seulement sur les moments où tu as réussi ce que tu désirais — et cette force t'aidera à obtenir ce que tu veux. »

« A une époque j'ai désiré être charpentier, ensuite j'ai voulu être un prophète envoyé pour le salut d'Israël, pensa Elie. Les anges descendaient des cieux, et le Seigneur me parlait. Et puis j'ai compris qu'Il n'était pas juste et que Ses motifs seraient toujours au-delà de mon entendement. »

Le berger cria à sa femme qu'il n'allait pas repartir — tout compte fait, il était déjà allé à pied jusqu'à Akbar et il n'avait pas le courage de refaire le chemin.

« Merci de nous accueillir, dit Elie.

— Ça ne coûte rien de vous abriter pour une nuit. »

148

L'enfant intervint dans la conversation :

« Nous voulons retourner à Akbar.

— Attendez jusqu'à demain. Les habitants de la cité sont en train de la saccager, et il n'y a nulle part où dormir. »

Le gamin regarda le sol, se mordit les lèvres et, une fois de plus, se retint de pleurer. Le berger les conduisit à l'intérieur, rassura sa femme et ses enfants et passa le reste de la journée à parler du temps pour les distraire tous les deux.

Le lendemain, ils se réveillèrent tôt, prirent un repas que leur avait préparé la femme du berger et allèrent jusqu'à la porte de la maison.

« Je te souhaite longue vie et prospérité à ton troupeau, dit Elie. J'ai mangé ce dont mon corps avait besoin, et mon âme a appris ce que j'ignorais encore. Que Dieu n'oublie jamais ce que vous avez fait pour nous, et que vos enfants ne soient jamais des étrangers sur une terre étrangère.

— Je ne sais à quel Dieu tu fais allusion ; ils sont nombreux, les habitants de la Cinquième Montagne », dit le berger durement. Puis aussitôt, changeant de ton : « Rappelle-toi les bonnes choses que tu as réalisées. Elles te donneront du courage.

— J'en ai fait bien peu, et aucune grâce à mes qualités.

— Alors il est temps de faire davantage.

— J'aurais peut-être pu éviter l'invasion. »

Le berger rit :

« Même si tu avais été le gouverneur d'Akbar, tu n'aurais pas pu empêcher l'inévitable.

— Le gouverneur aurait peut-être dû attaquer les Assyriens quand ils sont arrivés dans la vallée avec quelques troupes. Ou négocier la paix avant que la guerre n'éclate.

— Tout ce qui aurait pu arriver mais n'est pas arrivé, le vent l'emporte et il n'en reste nulle trace, dit le berger. La vie est faite de nos attitudes. *Et il est des choses que les dieux nous obligent à vivre.* Peu importe la raison qui est la leur, et faire tout notre possible pour les éviter ne sert à rien.

— Pourquoi ?

— Demande à un prophète israélite qui vivait à Akbar. Il paraît qu'il a réponse à tout. »

L'homme se dirigea vers l'enclos. « Je dois mener mon troupeau au pâturage. Hier, les bêtes ne sont pas sorties et elles sont impatientes. »

Il prit congé d'un signe de tête et s'éloigna avec ses brebis.

L'enfant et l'homme avançaient dans la vallée.

« Tu marches lentement, disait le gamin. Tu as peur de ce qui pourra t'arriver.

— Je n'ai peur que de moi, répondit Elie. Ils ne peuvent rien me faire, car mon cœur n'existe plus.

— Le Dieu qui m'a fait revenir de la mort est encore vivant. Il peut ramener ma mère, si tu accomplis la même chose pour la cité.

— Oublie ce Dieu. Il est loin, et Il ne réalise plus les miracles que nous attendons de Lui. »

Le berger avait raison. Désormais, il fallait reconstruire son propre passé, oublier qu'un jour on jugerait un prophète qui devait libérer Israël mais qui avait échoué dans sa mission de sauver une simple cité.

Cette pensée lui procura un étrange sentiment d'euphorie. Pour la première fois de sa vie, il se sentit libre, prêt à faire ce qu'il voulait, quand il voulait. Il n'entendrait plus les anges, mais en contrepartie il était libre de retourner en Israël, de reprendre son travail de charpentier, de voyager jusqu'en Grèce pour y suivre l'enseignement des sages, ou de gagner avec les navigateurs phéniciens les contrées de l'autre côté de la mer.

Mais auparavant, il devait se venger. Il avait consacré les meilleures années de sa jeunesse à un Dieu sourd qui lui donnait sans cesse des ordres tout en faisant toujours les choses à Sa manière. Il avait appris à accepter Ses décisions et à respecter Ses desseins. Mais sa fidélité avait été récompensée par l'abandon, son dévouement ignoré, ses efforts pour accomplir la Volonté suprême avaient abouti à la mort de la seule femme qu'il avait aimée dans sa vie.

« Tu as toute la force du monde et des étoiles », dit Elie dans sa langue natale, afin que l'enfant ne comprît pas le sens de ses paroles. « Tu peux détruire une cité, un pays, comme nous détruisons les insectes. Alors, envoie le feu du ciel et mets fin à mes jours tout de suite, sinon j'irai contre Ton œuvre. »

Akbar apparut au loin. Il prit la main du gamin et la serra de toutes ses forces.

« Désormais, jusqu'à ce que nous franchissions les portes de la cité, je marcherai les yeux fermés ; il faut que tu me guides, dit-il à l'enfant. Si je meurs en cours de route, fais ce que tu m'as demandé de faire : reconstruis Akbar, même si pour cela il te faut d'abord grandir, puis apprendre à couper le bois ou à tailler la pierre. »

L'enfant resta silencieux. Elie ferma les yeux et se laissa guider. Il écoutait le bruit du vent et le son de ses pas sur le sable.

Il se rappela Moïse. Après qu'il eut libéré et conduit le peuple élu dans le désert, surmontant d'énormes difficultés, Dieu l'avait empêché d'entrer en Canaan. Alors, Moïse avait dit : « *Permets que je passe de l'autre côté, et que je voie le bon pays qui est au-delà du Jourdain.* »

Mais le Seigneur s'était indigné de sa requête. Et il avait répondu : « *Assez. Cesse de me parler de cela. Lève les yeux vers l'ouest et vers le nord, vers le sud et vers l'est ; regarde de tous tes yeux car tu ne passeras pas le Jourdain que voici.* »

Ainsi le Seigneur avait-il récompensé Moïse pour

sa longue et rude tâche : il ne lui avait pas permis de poser le pied en Terre promise. Que serait-il arrivé s'il avait désobéi ?

Elie tourna de nouveau sa pensée vers les cieux.

« Seigneur, cette bataille n'a pas eu lieu entre les Assyriens et les Phéniciens, mais entre Toi et moi. Tu ne m'as pas averti de notre guerre singulière et — comme toujours — Tu as gagné et fait accomplir Ta volonté. Tu as détruit la femme que j'ai aimée et la cité qui m'a accueilli quand j'étais loin de ma patrie. »

Le vent souffla plus fort à ses oreilles. Elie eut peur, mais il continua :

« Il m'est impossible de faire revenir la femme, mais je peux changer le destin de Ton œuvre de destruction. Moïse a accepté Ta volonté, et il n'a pas franchi le fleuve. Moi, je poursuivrai : tue-moi sur-le-champ, car, si Tu me laisses arriver jusqu'aux portes de la cité, je reconstruirai ce que Tu as voulu faire disparaître de la surface de la terre. Et j'irai contre Ta décision. »

Il se tut. Il fit le vide dans son esprit et attendit la mort. Pendant très longtemps, il se concentra seulement sur le son des pas dans le sable ; il ne voulait pas entendre la voix des anges ou les menaces du Ciel. Son cœur était libre et il n'avait plus peur de ce qui pourrait lui arriver. Cependant, dans les profondeurs de son âme, quelque chose commença à le perturber — comme s'il avait oublié un élément d'importance.

Longtemps après, l'enfant s'arrêta et secoua le bras d'Elie.

« Nous sommes arrivés », dit-il.

Il ouvrit les yeux. Le feu du ciel n'était pas descendu sur lui et les murailles en ruine d'Akbar l'entouraient.

*

Il regarda l'enfant qui lui tenait les mains comme s'il craignait qu'il ne s'échappât. L'aimait-il ? Il l'ignorait. Mais ces réflexions pouvaient être remises à

plus tard ; il avait maintenant une tâche à accomplir
— la première depuis des années qui ne lui fût pas
imposée par Dieu.

De là où ils se tenaient, ils pouvaient sentir l'odeur
de brûlé. Des charognards tournoyaient dans le ciel,
attendant le moment propice pour dévorer les
cadavres de sentinelles qui pourrissaient sur le sol.
Elie prit l'épée à la ceinture d'un soldat mort. Dans
la confusion de la nuit précédente, les Assyriens
avaient oublié de ramasser les armes qui se trouvaient hors de la cité.

« Pourquoi prends-tu cette épée ? demanda
l'enfant.

— Pour me défendre.

— Les Assyriens sont partis.

— Il est tout de même bon d'en avoir une sur moi.
Nous devons nous tenir prêts. »

Sa voix tremblait. Il était impossible de savoir ce
qui se passerait lorsqu'ils franchiraient la muraille à
moitié démolie, mais il était prêt à tuer quiconque
tenterait de l'humilier.

« J'ai été détruit comme cette cité, dit-il à l'enfant.
Mais, de même que cette cité, je n'ai pas encore terminé ma mission. »

Le gamin sourit.

« Tu parles comme autrefois, dit-il.

— Ne te laisse pas abuser par les mots. Avant,
j'avais l'objectif de chasser du trône Jézabel et de
rendre Israël au Seigneur, mais maintenant qu'Il
nous a oubliés, nous aussi nous devons L'oublier. Ma
mission consiste à accomplir ce que tu me
demandes. »

L'enfant le regarda, méfiant :

« Sans Dieu, ma mère ne reviendra pas d'entre les
morts. »

Elie lui caressa la tête.

« Seul le corps de ta mère s'en est allé. Elle est toujours parmi nous et, comme elle nous l'a dit, elle est
Akbar. Nous devons l'aider à retrouver sa beauté. »

*

La cité était quasi déserte. Des vieux, des femmes et des enfants erraient dans les rues — répétant la scène qu'il avait vue durant la nuit de l'invasion. Ils semblaient ne pas savoir quoi faire, quoi décider.

Chaque fois qu'ils croisaient quelqu'un, l'enfant remarquait qu'Elie serrait de toutes ses forces la poignée de l'épée. Mais les gens leur manifestaient de l'indifférence : la plupart reconnaissaient le prophète d'Israël, certains le saluaient de la tête, et personne ne lui adressait la moindre parole — même de haine.

« Ils ont perdu jusqu'au sentiment de la colère », pensa-t-il, regardant vers la Cinquième Montagne, dont le sommet restait couvert de ses éternels nuages. Alors il se rappela les paroles du Seigneur :

« Je jetterai vos cadavres sur les cadavres de vos dieux ; mon âme se lassera de vous. Votre pays sera dévasté et vos cités seront désertées.

Et ceux d'entre vous qui resteront, je leur mettrai dans le cœur une telle anxiété que le bruit d'une feuille qui bouge les poursuivra.

Et ils tomberont sans que personne ne les poursuive. »

« Voilà ce que Tu as fait, Seigneur : Tu as tenu Ta parole, et les morts vivants continuent d'errer sur la terre. Et Akbar est la cité choisie pour les abriter. »

Ils gagnèrent tous deux la place principale, s'assirent sur des décombres et regardèrent alentour. La destruction semblait avoir été plus rigoureuse et implacable qu'il ne l'avait pensé ; la plupart des toits s'étaient écroulés, la saleté et les insectes prenaient possession de tout.

« Il faut enlever les morts, dit-il. Ou bien la peste entrera dans la cité par la grande porte. »

L'enfant gardait les yeux baissés.

« Lève la tête, dit Elie. Nous devons beaucoup travailler pour que ta mère soit contente. »

Mais le gamin n'obéit pas ; il commençait à comprendre que, quelque part dans ces ruines, se trouvait le corps qui lui avait donné la vie, et que ce corps était dans le même état que tous les autres épars autour de lui.

Elie n'insista pas. Il se leva, prit un cadavre sur ses épaules et le porta au centre de la place. Il ne parvenait pas à se rappeler les recommandations du Seigneur sur l'enterrement des morts ; tout ce qu'il devait faire, c'était empêcher que ne survînt la peste, et la seule solution était de les incinérer.

Il travailla ainsi toute la matinée. L'enfant ne quitta pas cet endroit et ne leva pas les yeux un instant, mais il tint la promesse qu'il avait faite à sa mère : pas une larme ne tomba sur le sol d'Akbar.

Une femme s'arrêta et resta un moment à observer l'activité d'Elie.

« L'homme qui résolvait les problèmes des vivants débarrasse les corps des morts, remarqua-t-elle.

— Où sont donc les hommes d'Akbar ? demanda Elie.

— Ils sont partis et ont emporté le peu qui restait. Il n'y a plus rien qui vaille la peine de s'attarder ici. Les seuls à n'avoir pas quitté la cité sont ceux qui étaient incapables de le faire : les vieux, les veuves et les orphelins.

— Mais ils étaient ici depuis des générations ! On ne peut pas renoncer aussi facilement.

— Essaie d'expliquer cela à quelqu'un qui a tout perdu.

— Aide-moi, dit Elie tout en prenant un des corps sur son dos puis en le mettant sur le tas. Nous allons les incinérer pour que le dieu de la peste ne vienne pas nous rendre visite. Il a horreur de l'odeur de la chair qui brûle.

— Que vienne le dieu de la peste, répliqua la femme. Et qu'il nous emporte tous, le plus vite possible. »

Elie continua son travail. La femme s'assit à côté

de l'enfant et le regarda faire. Quelque temps après, elle s'approcha de nouveau.

« Pourquoi désires-tu sauver une cité condamnée ?

— Si je m'arrête pour réfléchir, je me retrouverai incapable d'agir comme je le veux », répondit-il.

Le vieux berger avait raison : oublier son passé d'incertitudes et se créer une nouvelle histoire était la seule issue. L'ancien prophète était mort avec la femme dans l'incendie de sa maison ; maintenant, il était un homme sans foi en Dieu, habité de nombreux doutes. Mais il était en vie, même après avoir bravé la malédiction divine. S'il voulait poursuivre sa route, il devait suivre ses conseils.

La femme choisit un corps plus léger et le traîna par les pieds jusqu'au tas qu'Elie avait commencé.

« Ce n'est pas par peur du dieu de la peste, dit-elle. Ni pour Akbar, puisque les Assyriens reviendront bientôt. C'est pour le gamin assis là, tête basse ; il doit comprendre qu'il a encore la vie devant lui.

— Merci, dit Elie.

— Ne me remercie pas. Quelque part dans ces ruines, nous trouverons le corps de mon fils. Il avait à peu près le même âge que ce gamin. »

Elle mit sa main sur son visage et pleura abondamment. Elie la prit délicatement par le bras.

« La douleur que toi et moi ressentons ne passera jamais, mais le travail nous aidera à la supporter. La souffrance n'a pas la force de meurtrir un corps fatigué. »

Ils consacrèrent la journée entière à cette tâche macabre, ramasser et empiler les morts ; la plupart étaient des jeunes gens que les Assyriens avaient pris pour des membres de l'armée d'Akbar. Mais plus d'une fois il reconnut des amis, et il pleura, sans toutefois interrompre sa besogne.

*

A la fin de l'après-midi, ils étaient épuisés. Pourtant, le travail réalisé était loin de suffire ; et aucun autre habitant d'Akbar ne leur avait prêté main-forte.

Ils revinrent tous les deux près de l'enfant. Pour la première fois, il leva la tête.

« J'ai faim, dit-il.

— Je vais chercher quelque chose, répondit la femme. Il y a suffisamment de nourriture cachée dans les habitations d'Akbar : les gens s'étaient préparés à un siège prolongé.

— Apporte de la nourriture pour toi et moi, parce que nous prenons soin de la cité à la sueur de notre front, répliqua Elie. Mais si ce petit veut manger, il devra se débrouiller tout seul. »

La femme comprit ; elle aurait agi de la même manière avec son fils. Elle se rendit jusqu'à l'endroit où auparavant s'élevait sa maison ; les pillards avaient quasiment tout retourné à la recherche d'objets de valeur, et sa collection de vases, créés par les grands maîtres verriers d'Akbar, gisait en morceaux sur le sol. Mais elle trouva les fruits secs et la farine qu'elle avait stockés.

Elle retourna sur la place et partagea sa nourriture avec Elie. L'enfant ne dit rien.

Un vieux s'approcha :

« J'ai vu que vous aviez passé la journée entière à ramasser les corps. Vous perdez votre temps. Ne savez-vous pas que les Assyriens reviendront, une fois Tyr et Sidon conquises ? Que le dieu de la peste vienne donc s'installer ici, pour les détruire aussi.

— Nous ne faisons pas cela pour eux, ni pour nous-mêmes, répliqua Elie. Elle travaille dans le but d'enseigner à un enfant qu'il existe un avenir. Et moi, je le fais pour montrer qu'un passé n'est plus.

— Ainsi, le prophète n'est plus une menace pour la grande princesse de Tyr : quelle surprise ! Jézabel gouvernera Israël jusqu'à la fin de ses jours, et nous aurons toujours un endroit où nous réfugier, si les Assyriens ne sont pas généreux avec les vaincus. »

Elie resta silencieux. Le nom qui autrefois lui inspirait tant de haine sonnait maintenant d'une manière étrangement lointaine.

« Akbar sera reconstruite, de toute façon, insista le vieillard. Ce sont les dieux qui choisissent les lieux où l'on élève les cités, et ils ne vont pas l'abandonner ; mais nous pouvons laisser ce travail aux générations futures.

— Nous pouvons. Mais nous n'allons pas le faire. »

Elie tourna le dos au vieil homme, mettant fin à la conversation.

*

Ils dormirent tous les trois à la belle étoile. La femme prit l'enfant dans ses bras et remarqua que la faim faisait gronder son estomac. Elle pensa lui donner un peu de nourriture ; mais elle changea aussitôt d'avis : la fatigue physique diminuait réellement la douleur, et cet enfant, qui paraissait souffrir beaucoup, devait s'occuper à quelque chose. La faim le persuaderait peut-être de travailler.

Le lendemain, Elie et la femme reprirent leur ouvrage. Le vieillard qui s'était approché la veille revint les voir.

« Je n'ai rien à faire et je pourrais vous aider, dit-il. Mais je suis trop faible pour porter les corps.

— Alors, rassemble le petit bois et les briques. Tu nettoieras les cendres. »

Le vieux se mit au travail.

*

Quand le soleil atteignit le zénith, Elie s'assit par terre, épuisé. Il savait que son ange était à ses côtés mais il ne pouvait plus l'entendre. « A quoi bon ? Il a été incapable de m'aider quand j'en avais besoin, maintenant je ne veux pas de ses conseils ; tout ce que je dois faire, c'est laisser cette cité en ordre, montrer à Dieu que je suis capable de L'affronter, et ensuite partir où je le désirerai. »

Jérusalem n'était pas loin, à sept jours de marche seulement, sans passages difficiles, mais là-bas il était recherché comme traître. Il valait peut-être mieux aller à Damas, ou trouver un emploi de scribe dans une cité grecque.

Il sentit qu'on le touchait. Il se retourna et vit l'enfant, un petit vase à la main.

« Je l'ai trouvé dans une maison », dit le gamin, et il le lui tendit.

Il était plein d'eau. Elie but jusqu'à la dernière goutte.

« Mange quelque chose, dit-il. Tu travailles, tu mérites ta récompense. »

Pour la première fois depuis la nuit de l'invasion, un sourire apparut sur les lèvres du gamin, qui se précipita vers l'endroit où la femme avait laissé les fruits et la farine.

Elie se remit au travail ; il entrait dans les maisons en ruine, écartait les décombres, prenait les corps et les portait jusqu'au tas amoncelé au centre de la place. Le pansement que le berger lui avait fait au bras était tombé, mais cela n'avait pas d'importance ; il devait se prouver à lui-même qu'il était assez fort pour reconquérir sa dignité.

Le vieux, qui maintenant rassemblait les ordures répandues sur la place, avait raison ; d'ici peu, les ennemis seraient de retour, récoltant les fruits de ce qu'ils n'avaient pas semé. Elie épargnait du travail aux assassins de la seule femme qu'il avait aimée de toute sa vie, puisque les Assyriens, étant superstitieux, reconstruiraient Akbar de toute manière. D'après leurs croyances, les dieux avaient disposé les cités selon un ordre bien précis, en harmonie avec les vallées, les animaux, les fleuves, les mers. Dans chacune d'elles, ils avaient conservé un lieu sacré où se reposer durant leurs longs voyages de par le monde. Lorsqu'une cité était détruite, il y avait toujours un grand risque que les cieux ne tombent sur la terre.

La légende racontait que le fondateur d'Akbar,

venant du nord, était passé par là, voilà des siècles. Il décida de dormir sur place et, pour marquer l'endroit où il avait laissé ses affaires, il enfonça une baguette de bois dans le sol. Le lendemain, comme il ne réussissait pas à l'arracher, il comprit la volonté de l'univers ; il marqua d'une pierre l'endroit où le miracle s'était produit et découvrit une source non loin de là. Peu à peu, des tribus s'installèrent à proximité de la pierre et du puits : Akbar était née.

Le gouverneur avait expliqué une fois à Elie que, selon la tradition phénicienne, toute cité était le *troisième point*, l'élément de liaison entre la volonté des cieux et celle de la terre. L'univers faisait que la semence se transformât en plante, le sol lui permettait de se développer, les hommes la cueillaient et la portaient à la cité, où ils consacraient aux dieux les offrandes avant de les abandonner sur les montagnes sacrées. Même s'il n'avait pas beaucoup voyagé, Elie savait que de nombreuses nations dans le monde partageaient cette vision.

Les Assyriens avaient peur de priver de nourriture les dieux de la Cinquième Montagne ; ils ne désiraient pas mettre fin à l'équilibre de l'univers.

« Pourquoi pensé-je tout cela si cette lutte est une lutte entre ma volonté et celle du Seigneur qui m'a laissé seul au beau milieu de mes tribulations ? »

L'impression qu'il avait eue la veille au moment où il bravait Dieu revint. Il oubliait un élément important, et il avait beau chercher dans sa mémoire, il ne parvenait pas à s'en souvenir.

Un autre jour passa. ils avaient déjà rassemblé la plupart des corps, quand une femme inconnue s'approcha.

« Je n'ai rien à manger, dit-elle.

— Nous non plus, répliqua Elie. Hier et aujourd'hui nous avons partagé en trois la part destinée à une personne. Va voir où l'on peut trouver des aliments et tiens-moi au courant.

— Comment le découvrir ?

— Demande aux enfants. Ils savent tout. »

Depuis qu'il lui avait offert de l'eau, le gamin paraissait reprendre un peu goût à la vie. Elie l'avait envoyé ramasser les ordures et les débris avec le vieux, mais il n'avait pas réussi à le faire travailler très longtemps ; maintenant il jouait en compagnie d'autres enfants dans un coin de la place.

« Cela vaut mieux. Il aura bien le temps de suer, une fois adulte. » Mais il ne regrettait pas de lui avoir fait endurer la faim une nuit entière, sous prétexte qu'il devait travailler ; s'il l'avait traité en pauvre orphelin, victime de la méchanceté des guerriers assyriens, jamais il ne serait sorti de la dépression dans laquelle il était plongé lorsqu'ils étaient revenus dans la cité. Dorénavant il avait l'intention de le laisser quelques jours tout seul trouver ses propres réponses à ce qui s'était passé.

« Comment les enfants peuvent-ils savoir quelque chose ? insista la femme qui lui avait demandé à manger.

— Vois par toi-même. »

La femme et le vieux qui aidaient Elie la virent discuter avec les enfants qui jouaient dans la rue. Ils lui dirent quelques mots, elle se retourna, sourit et disparut au coin de la place.

« Comment as-tu découvert que les enfants savaient ? demanda le vieux.

— Parce que j'ai été gamin, et je sais que les enfants n'ont pas de passé, répondit-il, se rappelant de nouveau la conversation avec le berger. Ils ont été horrifiés par la nuit de l'invasion mais ils ne s'en soucient déjà plus ; la cité est transformée en un immense parc où ils peuvent aller et venir sans être dérangés. Tôt ou tard, ils devaient bien tomber sur la nourriture stockée par les habitants d'Akbar pour soutenir le siège.

« Un enfant peut toujours enseigner trois choses à un adulte : être content sans raison, s'occuper tou-

jours à quelque chose, et savoir exiger — de toutes
ses forces — ce qu'il désire. C'est à cause de ce gosse
que je suis revenu à Akbar. »

*

Cet après-midi-là, d'autres vieillards et d'autres
femmes participèrent au ramassage des morts. Les
enfants éloignaient les charognards et apportaient
des morceaux de bois et de tissu. Quand la nuit
tomba, Elie mit feu à la montagne de corps. Les survivants d'Akbar contemplèrent en silence la fumée
qui s'élevait vers les cieux.

Sa tâche terminée, Elie s'effondra de fatigue. Mais
avant de dormir, il éprouva de nouveau la sensation
qu'il avait eue le matin même : un élément capital
luttait désespérément pour lui revenir en mémoire.
Ce n'était rien qu'il eût appris pendant le temps qu'il
avait passé à Akbar, mais une histoire ancienne, qui
semblait donner sens à tout ce qui était en train de
se produire.

« *Cette nuit-là, un homme lutta avec Jacob jusqu'au
lever du jour. Voyant qu'il ne pouvait l'emporter sur
lui, il lui dit :* "Laisse-moi partir."

Jacob répondit : "Je ne te laisserai pas, que tu ne
m'aies béni."

Alors l'homme lui dit : « Comme un prince, tu as
lutté avec Dieu. Comment t'appelles-tu ? "

Jacob dit son nom, et l'homme répondit : "Désormais, tu t'appelleras Israël." »

162

Elie se réveilla d'un bond et regarda le firmament. Voilà l'histoire qui manquait !

Longtemps auparavant, alors que le patriarche Jacob avait installé son camp, quelqu'un entra dans sa tente au cours de la nuit et lutta avec lui jusqu'au lever du soleil. Jacob accepta le combat, bien qu'il sût que son adversaire était le Seigneur. A l'aube, il n'était toujours pas vaincu, et le combat ne prit fin que lorsque Dieu accepta de le bénir.

L'histoire s'était transmise de génération en génération afin que personne ne l'oubliât jamais : *quelquefois il était nécessaire de lutter avec Dieu*. Tout être humain, à un moment donné, voyait une tragédie traverser sa vie ; ce pouvait être la destruction d'une cité, la mort d'un enfant, une accusation sans preuve, une maladie qui le laissait invalide à tout jamais. A cet instant, Dieu le mettait au défi de L'affronter et de répondre à Sa question : « Pourquoi t'accrocher autant à une existence si courte et si pleine de souffrances ? Quel est le sens de ta lutte ? »

L'homme qui ne savait répondre se résignait. Mais celui qui cherchait un sens à l'existence trouvait que Dieu avait été injuste, et il bravait le destin. C'est alors qu'un autre feu descendait des cieux, non pas celui qui tue, mais celui qui détruit les antiques murailles et donne à chaque être humain ses véritables possibilités. Les lâches ne laissent jamais cette flamme embraser leur cœur — tout ce qu'ils désirent, c'est que la situation redevienne vite ce qu'elle était auparavant, afin qu'ils puissent continuer de vivre et de penser comme ils y étaient accoutumés. En revanche, les courageux mettent le feu à ce qui était vieux, dépassé, et, même au prix d'une grande souffrance intérieure, ils abandonnent tout, y compris Dieu, et vont de l'avant.

« Les courageux sont toujours têtus. »

Du ciel, le Seigneur sourit de contentement : c'était cela qu'Il voulait, que chacun prît en main la responsabilité de sa propre vie. Finalement, il avait donné à ses enfants le plus grand de tous les dons : la capacité de choisir et de décider de leurs actes.

Seuls les hommes et les femmes ayant le feu sacré avaient le courage de L'affronter. Et eux seuls connaissaient la voie du retour vers Son amour, car ils comprenaient enfin que la tragédie n'était pas une punition, mais un défi.

Elie revit chacun de ses pas ; depuis qu'il avait quitté la charpenterie, il avait accepté sa mission sans discuter. Même si elle était juste — et il pensait qu'elle l'était —, il n'avait jamais eu l'occasion de regarder ce qui se passait sur les chemins qu'il s'était refusé à parcourir par peur de perdre sa foi, son dévouement, sa volonté. Il considérait qu'il était très risqué de prendre le chemin des gens ordinaires — il pouvait finir par s'y habituer et aimer ce qu'il voyait. Il ne comprenait pas qu'il était lui aussi comme tout le monde, même s'il entendait des anges et recevait de temps en temps des ordres de Dieu ; il était tellement convaincu de savoir ce qu'il voulait qu'il s'était comporté de la même manière que ceux qui n'avaient jamais pris une décision importante de leur vie.

Il avait échappé au doute, à la défaite, aux moments d'indécision. Mais le Seigneur était généreux, et Il l'avait conduit à l'abîme de l'inévitable pour lui montrer que l'homme a besoin de *choisir* — et non d'*accepter* — son destin.

Bien des années auparavant, par une nuit semblable à celle-ci, Jacob n'avait pas laissé Dieu partir avant qu'Il ne l'ait béni. C'est alors que le Seigneur lui avait demandé : « *Comment t'appelles-tu ?* »

Telle était la question : avoir un nom. Une fois que Jacob eut répondu, Dieu l'avait baptisé *Israël*. Chacun a un nom au berceau, mais il doit apprendre à baptiser sa vie du mot qu'il a choisi pour lui donner un sens.

« Je suis *Akbar* », avait-elle dit.

Il avait fallu la destruction de la cité et la perte de la femme aimée pour qu'Elie comprît qu'il avait besoin d'un nom. Et, à l'instant même, il donna à sa vie le nom de *Libération*.

Il se leva et regarda la place devant lui : la fumée montait encore des cendres de ceux qui avaient perdu la vie. En mettant le feu à ces corps, il avait bravé une coutume très ancienne de son pays qui exigeait que les gens fussent enterrés selon les rites. Il avait lutté avec Dieu et la tradition en décidant l'incinération, mais il sentait qu'il n'avait pas péché, car il fallait une solution nouvelle à un problème nouveau. Dieu était infini dans Sa miséricorde, et implacable dans Sa rigueur à l'égard de ceux qui n'ont pas le courage d'oser.

Il parcourut de nouveau la place du regard : quelques survivants n'étaient pas encore allés se coucher et ils gardaient les yeux fixés sur les flammes, comme si ce feu avait consumé aussi leurs souvenirs, leur passé, les deux cents ans de paix et d'inertie d'Akbar. L'époque de la peur et de l'attente était révolue : il ne restait désormais que la reconstruction ou la défaite.

Comme Elie, eux aussi pouvaient se choisir un nom. *Réconciliation, Sagesse, Amant, Pèlerin*, il y avait autant de choix que d'étoiles dans le ciel, mais chacun devait donner un nom à sa vie.

Elie se leva et pria :

« J'ai lutté contre Toi, Seigneur, et je n'ai pas honte. Ainsi, j'ai découvert que je suis sur mon chemin parce que je le désire, non parce que cela m'a été imposé par mes parents, par les traditions de mon pays, ou par Toi-même.

« Vers Toi, Seigneur, j'aimerais revenir en cet instant. Je veux T'offrir toute la force de ma volonté, et non la lâcheté de celui qui n'a pas su choisir un chemin différent. Cependant, pour que Tu me confies Ton importante mission, je dois poursuivre cette bataille contre Toi, jusqu'à ce que Tu me bénisses. »

Reconstruire Akbar. Ce qu'Elie prenait pour un défi à Dieu était, en vérité, ses retrouvailles avec Lui.

La femme qui avait réclamé de la nourriture reparut le lendemain matin. Elle était accompagnée d'autres femmes.

« Nous avons découvert plusieurs dépôts, dit-elle. Comme beaucoup de gens sont morts et que beaucoup d'autres ont fui avec le gouverneur, nous avons des réserves pour un an.

— Trouve de vieilles personnes pour superviser la distribution des aliments, ordonna Elie. Elles ont l'expérience de l'organisation.

— Les vieux n'ont pas envie de vivre.

— Prie-les de venir de toute façon. »

La femme se préparait à partir quand Elie la retint :

« Tu sais écrire en te servant des lettres ?

— Non.

— J'ai appris, et je peux t'enseigner. Cela te sera utile pour m'aider à administrer la cité.

— Mais les Assyriens vont revenir.

— Quand ils arriveront, ils auront besoin de notre aide pour gérer les affaires de la cité.

— Pourquoi faire cela pour l'ennemi ?

— Fais-le pour que chacun puisse donner un nom à sa vie. L'ennemi n'est qu'un prétexte pour mettre à l'épreuve notre force. »

Les vieux vinrent, ainsi qu'il l'avait prévu.

« Akbar a besoin de votre aide, leur dit Elie. Et devant cela, vous ne pouvez pas vous offrir le luxe d'être vieux ; nous avons besoin de la jeunesse que vous aviez jadis et que vous avez perdue.

— Nous ne savons pas où la retrouver, répondit l'un d'eux. Elle a disparu avec les rides et les désillusions.

— Ce n'est pas vrai. Vous n'avez jamais eu d'illusions, et c'est pour cette raison que la jeunesse se cache. Il est temps de la retrouver, puisque nous avons un rêve commun : reconstruire Akbar.

— Comment pouvons-nous réaliser quelque chose d'impossible ?

— Avec enthousiasme. »

Les yeux voilés par la tristesse et le découragement voulaient briller de nouveau. Ce n'étaient plus les habitants bons à rien qui allaient assister aux jugements en quête d'un sujet de conversation pour la fin de l'après-midi ; ils avaient maintenant devant eux une mission importante, ils étaient nécessaires.

Les plus résistants séparèrent les matériaux encore utilisables des maisons qui avaient été très endommagées et s'en servirent pour remettre en état celles qui tenaient encore debout. Les plus âgés aidèrent à disperser dans les champs les cendres des cadavres incinérés, afin qu'on se rappelât les morts de la cité lors de la prochaine récolte ; d'autres se chargèrent de séparer les grains emmagasinés dans toute la cité dans le plus grand désordre, de fabriquer le pain et de tirer l'eau du puits.

Deux nuits plus tard, Elie réunit tous les habitants sur la place, nettoyée maintenant de la plus grande partie des décombres. On alluma des torches et il prit la parole :

« Nous n'avons pas le choix. Nous pouvons laisser l'étranger faire ce travail, mais alors cela signifie que nous renonçons à la seule chance que nous offre une tragédie : celle de reconstruire notre vie.

« Les cendres des morts que nous avons incinérés il y a quelques jours vont nourrir des plantes qui naîtront au printemps. Le fils perdu la nuit de l'invasion s'est changé en de nombreux enfants qui courent librement dans les rues détruites et s'amusent à envahir des lieux interdits et des maisons qu'ils n'avaient jamais connues. Jusqu'à présent, seuls les enfants ont été capables de surmonter les événements parce qu'ils n'ont pas de passé — pour eux, tout ce qui compte est le moment présent. Alors, essayons d'agir comme eux.

— Un homme peut-il éteindre dans son cœur la douleur d'une perte ? demanda une femme.

— Non. Mais il peut se réjouir d'avoir gagné quelque chose. »

Elie se retourna et montra la cime de la Cinquième Montagne, toujours couverte de nuages. La destruction des murailles la rendait visible du centre de la place.

« Je crois en un Seigneur unique, mais vous, vous pensez que les dieux habitent dans ces nuages, au sommet de la Cinquième Montagne. Je ne veux pas discuter maintenant pour savoir si mon Dieu est plus fort ou plus puissant que les vôtres ; je ne veux pas évoquer nos différences, mais nos ressemblances. La tragédie nous a réunis en un sentiment commun : le désespoir. Pourquoi est-ce arrivé ? Parce que nous pensions que tout avait trouvé une réponse et une solution dans nos âmes, et nous ne pouvions accepter le moindre changement.

« Vous et moi, nous appartenons à des nations commerçantes, mais nous savons aussi nous comporter en guerriers, poursuivit-il. Et un guerrier est toujours conscient du motif pour lequel cela vaut la peine de lutter. Il n'entreprend pas des combats dénués d'intérêt, et il ne perd jamais son temps en provocations.

« Un guerrier accepte la défaite. Il ne la traite pas comme un événement indifférent, ni ne tente de la transformer en victoire. La douleur de la perte le rend amer, il souffre de la froideur et la solitude le désespère. Une fois qu'il est passé par tout cela, il lèche ses blessures et prend un nouveau départ. Un guerrier sait que la guerre est faite de nombreuses batailles ; il va de l'avant.

« Des tragédies surviennent. Nous pouvons en découvrir la raison, en rendre les autres coupables, imaginer combien nos vies auraient été différentes sans elles. Mais rien de tout cela n'a d'importance : elles sont arrivées, point. Dès lors, nous devons oublier la peur qu'elles ont suscitée et entreprendre la reconstruction.

« Chacun de vous se donnera désormais un nom nouveau. Ce sera un nom sacré, qui synthétise tout ce pour quoi vous avez rêvé de vous battre. Je me suis choisi le nom de *Libération.* »

La place resta silencieuse un certain temps. Alors, la femme qui la première avait aidé Elie se leva.

« Mon nom est *Retrouvailles,* dit-elle.

— Je m'appelle *Sagesse* », déclara un vieux.

Le fils de la veuve qu'Elie avait tant aimée s'écria : « Mon nom est *Alphabet.* »

Les gens éclatèrent de rire. Honteux, l'enfant se rassit.

« Comment peut-on s'appeler *Alphabet* ? » cria un autre enfant.

Elie aurait pu intervenir mais il était bon que le garçon apprît à se défendre tout seul.

« Parce que c'est ce que faisait ma mère, dit le gamin. Chaque fois que je regarderai les lettres dessinées, je penserai à elle. »

Cette fois, personne ne rit. Un à un, les orphelins, les veuves et les vieillards d'Akbar annoncèrent leur nom et leur nouvelle identité. La cérémonie terminée, Elie conseilla à tout le monde de se coucher tôt : ils devaient se remettre au travail le lendemain matin.

Il prit l'enfant par la main et ils regagnèrent l'endroit de la place où ils avaient étendu quelques tissus en forme de tente.

A partir de cette nuit-là, il lui enseigna l'écriture de Byblos.

Les jours devinrent des semaines, et Akbar changeait de visage. L'enfant avait rapidement appris à dessiner les lettres et il parvenait désormais à créer des mots qui avaient un sens. Elie le chargea d'écrire sur des tablettes d'argile l'histoire de la reconstruction de la cité.

Les plaques d'argile étaient cuites dans un four improvisé, transformées en céramique et soigneusement archivées par un couple de vieillards. Lors des réunions qui se tenaient chaque soir, Elie demandait aux vieux de raconter ce qu'ils avaient vu dans leur enfance et il enregistrait le plus grand nombre d'histoires possible.

« Nous conserverons la mémoire d'Akbar dans un matériau que le feu ne peut détruire, expliquait-il. Un jour, nos enfants et petits-enfants sauront que la défaite n'a pas été acceptée et que l'inévitable a été surmonté. Cela peut leur servir d'exemple. »

Toutes les nuits, après l'étude avec le gamin, Elie marchait dans la cité déserte, il allait jusqu'au début de la route menant à Jérusalem, songeait à partir, puis y renonçait.

Le poids de sa tâche l'obligeait à se concentrer sur le présent. Il savait que les habitants d'Akbar comptaient sur lui pour la reconstruction ; il les avait déçus une fois, le jour où il s'était montré incapable d'empêcher la mort de l'espion, et d'éviter la guerre. Pourtant, Dieu offre toujours une seconde chance à ses enfants, et il devait saisir l'opportunité nouvelle. En outre, il s'attachait de plus en plus à l'enfant ; il voulait lui enseigner non seulement les caractères de Byblos, mais la foi dans le Seigneur et la sagesse de ses ancêtres.

Cependant, il n'oubliait pas que, dans son pays, régnaient une princesse et un dieu étranger. Il n'y avait plus d'anges tenant des épées de feu ; il était libre de partir quand il voulait et de faire ce que bon lui semblait.

Toutes les nuits, il songeait à s'en aller. Et toutes les nuits, il levait les mains vers le ciel et priait :

« Jacob a lutté la nuit entière et il a été béni à l'aurore. J'ai lutté contre Toi pendant des jours, des mois, et Tu refuses de m'écouter. Mais si Tu regardes autour de Toi, Tu sauras que je suis en train de vaincre : Akbar se relève de ses ruines et je vais reconstruire ce que Toi, en te servant des épées des Assyriens, Tu as transformé en cendres et en poussière.

« Je lutterai avec Toi jusqu'à ce que Tu me bénisses, et que Tu bénisses les fruits de mon travail. Un jour, Tu devras me répondre. »

*

Femmes et enfants apportaient l'eau dans les champs et luttaient contre la sécheresse qui paraissait sans fin. Un jour que le soleil implacable brillait de toute sa force, Elie entendit ce commentaire :

« Nous travaillons sans arrêt, nous ne pensons plus aux douleurs de cette nuit-là, et nous oublions même que les Assyriens reviendront dès qu'ils auront fini de mettre à sac Tyr, Sidon, Byblos et toute la Phénicie. Cela nous a fait du bien.

« Cependant, parce que nous sommes très concentrés sur la reconstruction de la cité, rien ne semble changer ; nous ne voyons pas le résultat de notre effort. »

Elie médita quelque temps sur ces paroles. Il exigea désormais que, au terme de chaque journée de travail, les gens se réunissent au pied de la Cinquième Montagne pour contempler ensemble le coucher du soleil.

Ils étaient en général tellement fatigués qu'ils échangeaient à peine un mot, mais ils découvraient combien il était important de laisser sa pensée errer sans but, comme les nuages dans le ciel. Ainsi, l'anxiété abandonnait leur cœur et tous retrouvaient la force et l'inspiration nécessaires pour le lendemain.

A son réveil, Elie annonça qu'il n'irait pas travailler.

« Aujourd'hui, dans mon pays, on célèbre le jour du Pardon.

— Il n'y a pas de péché dans ton âme, remarqua une femme. Tu as fait de ton mieux.

— Mais la tradition doit être maintenue. Et je la respecterai. »

Les femmes allèrent porter l'eau dans les champs, les vieux retournèrent à leur tâche, élever des murs et façonner des portes et des fenêtres en bois. Les enfants aidaient à mouler les petites briques d'argile qui, plus tard, seraient cuites dans le feu. Elie les contempla, une joie immense dans le cœur. Ensuite, il quitta Akbar et se rendit dans la vallée.

Il marcha sans but, faisant les prières qu'il avait apprises enfant. Le soleil n'était pas encore complètement levé et, de là où il se trouvait, il voyait l'ombre gigantesque de la Cinquième Montagne recouvrir une partie de la vallée. Il eut un horrible pressentiment : cette lutte entre le Dieu d'Israël et les dieux des Phéniciens allait se prolonger durant des générations et des millénaires.

*

Il se rappela qu'un soir il était monté jusqu'au sommet de la montagne et qu'il avait conversé avec un ange ; mais, depuis qu'Akbar avait été détruite, plus jamais il n'avait entendu les voix venant du ciel.

« Seigneur, aujourd'hui c'est le jour du Pardon, et la liste des péchés que j'ai commis envers Toi est longue », dit-il en se tournant en direction de Jérusalem. « J'ai été faible, parce que j'ai oublié ma propre force. J'ai été compatissant quand j'aurais dû être dur. Je n'ai pas choisi, de crainte de prendre de mauvaises décisions. J'ai renoncé avant l'heure, et j'ai blasphémé lorsque j'aurais dû remercier.

« Cependant, Seigneur, Tes péchés envers moi

forment aussi une longue liste. Tu m'as fait souffrir plus que nécessaire, emportant de ce monde quelqu'un que j'aimais. Tu as détruit la cité qui m'a accueilli, Tu as fait échouer ma quête, Ta dureté m'a presque fait oublier l'amour que j'ai pour Toi. Pendant tout ce temps, j'ai lutté avec Toi, et Tu n'admets pas la dignité de mon combat.

« Si nous comparons la liste de mes péchés et la liste des Tiens, Tu verras que Tu as une dette envers moi. Mais, comme aujourd'hui c'est le jour du Pardon, Tu me pardonnes et je Te pardonne, pour que nous puissions continuer à marcher ensemble. »

A ce moment le vent souffla, et il sentit que son ange lui parlait : « Tu as bien fait, Elie. Dieu a accepté ton combat. »

Des larmes coulèrent de ses yeux. Il s'agenouilla et embrassa le sol aride de la vallée.

« Merci d'être venu, parce que j'ai encore un doute : n'est-ce pas un péché d'agir ainsi ? »

L'ange répondit :

« Quand un guerrier lutte avec son instructeur, l'offense-t-il ?

— Non, c'est la seule manière d'apprendre la technique dont il a besoin.

— Alors continue jusqu'à ce que le Seigneur t'appelle et te renvoie en Israël, reprit l'ange. Lève-toi et continue à prouver que ta lutte a un sens, parce que tu as su traverser le courant de l'Inévitable. Beaucoup y naviguent et font naufrage ; d'autres sont rejetés vers des lieux qui ne leur étaient pas destinés. Mais toi, tu affrontes la traversée avec dignité, tu sais contrôler la direction de ton bateau et tu t'efforces de transformer la douleur en action.

— Dommage que tu sois aveugle, dit Elie. Sinon tu verrais comme les orphelins, les veuves et les vieillards ont été capables de reconstruire une cité. Bientôt, tout redeviendra comme avant.

— J'espère que non, répliqua l'ange. Finalement, ils ont payé le prix fort pour que leurs vies changent. »

Elie sourit. L'ange avait raison.

« J'espère que tu te comporteras comme les

hommes à qui l'on offre une seconde chance : ne commets pas deux fois la même erreur. N'oublie jamais la raison de ta vie.

— Je n'oublierai pas », répondit-il, content que l'ange fût revenu.

Les caravanes n'empruntaient plus le chemin de la vallée ; les Assyriens avaient dû détruire les routes et modifier les voies commerciales. Chaque jour, des enfants montaient dans la seule tour des remparts qui avait échappé à la destruction ; ils étaient chargés de surveiller l'horizon et d'avertir au cas où les guerriers ennemis reviendraient.

Elie projetait de les recevoir avec dignité et de leur remettre le commandement. Alors, il pourrait partir.

Mais, chaque jour qui passait, il sentait qu'Akbar faisait partie de sa vie. Sa mission n'était peut-être pas de chasser Jézabel du trône, mais de rester là, avec ces gens, jusqu'à sa mort, jouant l'humble rôle de serviteur du conquérant assyrien. Il aiderait à rétablir les voies commerciales, il apprendrait la langue de l'ennemi et, dans ses moments de repos, il pourrait s'occuper de la bibliothèque qui s'enrichissait de plus en plus.

Ce que l'on avait pris, une certaine nuit perdue dans le temps, pour la fin d'une cité signifiait maintenant la possibilité de la rendre encore plus belle. Les travaux de reconstruction comprenaient l'élargissement des rues, l'installation de toits plus résistants, et un ingénieux système pour porter l'eau du puits jusqu'aux endroits les plus éloignés. Son âme aussi se renouvelait ; chaque jour, il apprenait, des vieux, des enfants, des femmes, quelque chose de nouveau. Ce groupe — qui n'avait pas abandonné Akbar en raison de l'impossibilité absolue où il était de le faire — formait maintenant une équipe disciplinée et compétente.

« Si le gouverneur avait su qu'ils étaient aussi utiles, il aurait inventé un autre type de défense, et Akbar n'aurait pas été détruite. »

Elie réfléchit un peu et comprit qu'il se trompait. Akbar devait être détruite, pour que tous puissent réveiller en eux les forces qui dormaient.

Des mois passèrent, et les assyriens ne donnaient pas signe de vie. Akbar était maintenant quasi prête et Elie pouvait songer à l'avenir ; les femmes récupéraient les morceaux d'étoffe et en confectionnaient des vêtements. Les vieux réorganisaient les demeures et s'occupaient de l'hygiène de la cité. Les enfants aidaient quand on les sollicitait mais, en général, ils passaient la journée à jouer : c'est la principale obligation des enfants.

Elie vivait avec le gamin dans une petite maison en pierre, reconstruite sur le terrain de ce qui avait été autrefois un dépôt de marchandises. Chaque soir, les habitants d'Akbar s'asseyaient autour d'un feu sur la place principale et racontaient des histoires qu'ils avaient entendues au cours de leur vie ; avec l'enfant, il notait tout sur les tablettes qu'ils faisaient cuire le lendemain. La bibliothèque grossissait à vue d'œil.

La femme qui avait perdu son fils apprenait elle aussi les caractères de Byblos. Quand il vit qu'elle savait créer des mots et des phrases, il la chargea d'enseigner l'alphabet au reste de la population ; ainsi, lorsque les Assyriens reviendraient, ils pourraient servir d'interprètes ou de professeurs.

« C'était justement cela que le prêtre voulait éviter », dit un après-midi un vieux qui s'était appelé *Océan*, car il désirait avoir l'âme aussi vaste que la mer. « Que l'écriture de Byblos survécût et menaçât les dieux de la Cinquième Montagne.

— Qui peut éviter l'inévitable ? » rétorqua-t-il.

Les gens travaillaient le jour, assistaient ensemble au coucher du soleil et contaient des histoires à la veillée.

Elie était fier de son œuvre. Et il l'aimait de plus en plus.

*

Un enfant chargé de la surveillance descendit en courant.

« J'ai vu de la poussière à l'horizon ! dit-il, excité. L'ennemi est de retour ! »

Elie monta dans la tour et constata que l'information était exacte. Il calcula qu'ils arriveraient aux portes d'Akbar le lendemain.

L'après-midi, il prévint les habitants qu'ils ne devraient pas assister au coucher du soleil mais se retrouver sur la place. La journée de travail terminée, il rejoignit l'assemblée et remarqua que les gens avaient peur.

« Aujourd'hui nous ne raconterons pas des histoires du passé, et nous n'évoquerons pas les projets d'Akbar, dit-il. Nous allons parler de nous-mêmes. »

Personne ne dit mot.

*

« Il y a quelque temps, la pleine lune a brillé dans le ciel. Ce jour-là, il est arrivé ce que tous nous pressentions, mais que nous ne voulions pas accepter : Akbar a été détruite. Lorsque l'armée assyrienne s'est retirée, nos meilleurs hommes étaient morts. Les rescapés ont vu qu'il ne valait pas la peine de rester ici et ils ont décidé de s'en aller. Seuls sont restés les vieillards, les veuves et les orphelins, c'est-à-dire les bons à rien.

« Regardez autour de vous ; la place est plus belle que jamais, les bâtiments sont plus solides, la nourriture est partagée, et tous apprennent l'écriture inventée à Byblos. Quelque part dans cette cité se trouve une collection de tablettes sur lesquelles nous avons inscrit nos histoires, et les générations futures se rappelleront ce que nous avons fait.

« Aujourd'hui, nous savons que les vieux, les orphelins et les veuves sont partis aussi. Ils ont laissé place à une bande de jeunes gens de tous âges, pleins d'enthousiasme, qui ont donné un nom et un sens à leur vie.

« A chaque moment de la reconstruction, nous savions que les Assyriens allaient revenir. Nous savions qu'un jour il nous faudrait leur livrer notre cité et, avec elle, nos efforts, notre sueur, notre joie de la voir plus belle qu'avant. »

La lumière du feu illumina les larmes qui coulaient des visages. Même les enfants, qui d'habitude jouaient pendant les réunions nocturnes, étaient attentifs à ses paroles. Elie poursuivit :

« Cela n'a pas d'importance. Nous avons accompli notre devoir envers le Seigneur, car nous avons accepté Son défi et l'honneur de Sa lutte. Avant cette nuit-là, Il insistait auprès de nous, disant : "Marche !" Mais nous ne l'écoutions pas. Pourquoi ?

« Parce que chacun de nous avait déjà décidé de son propre avenir : je pensais chasser Jézabel du trône, la femme qui maintenant s'appelle *Retrouvailles* voulait que son fils fût navigateur, l'homme qui aujourd'hui porte le nom de *Sagesse* désirait simplement passer le reste de ses jours à boire du vin sur la place. Nous étions habitués au mystère sacré de la vie et nous ne lui accordions plus d'importance.

« Alors le Seigneur s'est dit : "Ils ne veulent pas marcher ? Alors ils vont rester arrêtés très longtemps !"

« Et là, seulement, nous avons compris Son message. L'acier de l'épée assyrienne a emporté nos jeunes gens, et la lâcheté s'est emparée des adultes. Où qu'ils soient à cette heure, ils sont encore arrêtés ; ils ont accepté la malédiction de Dieu.

« Mais nous, nous avons lutté contre le Seigneur. Comme nous avons lutté avec les hommes et les femmes que nous aimions durant notre vie, parce que c'est le combat qui nous bénit et qui nous fait grandir. Nous avons saisi l'opportunité de la tragédie et nous avons accompli notre devoir envers Lui, prouvant que nous étions capables d'obéir à l'ordre de *marcher*. Même dans les pires circonstances, nous sommes allés de l'avant.

« Il y a des moments où Dieu exige obéissance. Mais il y a des moments où Il désire tester notre volonté et nous met au défi de comprendre Son amour. Nous avons compris cette volonté quand les murailles d'Akbar se sont écroulées : elles ont ouvert notre horizon et laissé chacun de nous voir de quoi il était capable. Nous avons cessé de réfléchir à la vie, et nous avons décidé de la vivre. Le résultat a été bon. »

Elie remarqua que les yeux se mettaient à briller. Les gens avaient compris.

« Demain, je livrerai Akbar sans lutte ; je suis libre de partir quand je veux, car j'ai accompli ce que le Seigneur attendait de moi. Cependant, mon sang, ma sueur et mon unique amour sont dans le sol de cette cité, et j'ai décidé de passer ici le reste de mes jours, pour empêcher qu'elle ne soit de nouveau détruite. Que chacun prenne la décision qu'il voudra, mais n'oubliez jamais ceci : vous êtes bien meilleurs que vous ne le pensiez.

« Vous avez saisi la chance que la tragédie vous a donnée ; tout le monde n'en est pas capable. »

Elie se leva et annonça que la réunion était close. Il avertit l'enfant qu'il allait rentrer tard et lui conseilla de se coucher sans l'attendre.

*

Il alla jusqu'au temple, le seul monument ayant échappé à la destruction ; ils n'avaient pas eu besoin de le reconstruire, bien que les statues des dieux aient été emportées par les Assyriens. Respectueusement, il toucha la pierre qui marquait l'endroit où, selon la tradition, un ancêtre avait enfoncé une baguette dans le sol et n'était pas parvenu à la retirer.

Il songea que, dans son pays, Jézabel avait édifié des monuments comme celui-ci et qu'une partie de son peuple se prosternait pour adorer Baal et ses divinités. De nouveau, le pressentiment traversa son âme : la guerre entre le Seigneur d'Israël et les dieux des Phéniciens durerait très longtemps, bien au-delà de ce que son imagination pouvait atteindre. Comme dans une vision, il entrevit les étoiles qui croisaient le soleil et répandaient dans les deux pays la destruction et la mort. Des hommes qui parlaient des langues inconnues chevauchaient des animaux d'acier et s'affrontaient en duel au milieu des nuages.

« Ce n'est pas cela que tu dois voir maintenant, car le temps n'est pas encore venu, lui dit son ange. Regarde par la fenêtre. »

Elie obéit. Dehors, la pleine lune illuminait les maisons et les rues d'Akbar, et, bien qu'il fût tard, il pouvait entendre les conversations et les rires de ses habitants. Malgré le retour des Assyriens, ce peuple avait encore envie de vivre, il était prêt à affronter une nouvelle étape de son existence.

Alors, il aperçut une silhouette et il sut que c'était la femme qu'il avait tant aimée et qui maintenant marchait de nouveau orgueilleusement dans la cité. Il sourit et sentit qu'elle touchait son visage.

« Je suis fière, semblait-elle dire. Akbar demeure vraiment belle. »

Il eut envie de pleurer mais il se rappela l'enfant qui jamais n'avait laissé couler une larme pour sa mère. Il contrôla ses pleurs et se remémora les plus beaux moments de l'histoire qu'ils avaient vécue ensemble — depuis la rencontre aux portes de la cité jusqu'à l'instant où elle avait écrit le mot « amour » sur une tablette d'argile. Il revit sa robe, ses cheveux, l'arête fine de son nez.

« Tu m'as dit que tu étais Akbar. Alors j'ai pris soin de toi, je t'ai guérie de tes blessures, et maintenant je te rends à la vie. Sois heureuse avec tes nouveaux compagnons. Et je voudrais te dire une chose : moi aussi j'étais Akbar, et je ne le savais pas. »

Il avait la certitude qu'elle souriait.

« Le vent du désert, il y a très longtemps, a effacé nos pas sur le sable. Mais, à chaque seconde de mon existence, je pense à ce qui s'est passé, et tu marches encore dans mes rêves et dans ma réalité. Merci d'avoir croisé mon chemin. »

Il s'endormit là, dans le temple, sentant que la femme lui caressait les cheveux.

Le chef des marchands aperçut un groupe de gens en guenilles au milieu de la route. Il crut que c'étaient des brigands et demanda à tous les membres de la caravane de s'emparer de leurs armes.

« Qui êtes-vous ? interrogea-t-il.

— Nous sommes le peuple d'Akbar », répondit un barbu, les yeux brillants. Le chef de la caravane remarqua qu'il parlait avec un accent étranger.

« Akbar a été détruite. Nous sommes chargés par le gouvernement de Tyr et de Sidon de localiser son puits, afin que les caravanes puissent de nouveau emprunter cette vallée. Les communications avec le reste du pays ne peuvent rester interrompues pour toujours.

— Akbar existe encore, répliqua l'homme. Où sont les Assyriens ?

— Le monde entier sait où ils sont, répondit en riant le chef de la caravane. Ils rendent plus fertile le sol de notre pays et il y a longtemps qu'ils nourrissent nos oiseaux et nos bêtes sauvages.

— Mais c'était une armée puissante.

— Une armée n'a aucun pouvoir, si l'on sait quand elle va attaquer. Akbar a fait prévenir qu'ils approchaient et Tyr et Sidon ont organisé une embuscade à l'autre bout de la vallée. Ceux qui ne sont pas morts au combat ont été vendus comme esclaves par nos navigateurs. »

Les gens en haillons applaudissaient et s'embrassaient, pleurant et riant en même temps.

« Qui êtes-vous ? répéta le marchand. Qui es-tu ? demanda-t-il en indiquant le chef.

— Nous sommes les jeunes guerriers d'Akbar »,
lui fut-il répondu.

La troisième récolte avait commencé, et Elie était
le gouverneur d'Akbar. Il y avait eu beaucoup de
résistance au début — l'ancien gouverneur voulait
revenir occuper son poste, ainsi que l'ordonnait la
tradition. Mais les habitants de la cité avaient refusé
de le recevoir et menacé pendant des jours d'empoi-
sonner l'eau du puits. L'autorité phénicienne avait
finalement cédé à leurs requêtes — au bout du
compte, Akbar n'avait pas tant d'importance, sinon
pour l'eau qu'elle procurait aux voyageurs, et le gouvernement d'Israël était aux mains d'une princesse
de Tyr. En concédant le poste de gouverneur à un
Israélite, les gouvernants phéniciens pouvaient bâtir
une alliance commerciale plus solide.
 La nouvelle parcourut toute la région, portée par
les caravanes de marchands qui s'étaient remises à
circuler. Une minorité en Israël considérait Elie
comme le pire des traîtres, mais Jézabel se charge-
rait en temps voulu d'éliminer cette résistance, et la
paix reviendrait dans la région. La princesse était
satisfaite parce que l'un de ses pires ennemis était
devenu son meilleur allié.

*

 La rumeur d'une nouvelle invasion assyrienne se
répandit et on releva les murailles d'Akbar. On mit
au point un nouveau système de défense, avec des
sentinelles et des garnisons disséminées entre Tyr et
Akbar ; de cette manière, si l'une des cités était assié-
gée, l'autre pourrait dépêcher des troupes par terre
et assurer le ravitaillement par mer.
 La région prospérait à vue d'œil : le nouveau gou-

verneur israélite avait instauré un rigoureux contrôle des taxes et des marchandises, fondé sur l'écriture. Les vieux d'Akbar s'occupaient de tout, utilisaient les nouvelles techniques et résolvaient patiemment les problèmes qui surgissaient.

Les femmes partageaient leur temps entre leur labeur et le tissage. Pendant la période d'isolement de la cité, pour remettre en état le peu de tissus qui leur restaient, elles avaient été obligées d'inventer de nouveaux motifs de broderie ; lorsque les premiers marchands arrivèrent, ils furent enchantés par les dessins et passèrent de nombreuses commandes.

Les enfants avaient appris l'écriture de Byblos ; Elie était certain que cela leur serait utile un jour.

Comme toujours avant la récolte, il se promenait dans la campagne et il remerciait le Seigneur cet après-midi-là des innombrables bénédictions qu'il avait reçues pendant toutes ces années. Il vit les gens tenant les paniers chargés de grain, les enfants jouant tout autour. Il leur fit signe et ils lui répondirent.

Un sourire sur le visage, il se dirigea vers la pierre où, très longtemps auparavant, il avait reçu une tablette d'argile portant le mot « amour ». Il venait tous les jours visiter cet endroit, pour assister au coucher du soleil et se rappeler chaque instant qu'ils avaient passé ensemble.

« *La parole du Seigneur fut adressée à Elie, la troisième année :*
"Va, montre-toi à Achab, je vais donner de la pluie sur la surface du sol." »

De la pierre sur laquelle il était assis, Elie vit le monde trembler autour de lui. Le ciel devint noir pendant un moment, puis très vite le soleil se remit à briller.

Il vit la lumière. Un ange du Seigneur se tenait devant lui.

« Que s'est-il passé ? demanda Elie, effrayé. Dieu a-t-Il pardonné à Israël ?

— Non, répondit l'ange. Il veut que tu retournes libérer ton peuple. Ton combat avec Lui est terminé et, à cet instant, Il t'a béni. Il t'a donné la permission de poursuivre Son travail sur cette terre. »

Elie était abasourdi.

« Maintenant, justement quand mon cœur vient de retrouver la paix ?

— Rappelle-toi la leçon qui t'a été enseignée une fois. Et rappelle-toi les paroles que le Seigneur adressa à Moïse :

"Souviens-toi du chemin sur lequel le Seigneur t'a guidé, pour t'humilier, pour te mettre à l'épreuve, pour savoir ce qui était dans ton cœur.

Quand tu auras mangé à satiété, quand tu auras construit de belles maisons pour y habiter, quand ton troupeau et ton bétail se seront multipliés, garde-toi de devenir orgueilleux et d'oublier le Seigneur ton Dieu." »

Elie se tourna vers l'ange.

« Et Akbar ? demanda-t-il.

— Elle peut vivre sans toi, car tu as laissé un héritier. Elle survivra de nombreuses années. »

L'ange du Seigneur disparut.

Elie et l'enfant arrivèrent au pied de la Cinquième Montagne. Les broussailles avaient poussé entre les pierres des autels ; depuis la mort du grand prêtre, plus personne ne venait ici.

« Nous allons monter, dit-il.

— C'est interdit.

— Oui, c'est interdit. Mais ce n'est pas dangereux pour autant. »

Il le prit par la main, et ils commencèrent à monter en direction du sommet. Ils s'arrêtaient de temps en temps et regardaient la vallée en contrebas ; la sécheresse avait marqué le paysage et, à l'exception des champs cultivés autour d'Akbar, le reste semblait un désert aussi rude que les terres d'Egypte.

« J'ai entendu mes amis dire que les Assyriens allaient revenir, dit le gamin.

— Peut-être, mais ce que nous avons fait valait la peine ; c'est la manière que Dieu a choisie pour que nous apprenions.

— Je ne sais pas s'Il se donne beaucoup de mal pour nous, remarqua l'enfant. Il n'avait pas besoin d'être aussi sévère.

— Il a dû essayer par d'autres moyens, jusqu'à ce qu'Il découvre que nous ne L'écoutions pas. Nous étions trop habitués à nos existences, et nous ne lisions plus Ses paroles.

— Où sont-elles écrites ?

— Dans le monde autour de toi. Il suffit de faire attention à ce qui se passe dans ta vie, et tu vas découvrir où, à chaque moment du jour, Il cache Ses paroles et Sa volonté. Essaie d'accomplir ce qu'Il demande : c'est ta seule raison d'être en ce monde.

— Si je les découvre, je les écrirai sur les tablettes d'argile.

— Fais-le. Mais écris-les surtout dans ton cœur ; là, elles ne pourront pas être brûlées ou détruites, et tu les emporteras où que tu ailles. »

Ils marchèrent encore un moment. Les nuages étaient maintenant tout proches.

« Je ne veux pas entrer là-dedans, dit l'enfant en les montrant du doigt.

— Ils ne te causeront aucun mal : ce ne sont que des nuages. Viens avec moi. »

Il le prit par la main, et ils montèrent. Peu à peu, ils pénétrèrent dans le brouillard ; l'enfant se serra contre lui sans mot dire, même si, de temps en temps, Elie tentait d'engager la conversation. Ils marchèrent parmi les rochers nus du sommet.

« Retournons », pria l'enfant.

Elie décida de ne pas insister, cet enfant avait déjà rencontré beaucoup de difficultés dans sa brève existence et connu la peur. Il fit ce qu'il demandait ; ils sortirent de la brume et de nouveau distinguèrent la vallée en bas.

« Un jour, cherche dans la bibliothèque d'Akbar ce que j'ai laissé écrit pour toi. Cela s'appelle *Le Manuel du guerrier de la lumière*.

— Je suis un guerrier de la lumière, répliqua l'enfant.

— Tu sais comment je m'appelle ? demanda Elie.

— *Libération*, répondit le gamin.

— Assieds-toi là près de moi, dit Elie en indiquant un rocher. Il m'est impossible d'oublier mon nom. Je dois poursuivre ma mission, même si, en ce moment, tout ce que je désire est rester avec toi. C'est pour cela qu'Akbar a été reconstruite ; pour nous enseigner qu'il faut aller de l'avant, aussi difficile que cela puisse paraître.

— Tu t'en vas.

— Comment le sais-tu ? demanda-t-il, surpris.

— Je l'ai écrit sur une tablette, hier soir. Quelque chose me l'a dit ; peut-être ma mère, ou bien un ange. Mais je le sentais déjà dans mon cœur. »

Elie caressa la tête de l'enfant.

« Tu as su lire la volonté de Dieu, dit-il, content. Alors je n'ai rien à t'expliquer.

— Ce que j'ai lu, c'était la tristesse dans tes yeux. Je n'ai pas eu de mal, certains de mes amis l'ont perçue aussi.

— Cette tristesse que vous avez lue dans mon regard est une partie de mon histoire. Mais une petite partie, qui ne va durer que quelques jours. Demain, quand je prendrai la direction de Jérusalem, elle aura perdu de sa force, et peu à peu elle disparaîtra. Les tristesses ne durent pas éternellement, lorsque nous marchons vers ce que nous avons toujours désiré.

— Faut-il toujours partir ?

— Il faut toujours savoir quand finit une étape de la vie. Si tu persistes à y demeurer au-delà du temps nécessaire, tu perds la joie et le sens du repos. Et tu risques d'être rappelé à l'ordre par Dieu.

— Le Seigneur est dur.

— Seulement avec Ses élus. »

*

Elie regarda Akbar tout en bas. Oui, Dieu pouvait parfois se montrer très dur, mais jamais au-delà de ce que chacun pouvait endurer : l'enfant ignorait que, à l'endroit où ils étaient assis, Elie avait reçu la visite d'un ange du Seigneur et qu'il avait appris comment le ramener d'entre les morts.

« Je vais te manquer ? demanda-t-il.

— Tu m'as dit que la tristesse disparaissait si nous allions de l'avant, répondit le gamin. Il reste beaucoup à faire pour rendre Akbar aussi belle que ma mère le mérite. Elle se promène dans ses rues.

— Reviens ici lorsque tu auras besoin de moi. Et regarde en direction de Jérusalem : j'y serai, cherchant à donner un sens à mon nom, *Libération*. Nos cœurs sont liés à tout jamais.

— C'est pour cela que tu m'as amené en haut de la Cinquième Montagne ? Pour que je puisse voir Israël ?

— Pour que tu voies la vallée, la cité, les autres montagnes, les rochers et les nuages. Le Seigneur avait coutume d'ordonner à Ses prophètes de se rendre sur les montagnes pour converser avec Lui. Je me suis toujours demandé pourquoi, et maintenant je comprends la réponse : du sommet, nous sommes capables de voir tout petit. Nos gloires et nos chagrins perdent leur importance. Ce que nous

186

avons gagné ou perdu est resté là en bas. Du haut de la montagne, tu peux voir comme le monde est vaste et comme l'horizon s'étend loin. »

L'enfant regarda tout autour. Du haut de la Cinquième Montagne, il percevait l'odeur de la mer qui baignait les plages de Tyr. Il entendait le vent du désert qui soufflait d'Egypte.

« Un jour, je gouvernerai Akbar, dit-il à Elie. Je connais ce qui est grand, mais je connais aussi chaque recoin de la cité. Je sais ce qu'il faut transformer.

— Alors, transforme-le. Ne laisse pas les choses se figer.

— Dieu ne pouvait-Il pas choisir une meilleure manière de nous montrer tout cela ? A un moment, j'ai pensé qu'Il était mauvais. »

Elie resta silencieux. Il se rappelait une conversation qu'il avait eue, des années auparavant, avec un prophète lévite, alors qu'ils attendaient que les soldats de Jézabel viennent les mettre à mort.

« Dieu peut-Il être mauvais ? insista l'enfant.

— Dieu est tout-puissant, répondit Elie. Il peut tout, et rien ne Lui est interdit ; sinon, cela signifierait qu'il existe quelqu'un de plus puissant et de plus grand que Lui pour l'empêcher de faire certaines choses. En ce cas, je préférerais adorer et révérer ce quelqu'un plus puissant. »

Il s'interrompit quelques instants, pour que le gamin pénètre bien le sens de ses propos. Puis il reprit :

« Cependant, dans Son infini pouvoir, Il a choisi de faire seulement le Bien. Si nous parvenons jusqu'à la fin de notre histoire, nous verrons que très souvent le Bien a l'apparence du Mal mais qu'il reste le Bien et fait partie du plan qu'Il a créé pour l'humanité. »

Il prit le garçon par la main et ils s'en retournèrent en silence.

*

Cette nuit-là, l'enfant dormit serré contre lui. Dès que le jour commença à poindre, Elie l'écarta délicatement de sa poitrine pour ne pas le réveiller.

Ensuite, il s'habilla du seul vêtement qu'il possédait et sortit. Sur le chemin, il ramassa un morceau de bois et s'en fit un bâton. Il avait l'intention de ne jamais s'en séparer : c'était le souvenir de son combat avec Dieu, de la destruction et de la reconstruction d'Akbar.

Sans regarder en arrière, il prit la direction d'Israël.

Epilogue

Cinq ans plus tard, l'Assyrie envahit de nouveau le pays, cette fois avec une armée plus professionnelle et des généraux plus compétents. Toute la Phénicie tomba sous la domination du conquérant étranger, à l'exception de Tyr et de Sarepta, que ses habitants dénommaient Akbar.

L'enfant se fit homme, gouverna la cité et fut considéré comme un sage par ses contemporains. Il mourut âgé, entouré des êtres qu'il chérissait, et disant toujours qu'« il fallait garder la cité belle et forte, parce que sa mère se promenait encore dans ces rues ». Grâce à un système de défense développé conjointement, Tyr et Sarepta ne furent occupées par le roi assyrien Sennachérib qu'en 701 avant Jésus-Christ, presque cent soixante ans après les faits relatés dans ce livre.

Mais les cités phéniciennes ne retrouvèrent jamais leur importance ; elles subirent dès lors une succession d'invasions — par les néo-Babyloniens, les Perses, les Macédoniens, les Séleucides, et enfin les Romains. Pourtant elles ont continué d'exister jusqu'à nos jours, parce que, selon la tradition antique, le Seigneur ne choisissait jamais par hasard les lieux qu'Il désirait voir habités. Tyr, Sidon et Byblos font toujours partie du Liban, qui est aujourd'hui encore un champ de bataille.

Elie retourna en Israël et réunit les prophètes sur le mont Carmel. Là, il leur demanda de se séparer en deux groupes : ceux qui adoraient Baal, et ceux qui croyaient dans le Seigneur. Suivant les instructions de l'ange, il offrit un bouvillon aux premiers et leur enjoignit de prier à grands cris leur dieu de recevoir le sacrifice. La Bible raconte :

« A midi, Elie se moqua d'eux et dit : "Criez plus fort, c'est un dieu ; peut-être qu'il médite, ou qu'il est en voyage, ou qu'il dort."

Ils crièrent plus fort et, selon leur coutume, se tailladèrent à coups de couteaux et de lances, mais il n'y eut ni voix, ni personne qui répondît, ni aucune réaction. »

Alors Elie saisit l'animal et l'offrit selon les instructions de l'ange du Seigneur. A ce moment, le feu du ciel descendit et *« dévora l'holocauste, le bois, les pierres »*. Quelques minutes plus tard, une pluie abondante tomba, mettant fin à quatre années de sécheresse.

A partir de cet instant, une guerre civile éclata. Elie fit exécuter les prophètes qui avaient trahi le Seigneur, et Jézabel le recherchait partout pour le faire mettre à mort. Mais il se réfugia sur le flanc ouest de la Cinquième Montagne, qui donnait vers Israël.

Des gens venus de Syrie envahirent le pays et tuèrent le roi Achab, époux de la princesse de Tyr, d'une flèche qui pénétra accidentellement par une ouverture de son armure. Jézabel se réfugia dans son palais et, après quelques soulèvements populaires, après l'ascension et la chute de plusieurs gouvernants, elle finit par être capturée. Elle préféra se jeter par la fenêtre plutôt que de se livrer aux hommes envoyés pour l'arrêter.

Elie demeura dans la montagne jusqu'à la fin de ses jours. La Bible raconte qu'un certain soir, tandis qu'il conversait avec Elisée, le prophète qu'il avait désigné comme son successeur, « *un char de feu et des chevaux de feu les séparèrent l'un de l'autre ; et Elie monta au ciel dans la tempête* ».

Quelque huit cents ans plus tard, Jésus invite Pierre, Jacques et Jean à gravir une montagne. L'évangéliste Matthieu raconte que « [Jésus] *fut transfiguré devant eux ; son visage resplendit comme le soleil et ses habits devinrent blancs comme la lumière. Et voici que leur apparurent Moïse et Elie qui s'entretenaient avec lui* ».

Jésus demande aux apôtres de ne pas raconter cette vision tant que le Fils de l'homme ne sera pas ressuscité des morts, mais ils rétorquent que cela ne se produira que lorsque Elie reviendra.

Matthieu (17, 10-13) relata la suite de l'histoire :

« *Et les disciples l'interrogèrent : "Pourquoi donc les scribes disent-ils qu'Elie doit venir d'abord ?"*

Jésus répondit alors : "Certes, Elie va venir et il rétablira tout ; mais, je vous le déclare, Elie est déjà venu et, au lieu de le reconnaître, ils ont fait de lui tout ce qu'ils ont voulu."

Alors les disciples comprirent qu'il leur parlait de Jean le Baptiste. »

Composition réalisée par JOUVE

Achevé d'imprimer en juillet 2007 en France sur Presse Offset par

C P I
Brodard & Taupin

La Flèche (Sarthe).
N° d'imprimeur : 40211 – N° d'éditeur : 85291
Dépôt légal 1re publication : octobre 1999
Édition 11 – juillet 2007
LIBRAIRIE GÉNÉRALE FRANÇAISE – 31, rue de Fleurus – 75278 Paris cedex 06.

31/4710/5